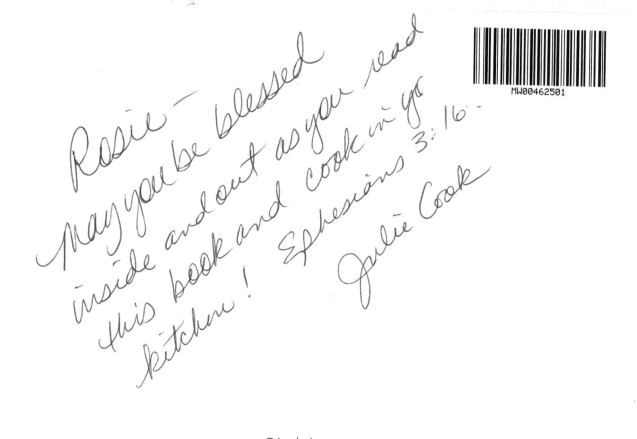

Rosie —
May you be blessed
inside and out as you read
this book and cook in your
kitchen! Ephesians 3:16 —
                    Julie Cook

Disclaimer:

Please note that the contents of this book in its entirety are for educational and culinary purposes only. The reader

assumes full responsibility for their health and understands that these statements have not been evaluated by the Food

and Drug Administration, nor are they to replace a doctor's advice. Although the authors have done their best to provide

accurate information and suggestions, please consult your doctor before undergoing a change in your diet. None of these

statements, products, or ingredients are intended to diagnose, treat, prevent, or cure disease.

Please enjoy this book with these facts in mind.

Published by Purpose Publishing LLC.
1503 Main Street #168 ❧ Grandview, Missouri
www.purposepublishing.com

ISBN: 978-0-9903010-8-0
Cover design by: Isella Vega
Editing by: Rae Lewis

Printed in the United States of America

This book is available at quantity discounts for bulk purchase.
Please contact Robin Cook at the following website:
www.cook2flourish.com

COOK 2 FLOURISH

by Robin Cook and Julie Cook

Setting the Table...

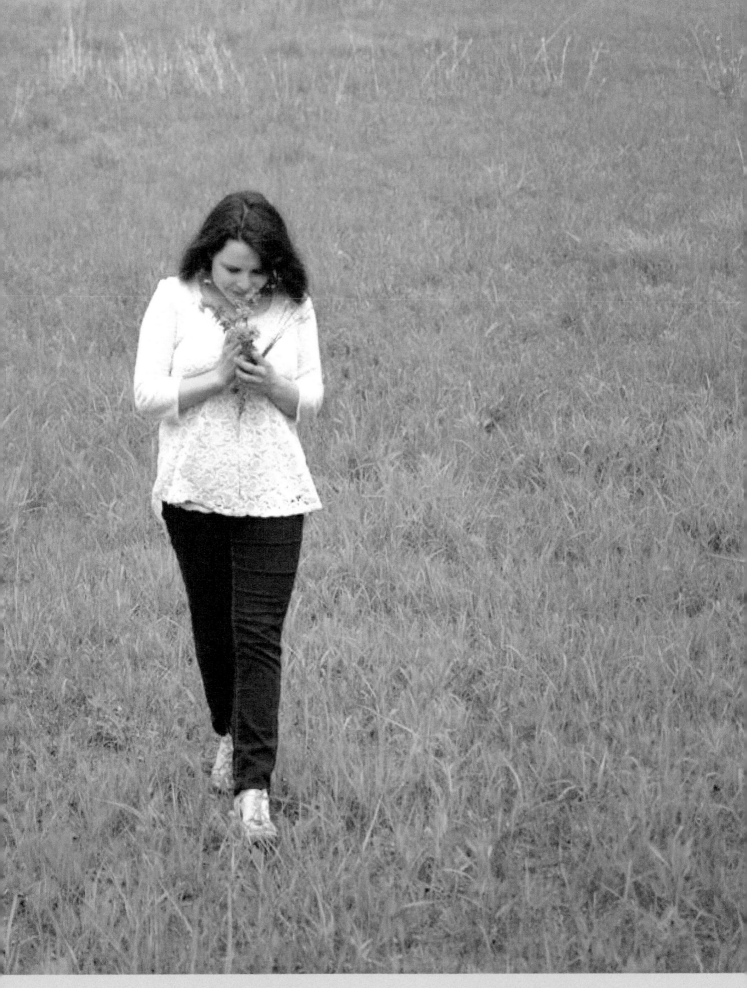

COOK 2 FLOURISH

Author's Story - Robin Cook

There is so much potential in each of our lives; God indeed has destined us all for great and mighty plans for His glory. I believe health is a foundation to this, for without health, we are hindered from accomplishing such a calling. In this cookbook, we endeavor to educate, equip and encourage you to cook the foods God created so you can Nourish 2 Flourish. Be prepared for some puns, gorgeous produce, and recipes filled with love and flavor. In all this, know that every step toward health is remarkable; start where you can and advance. Savor the bites, enjoy the times, make the most of every day, and honor the Lord!

This book is dedicated to my Lord and Savior, Jesus Christ, who gave His precious life for you and me and rose again. He has walked with me every step of the way in this health journey and provided the inspiration to create this cookbook. I never dreamed my mom's health crisis would be the seed bed for this cookbook, but God did! With deep gratitude for my beloved family: Del, Julie, Timo, PaPa, TeTe, Grandma and PePa must be acknowledged. Thank you for your love and support in this mission and for your patience with my trial and error recipes.

Many friends' hands I could not have done without, especially Ruthie, Joyce, Lauren, Katie, and my farmer friends: Terri, Karen, Mark, Jim, Rita, Jim and Ami.
Each of you have blessed me beyond measure. Thank you, and God bless you all!

~Robin Cook
Health Coach AADP, Certified Herbalist - Nourish 2 Flourish
Robin Cook is a holistic health coach and graduate of the Institute for Integrative Nutrition. In addition, she is an IN.FORM™ coach and Certified Herbalist, writing and teaching group wellness classes to encourage women how to take charge of their health and flourish.

Cook 2 Flourish Goals:

1. To educate you to transform your kitchen so you can transform your cooking, your health and your family

2. To equip you to eat deliciously while nourishing your body

3. To encourage you to continue on your health journey with renewed vigor and flavor

4. To help you discover delicious gluten and grain free foods

5. Provide inspirational notes throughout the book to keep you motivated

6. Present you with fresh ways to cook whole foods for vibrant health

Journey 2 Flourish: Preparing for health in mind, body and soul

Before we get into the pantry, I encourage you to ponder the following:

1. Vision.

Determine your health goals. Where are you now and where do you want to be? How can health help you get there? It is your "why" that will help you keep going.

"And the LORD answered me: 'Write the vision; make it plain on tablets, so he may run who reads it.'" Habbakuk 2:2 ESV
"Where there is no vision, the people perish: but he that keepeth the law, happy is he." Proverbs 29:18 KJV

2. Value.

Count the cost; are your goals worth it to you to make the necessary changes to be well and flourish? How will it affect your health if your current lifestyle doesn't change? What will propel you to maintain your healthy changes? Remember, YOU are worth it!

3. Support, support, support.

"Two people are better off than one, for they can help each other succeed. If one person falls, the other can reach out and help. But someone who falls alone is in real trouble." Ecceliastes 4:9 NLT

Likewise, by inviting the Lord into this often challenging journey, He will help you succeed. God desires for you to be in good health even as your soul prospers.

> *"Dear friend, I pray that you may enjoy good health and that all may go well with you, even as your soul is getting along well." 3 John 2 NIV (See also Psalms 103:3)*

Next, family and friends can be a tremendous support by encouraging you or serving as accountability. Hopefully, as they see your health being transformed, they will hunger for healthy change too.

Thirdly, you must support yourself. This may seem obvious, but it is vital; if you do not believe that you can change what you eat and be well, it will be very difficult to achieve the wellness you desire. Quoting Scripture and even praying to be transformed by the renewing of your mind (Romans 12:2, Ephesians 4:23) can be your keys to success.

4. Grace.

Not every day will be perfect in this lifestyle change journey. Be at peace and know that it is okay. Believe me, there have been some rather flat biscuits and less than appealing smoothies, but you can learn from every experience. As people we are not perfect, but God's mercies are new every morning (Lamentations 3:22-23).

If yesterday's plate had a cheeseburger jump on it and a half a tub of ice cream mysteriously disappear, forgive yourself and get back on track the next day. Health does not afford the luxury of guilt; it only slows our progress. May you have the grace and strength to overcome- the victory is yours through Christ Jesus (1 Corinthians 15:57)!

5. Joy.

One of my favorite phrases that has shaped my food philosophy is, *"Eat what God created and ENJOY."*

This simple, yet profound maxim is a reminder that healthy food is to be enjoyed. Brussels sprouts may not be your favorite food (yet), but learn to appreciate these unique, nourishing foods and begin to think of how they are influencing your body to flourish. Joy just may be one of the most underestimated antioxidants...

Swap 2 Flourish part 1: "Alteration, not Deprivation"

You are only as healthy as your kitchen is.

In order to nourish your body, you must have your fridge and pantry stocked with nourishing foods. When my family and I first began transitioning to healthier foods, it was all at once because it was a crisis situation. If my mom did not change her diet radically and rapidly, she may not have lived. For you, it may not be as severe, but the quicker you can transition, the quicker you will feel better, and the quicker cravings for the H.A.R.S.H. food can subside. (More on H.A.R.S.H. foods in a minute...)

Disclaimer: This may be traumatic for some people with certain foods. We can get attached to food emotionally, making it hard to give up, but your health is worth it, right? What is it worth for you to feel your best and feed your family food that will make them vibrant? Trust me, being the label reading queen (I've been called worse), I received some scowls and even witnessed a near tantrum as I told my mom that Cheez-its® should no longer loom in our pantry. Change is not easy, but in this case, it is necessary. Keep your goals in mind and visualize how your food is feeding or impeding your progress. Within a couple weeks, your taste buds will be changing and desiring the healthy foods!

Now for the good news... You see the word "swap" above? This is where the phrase "Alteration, not Deprivation" comes into play. Healthy eating can be delicious and satisfying; one of my goals in this cookbook is to help you make this a reality in your home. How does it work? I'm glad you're intrigued! Simply replace- or alter- your current pantry staples with the healthier, more nutrient rich counterparts. This way, you don't have to deprive yourself, and you can allow yourself to enjoy the more nourishing foods! How does that sound? This has been my vision since I began cooking for my family in 2006: how can I make fried chicken, chocolate cake... oh yes, and salad all taste good while simultaneously making us flourish? It's our joy for you to reap the harvest of the labor in the pages to come. May you be inspired, encouraged, and equipped to be transformed in this amazing health journey!

Swap 2 Flourish part 2 "H.A.R.S.H."

Are you ready to peer into the pantry? What should be inside it and how do you know what is truly healthy?

Meet the H.A.R.S.H. ingredients (and swiftly run away from them!):

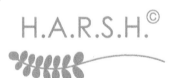

Avoid the foods that God didn't create:

H ------- Hydrogenated oils

A ------- Additives

R ------- Refined flour/ grains

S ------- Sugar

H ------- High Fructose Corn Syrup

H.A.R.S.H. foods are H.A.R.S.H. on our bodies! Rather, eat & enjoy what God has created; it is pleasing to the eye & good for food! Did you know? According to Harvard School of Public Health, several diseases are preventable, and eating a healthy, nutrient rich diet can help decrease the risk for such diseases. Whether it is to maintain a healthy weight, support brain health or heart health, what we put on our plates directly affects our health, so let's use our forks to help us flourish!

As unpleasant as it may be to talk about them, let's unwrap why they should not enter our mouths:

H: Hydrogenated oils

1. What are they?

• The oils that are processed by taking a liquid oil, subjecting it to extreme heat and injecting hydrogen gas into it. The result is a hardened (and toxic) fat.

2. What are they used in?

• Shortening, margarine, processed cheese, tortillas, crackers, chips, candies, and more.

3. Why don't they help us flourish?

• Unhealthy cholesterol influence- decreases HDL and increases LDL

• May discourage immune function

• Suppresses the body's anti-inflammatory mechanisms

4. Tips:

• These oils are called "trans fats," and read the ingredients because 0.5 grams of trans fats can be present without being listed on the nutrition facts. If you see hydrogenated oil or partially hydrogenated oil, do not partake! Many fried foods are submerged in hydrogenated oil, another reason to avoid fried foods.

5. What to use instead:

• Consider using grapeseed oil and avocado oil for medium to medium high heat cooking and roasting. Extra Virgin Coconut oil, butter, and ghee for low to medium cooking.

• Extra Virgin Olive Oil is excellent for salad dressing, dips, and drizzling on cooked foods.

Healthy Fats help allow nutrients into the body's cells and help with many other important brain and body functions. Fat is not your enemy, in fact, by eating more healthy fats instead of refined sugars, refined grains and toxic fats, your body will be able to burn fat instead of burning sugar- that is a good thing! When we feed on the healthy fats, our cells will be supple and receptive to communication with each other and open to receive incoming nutrients and release waste.

Did you know that the brain is approximately 60% fat? Omega 3 fatty acids are particularly important to brain health and protecting the body from too much inflammation. For a great source of omega 3 fatty acids consume salmon, walnuts and cold pressed flaxseed oil with lignans.

A: Additives

1. What are they?

• Aspartame, sucralose, acesulfame K (potassium), colorings, sulfites, nitrates, phosphates, pesticides, preservatives, MSG (and its other titles), BHT, hormones and antibiotics in meats, sulfur dioxide, and more.

2. Why don't they help us flourish?

• Each additive brings about a different toxic effect; artificial sweeteners can lead to a decline in brain function and trigger headaches, colorings/dyes have been linked to perpetuating behavior challenges in children, nitrates are chemicals in processed meat, MSG can cause fatigue and dampen the body's fullness signals, and sulfur dioxide can exacerbate respiratory challenges such as asthma.

3. What to use instead:

• In contrast to the cell-saddening assortment of additives, real whole foods contain antioxidants, vibrant colors and please the palate.

• Organic foods will help decrease the amount of pesticides, and organic meats will decrease the amount of hormones and antibiotics entering the body (your liver will be glad).

• Read your labels and enjoy the ingredients in this cookbook to add flavor and nutrition without the health-subtracting additives! You will find natural ways to color food, such as beet powder, in the recipes to come.

R: Refined Flour & Refined Grains

1. What are they?

• Refined flour and refined grains are synonymous with white bread and white bread products. Common ingredient names are: all purpose flour, wheat flour, enriched bleached flour, bromated flour, durum wheat, white rice, white rice flour, pearled barley, white pasta, semolina, etc.

• Unless it says "whole" in front of the grain's name, it is usually refined. The second red flag is if the product has less than 3 grams of fiber.

• Beware of gluten free products as well; they often are comprised of refined grains and starches that offer little nutrition and insufficient fiber to balance out the impending surge in blood sugar. Whole gluten free grains are best and are referenced throughout this book.

2. Why don't they help us flourish?

• God designed grains with 3 parts: the outer bran, the starchy endosperm, and the inner germ. Each part plays a roll; without each of these components, the body has a more difficult time assimilating the grain. (pun intended)

• Refined grains only contain the carb-rich endosperm. This contributes to blood sugar surges and crashes, which is unfriendly to energy levels and our waist lines.

• Excess grains in the diet can hinder weight management, hamper energy, and encourage inflammation in the body. Continual eating of wheat may be linked to gluten sensitivities. Listen to your body and see what is best for you.

• Some grains that contain gluten have been genetically altered in the past decades, which has contributed to gluten allergies and sensitivities. To avoid unpleasant acute symptoms and potential subtle chronic health consequences of gluten, many people have found that eating gluten free whole grains in moderation contributes to a healthy diet. Again, you can see what works best for your body... you may be surprised at what removing gluten can bring about- clearer thinking, calmer digestion, less joint pain, etc.

• Most all of our recipes are free of gluten or provide substitutions to make it gluten free so you can be full of health and vitality!

3. What to use instead:

Whole Grains with gluten*:	Whole grains without gluten:	Non-grain & gluten free:
• Whole wheat • Whole spelt • Whole barley • Whole Kamut® (khorasan) • Whole rye • Einkorn whole wheat	• Whole millet • Whole buckwheat groats • Organic quinoa • Organic brown rice • Organic wild rice • Gluten free oats, depending on tolerance	• Garbanzo bean flour • Organic coconut flour • Almond flour • Spaghetti squash • Spiralized vegetables

In moderation or as a transition food; better than using white flour, but still has the effects of gluten. Throughout this book you will see these leaf icons that will indicate if a recipe is gluten free or not. Be sure to verify that all the other ingredients in the recipe are agreeable to you, however.

Gluten Free

S: Sugar

First of all, in our modern society, processed sugar has become a commodity and consumed nearly incessantly at the cost of declining health and expanding waist lines. Fat has been the blame of weight gain, "don't eat fat because it will make you fat..." This sounds familiar, but it is a myth! The truth is that healthy fats satisfy and in proper amounts keep us slim. Refined sugars pack on the pounds with bitter consequences. Thankfully, God gave us naturally sweet foods such as berries, sweet potatoes, honey, stevia, dates, coconut nectar, and pure maple syrup for our enjoyment. You will find many references to these foods in our cookbook. As you begin changing your eating habits, you'll be shocked at how your taste buds change and begin to crave and appreciate the naturally sweet foods. Speaking from experience, I used to drink soda (gasp!) and after not having it a while, I accidently began to drink out of what I thought was my glass with iced tea and it was Coke®- what a nasty surprise! Your body will be forever grateful when you give it up! You CAN break the sugar addiction!

1. What is refined sugar?

• Common names of refined sugar are cane juice, corn syrup, dextrose, sucrose, brown sugar, white sugar, beet sugar, and so many more.

• Sugar is sly; you almost have to be a detective to find it! Cookies, pastries, breads, energy bars, granola bars, energy drinks, lemonade, sports drinks, ketchup, sauces, meats, seasonings, crackers, dressings, etc. often have sugar of one form or another. Read your labels, and note that every 4 grams of sugar equals one teaspoon.

2. Why doesn't it help us flourish?

• These are usually processed and isolated simple sugars that offer no nutrients yet supply calories and cause blood sugar to soar since no fiber is present to slow the sugar's release.

• The sugar cycle is like a revolving Ferris wheel; you eat a pastry or drink a soda, the sugar surges into your blood stream, you get a jolt of energy, insulin rushes in to save your body from the overload of sugar, your blood sugar crashes, your energy level plummets, and your brain says "I need a pick-me-up." Does this sound familiar? Unfortunately, we have all been here. It is time to get off the Ferris wheel, do you agree?

Note: if this cycle continues long enough, insulin resistance can result and silent inflammation can ensue, which may open the door to disease. Sugar isn't very sweet when we look at it this way.

• Further reasons to quell a high sugar intake: sugar has a negative effect on heart function, it can pack on belly fat, and it deregulates the body's fullness signal (leptin). Research has shown that high insulin levels (due to consumption of excess sugar) may cause heightened cancer risks, hasten the aging process, trigger inflammation, and more.

3. Notes & What to use instead:

• Admittedly, sugar is tricky to navigate around; there are many types of "natural sugars" and alternatives. To never have a sweet treat is unrealistic, yet finding a good source for a natural sweetener can be a challenge. We have done much research and have created these recipes in light of our health journey and studying.

• For some, a period of time without any sweetener may be best to re-adjust the taste buds and retrain the brain to be satisfied with healthy foods in the absence of sweets. A lack of protein in the diet or overgrowth of yeast such as candida can also contribute to sweet cravings, so listen to your body and adjust accordingly.

• Changing our perspective is key also; sweet foods are to be eaten and enjoyed in moderation. As King Solomon said, "Do you like honey? Don't eat too much, or it will make you sick!" Proverbs 25:16 NLT

• For years honey has been used as a sweetener, as have fruits and stevia. In this book we have chosen to use these sweeteners and a few choice others to naturally sweeten the foods in this book. Again, moderation and quality are imperative. Raw honey is less processed than pasteurized honey. Likewise, ultra refined stevia such as Truvia® is not the same as green stevia or organic stevia extract. Listen to your body and see what natural sweetener you respond best to and enjoy it in moderation as your health goals permit.

• By using these natural sweeteners that are far less refined, you will be getting more nutrients out of the sweetener. Plus, when you add these sweeteners into a dish that contains fiber and other nutrients, the blood sugar effect will be better than that of refined sugar with refined flour.

• Sweeteners included in these recipes: raw honey (preferably local and/ or organic), unrefined coconut sugar, raw coconut nectar, unsulfured black strap molasses (preferably organic), pure maple syrup grade B (preferably organic), organic dates, organic stevia extract (Stevita™ and Sweet Leaf Stevia® brands), prune puree, sweet potato puree and unsweetened applesauce.

H: High Fructose Corn Syrup

1. What is it?

· Another source of refined sugar, high fructose corn syrup saps the health right out of us!

2. Why doesn't it make us flourish?

· Being cheaper than regular white table sugar, high fructose corn syrup (HFCS) has been added to many processed foods in unprecedented, unhealthy amounts.

· These are some of the studied health effects of HFCS: causes blood sugar and insulin to soar, can contribute to leaky gut, causes the liver to produce more triglycerides, disturbs healthy metabolism making the body more vulnerable to weight gain, diabetes, etc.

3. Notes & what to replace it with:

· The extreme processing methods coupled with the genetically modified corn and its effects on the body render this ingredient poisonous. Please avoid it at all costs. Read the labels well and make as many homemade foods as you can to avoid this H.A.R.S.H. food. Many "foods" marketed to children and their parents can carry HFCS and certainly do not contribute to their well being and attention span. Rather, as already said, begin to embrace God's naturally sweetened food in effort to avoid the woes of this ingredient.

Flourish Forward Tips:
· ·

Many people notice that when they eliminate these potentially inflammatory foods, they think clearer, have more energy, experience improved digestion, and can manage weight better. If you have already removed H.A.R.S.H. ingredients from your eating, consider bulking up on the nutrient dense foods such as berries, kale, cauliflower, quinoa, organic animal proteins, etc. while decreasing:

1. (all H.A.R.S.H. ingredients)

2. Gluten- wheat, rye, barley, spelt, khorasan, einkorn, etc.

3. Grains (for a short time, if deemed necessary)

4. GMO's (Genetically Modified Organisms), especially wheat, corn and soy

5. Peanuts

6. Corn

7. Processed omega 6 fats (fried foods, packaged foods, vegetable oils, chips etc.)

8. Non-organic Dairy: butter, yogurt, milk, cottage cheese, cream cheese, cheese, ice cream...

This is not an all inclusive list, but you may wish to experiment replacing these foods with more whole foods and especially green vegetables and healthy fats to see how your body feels. For me, removing these foods has increased my energy levels, improved my digestion, and allowed me to think more clearly. Some people do just fine with dairy, but for example, when I omitted it from my diet, I no longer experienced the respiratory congestion that I had before. Yes, some of our recipes do call for dairy, and when we do use dairy it is organic and as unprocessed as possible. Dairy is a "treat" ingredient for me, not an everyday food.

Shop 2 Flourish:
....

So, what do you want in your pantry and fridge? Your grocery cart, pantry and fridge can either be your best health allies or your foes of flourishing. It is vital to stock your kitchen with the nourishing ingredients and supplies; when you have the healthy items on hand you will be set up for success. The more fresh foods you have, the better. The more alive your food is, the more alive you will be. It stands to reason that the least processed the food is, the more nutrients it has to offer you. Here are some of the Cook 2 Flourish staples:

Shop 2 Flourish: Pantry and Fridge Staples

Condiments and Pantry Staples- are your flavorings and foods favoring you? Many condiments and seasonings are loaded with hidden sugars, preservatives and other H.A.R.S.H. ingredients. Here are some common ingredients found in pantries with some suggestions for healthier alternatives. The more of them that you can make, the healthier, tastier, and cost effective they will be!

Tortillas	(Whole Grain Gluten Free wraps, Organic Brown Rice Tortillas, Whole Grain Spelt, Sprouted Whole Grain Wraps, Nori Seaweed Wraps, Cauliflower Flatbread p.270)
Crackers	(Crunch Master® whole grain gluten free crackers, Mary's Gone Crackers®)
Granola bars	(Soaked Oats p.69, Energy Balls p.70-71, Lara Bars®, Cascadian Farms™ protein bars)
Cereals	(Timo's Morning Oatmeal p.47, Pumpkin Pecan Quinoa p.49, Organic Oatmeal or Whole Grain Muesli, other cereals p.91)

Gum/mints	(Nature's Sunshine® Xylitol Peppermints p.29,71)
Chips	(Kale Chips p.75, Timo's Snack Mix p.91, Way Better Chips®, Organic Blue Corn Chips, Organic Corn Chips, Seaweed Chips)
Bread	(Veganic Sprouted Spelt Bread, Ezekiel 4:9® Bread, Canyon Bakehouse® Gluten Free 7 grain bread)
Jam	(St. Dalfour®, Polaner® All Fruit spread)
Dairy	(grass-fed or at least organic butter such as Kerry Gold™ butter, Kirkland™ Organic, Organic Valley® Organic butter, Organic Greek plain whole milk yogurt p.53, grass-fed organic cheese or organic cheese, use Greek yogurt for sour cream, organic cottage cheese, unsweetened almond milk without carrageenen p.57, Soft Serve Creamy Ice p.79, So Delicious® Dairy Free Coconut Milk No Sugar Added ice cream: vanilla bean, chocolate, mint chip and butter pecan)
Peanut butter	(Almond Butter, p. 73, organic peanut butter without sugar or hydrogenated oils) *most peanuts carry fungus/ mold
Boxed mixes	(Make your own from whole grain flours or garbanzo bean flour)
Mayonnaise	(Vegenaise® purple lid)
Salad dressing	(homemade, see salad section p.92)
Ketchup & BBQ sauce	(homemade p.251, Cucina Antica®, BBQ sauce sweet or spicy p.247)
Taco sauce	(Salsa Bravo p.249, salsa without sugar and natural flavoring [MSG])
Soy Sauce/ Sweet n Sour Sauce	(Bragg® liquid aminos, coconut aminos®)
Cheese Sauce	(Caul-it-Fredo sauce p.255, Mac N Cheese p.230)
Shortening/ Oil	(Extra-Virgin Coconut oil, grapeseed oil, avocado oil, grapeseed oil non-stick spray)

Shop 2 Flourish: Canned goods

1. Select BPA free canned goods whenever possible. One of my go-to brands is Muir Glen®. BPA can have undesired affects on hormones and be toxic to the body. Costco® frequently offers some BPA free canned goods such as black beans. The label will indicate if it is BPA free. The BPA seeps into the tomato products the most, so budget at least for BPA free tomatoes.

2. Read the label to check for added sugar. Can you believe that kidney beans often have added sugar in them?

3. As with other foods, organic is best if possible.

4. Unless you do your own canning, here are a couple of tips for purchasing canned goods:

- beans
- BPA free tomatoes
- pumpkin puree
- organic coconut milk
- black olives, without preservatives
- skipjack tuna or chunk light tuna in water for lower mercury (no flavoring or soy)
- wild sardines in olive oil
- canned wild salmon

Oils*:

For drizzling and dressings:

- organic 100% pure extra virgin olive oil
- Nature's Sunshine® flax seed oil with lignans
- herb infused extra virgin olive oils

For medium to medium high heat:

- grapeseed oil (least refined possible)
- pure avocado oil (least refined possible)
- or use broth p.128

For cooking on low to medium heat:

- organic extra virgin coconut oil
- toasted sesame oil
- or use broth p.128

some oils can take higher heats, but please make sure to protect all oils from smoking or burning and use lower heats when possible.

Jars:

- artichoke hearts in water**
- sundried tomatoes without sulfites in extra virgin olive oil**
- kalamata olives (without sulfites, flavors or preservatives)**
- organic salsa (without sugar or "natural flavors")-or- make our Salsa Bravo!**
- balsamic vinegar that does NOT have added sulfites or added caramel coloring.

(You would see this listed in the ingredient list.)

**once opened, these goods will be stored in the refrigerator*

Dry goods and Baking:

- Jovial® 100% organic whole grain einkorn pasta
- black bean pasta
- Mary's Gone Crackers®
- organic brown rice tortillas
- organic long grain brown rice
- organic wild rice
- organic whole chia seeds
- organic almond flour
- organic whole sprouted spelt flour
- organic old fashioned oats (certified gluten free, if desired)
- sprouted whole grain tortillas- such as Engine 2® or Food for Life®
- organic whole sprouted khorsan flour
- aluminum free baking powder
- pure organic vanilla, lemon & almond extract- not artificial. Our favorite is the organic alcohol free variety from Frontier® or Simply Organic®

- Crunch Master® Multi Grain crackers
- Flackers®
- organic blue corn chips
- Rudi's® gluten free tortillas
- whole buckwheat groats
- organic whole flaxseeds
- garbanzo bean flour
- organic coconut flour
- whole millet flour
- organic quinoa
- organic oat bran (certified gluten free, if desired)
- organic non-irradiated spices
- arrowroot powder

Shop 2 Flourish: Sweeteners and Flours

Making the transition to flourish in your health can come along with lots of changes and some trial and error. We have strived to give you practical and delicious recipes that will eliminate the guess work for you as you prepare tasty, nourishing alternatives to your family favorites. Here are a few notes about the ingredients that we have used for our baking:

Sweeteners:

- Stevia extract (powdered or liquid, we like Stevita™ and Sweet Leaf® brands):
  use 1 teaspoon per cup of white sugar being replaced.
- Raw honey: use 3⁄4 to 1 cup raw honey to 1 cup of white sugar being replaced.
- Unsulphured Blackstrap Molasses: use as an accent sweetener
- Raw Coconut Nectar: use in place of liquid sweeteners 1:1
- Unrefined Coconut Sugar: easiest sweetener to convert;
  1 cup unrefined coconut sugar to 1 cup white sugar being replaced.

From our personal research these are among the safest sweeteners to use but still need to be used in moderation. Having said that, remember Solomon's wisdom, "Do you like honey? Don't eat too much, or it will make you sick!" Proverbs 25:16 NLT

Flours:

- Whole Sprouted Spelt Flour (One Degree Organic Foods): use equal parts spelt to all purpose flour, but less liquid may be required.

- Whole Millet Flour: use in a mixture of other wholesome flours, light nutty taste

- Whole Buckwheat Flour: in a mixture of other wholesome flours, earthy taste

- Garbanzo Bean Flour: can be used in a mixture of other wholesome flours or approximately cup for cup all purpose flour (do not lick the batter- it'll taste beany!)

- Coconut Flour: very absorbent- use only 1/3 cup coconut flour to 1 cup all Purpose flour and extra eggs and liquid may be required (begin with the recipes we have included to familiarize yourself with it)

- Almond Flour: in a mixture of other wholesome flours or use cup for cup of all purpose flour. It can make baked goods more dense, so make sure not to pack the flour when measuring it.

- Love and Peas® protein powder (Sugar Free): not a true flour, but it can be used in place of 1/4 of the flour in a recipe (possibly more if you want to experiment) to give the baked goods more protein.

- Psyllium Husk fine powder: only used in our "Kan't Believe It's Not Bread" recipes, this flour is very absorbent and will require that you drink a lot of water after eating foods with it since it has a lot of fiber in it.

Depending on your gluten preference and if you are eating grains, you can decide what flours will work best for your cooking and baking needs. Admittedly, these flours do not all work exactly like all purpose flour but they provide a healthier alternative to make healthy breads and treats.

Please note that although there are many gluten free baking mixes and products on the market, often they contain fillers or starches that are devoid of fiber. By using the above flours, you will get more nutrients and fiber.

Shop 2 Flourish: Organic Fruits and Vegetables

Although "organic" may not be listed for every ingredient in our recipes, it is strongly encouraged to eat organic and non-GMO as much as possible. Besides the grocery store, many Farmer's Markets offer superb local, heirloom and organic produce to help you flourish! Visit www.ewg.org to view the least and most pesticide-laden foods.

Shop 2 Flourish: Meats

The higher up the food chain you eat, the more potential toxins you can intake. So, here is a list that shows in order of best protein choices to least desirable protein choices. Do the best you can, and make sure to be eating sufficient vegetables along with your protein for optimal digestion and energy.

Red Meat:	**Chicken:**

1. Grass fed & finished (organic)
2. Grass fed (organic)
3. Organic
4. No hormones or animal by-products*
   * make sure any feed is non GMO
	1. Pastured/local with organic feed
	2. Organic free range / cage free
	3. No added hormones or antibiotics*
	   * make sure any feed is non GMO

Fish:	**Eggs:**

1. Wild caught, fresh or frozen
2. Wild caught, canned
3. Whole Foods® farm raised
   * verify fish is not from China
   * if Tuna, get wild canned skipjack or chunk light tuna [eat in moderation]
   * avoid shellfish and fish that feed on the bottom- shrimp, tilapia, catfish, etc.
	1. Pastured/local with organic feed
	2. Organic free range
	3. Organic cage free
	4. Free range*
	   * make sure any feed is non GMO

Swap 2 Flourish: Cutting out the toxic utensils

As you are making this transition to healthier eating, it is important to note that toxins and unhealthy substances can not only come from our foods, but what our foods are cooked with and in. For a healthy kitchen environment, we admonish you to discontinue using the microwave, non-stick and Teflon® pans (pots, sauté pans, muffin tins, cookie sheets), non BPA plastic bags and containers, melamine, non-stick bleached parchment paper and in some cases aluminum foil.

There are many reasons, but many sources show non-stick ware to release hazardous gases and can impair hormonal balance. Some studies suggest that microwaves render the foods nutritionally poor and less flavorful. Whatever you do, do not microwave foods in plastic containers. Here's the good news, though, cooking healthily can involve some practical and enjoyable tools such as:

- Vegetable peelers for making vegetable "ribbons"
- High powered blender such as BlendTec® or a regular blender
- Spiralizer for making vegetables into fun pasta-like shapes
- Stainless Steel Pans (for cooking and re-heating)
- Unbleached Parchment Paper
- Glass bowls and storage containers
- Food processor
- Glass baking dishes
- Stoneware baking sheets and dishes
- Toaster Ovens (for cooking and re-heating)
- Unbleached parchment paper muffin liners
- Wooden or bamboo utensils
- Mini sized and full sized ceramic Crock-Pot® (for cooking and re-heating)
- BPA free plastic wrap and baggies (use as infrequently as possible and not with hot foods)

We have gone through a lot of nutrition; let's pause for a minute to consider:

1. How does this affect you and how can you use this information to change your lifestyle in a positive way?

2. If you change what's in your food, you can still eat your favorite foods, just prepare them with their healthier alternatives! This is what we call "Alteration, not Deprivation!"

3. This is not a diet (take a sigh of relief). In this book, we want to encourage you to take the education throughout this book so you can Nourish 2 Flourish. Do not be afraid of the healthy fats we use in the recipes and be creative with the assortment of veggies. If you do not follow each recipe verbatim, it is okay; you have freedom to swap out basil for parsley or blackberries for blueberries. Cooking is a science, but it is also a creative art- embrace it.

4. What the above H.A.R.S.H. list really boils down to is to eat what God created in the way He created it and enjoy. Everyone is different, too, so eat nutritiously and observe how your body responds and adjust accordingly. You may want to keep a food journal to track your progress.

Notes:

You have now read through some of the most health transforming information this book has to offer, now before you put it into practice in your kitchen, here are a few last keys:

• When you see the leaf icons, those are a guide to help you know what recipes are free of dairy, gluten and grains or a combination of them.

• When you see a recipe that has "eat in moderation" on the leaf icon, just know that it does contain dairy, gluten and or grains and is more of a "treat" food.

• Many recipes have the title "Caul-it___"; this is a play on words to tell you that cauliflower is our secret ingredient to make it taste like a carb-type food while having veggie benefits.

With all these things in mind, may you be blessed, inspired and strengthened to prepare these recipes and continue in your health journey! You CAN Nourish 2 Flourish!

Truth 2 Flourish no matter where you are in your journey:

Ezekiel 47:12 NIV : *"'Fruit trees of all kinds will grow on both banks of the river. Their leaves will not wither, nor will their fruit fail. Every month they will bear fruit, because the water from the sanctuary flows to them. Their fruit will serve for food and their leaves for healing.'"*

1 Peter 2:24 NIV : *"'He himself bore our sins' in his body on the cross, so that we might die to sins and live for righteousness; 'by his wounds you have been healed.'"*

1 Corinthians 6:19 NIV : *"Do you not know that your bodies are temples of the Holy Spirit, who is in you, whom you have received from God? You are not your own; you were bought at a price. Therefore honor God with your bodies."*

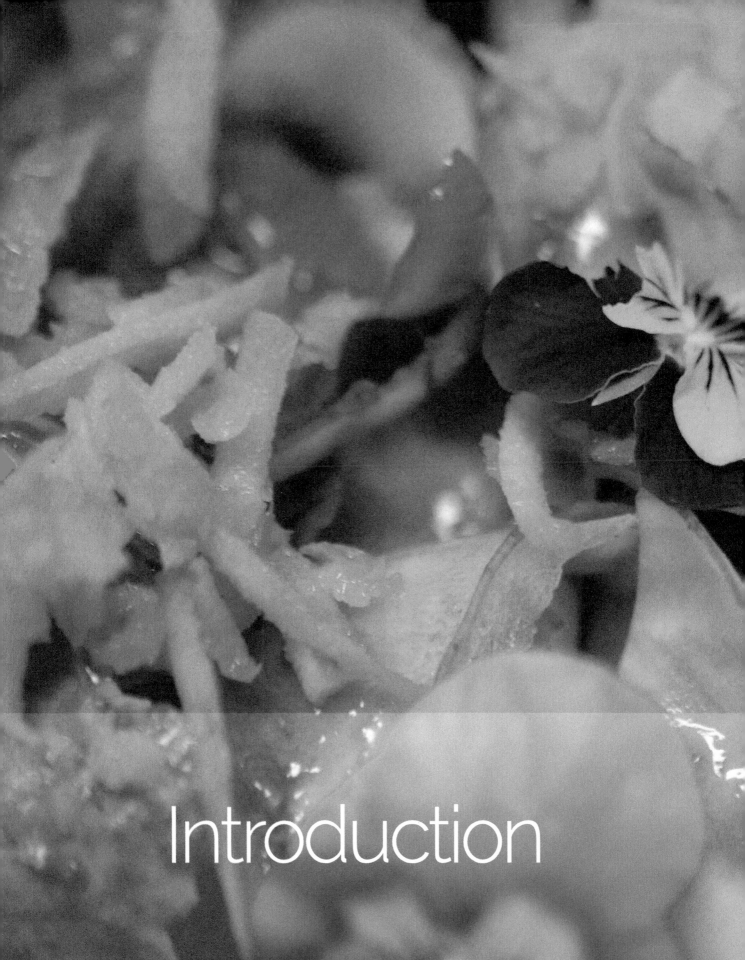

Introduction

COOK 2 FLOURISH

Author's Story - Julie Cook

I was overweight and worked many hours beside my husband in our busy jewelry store. I cared for our young children, my father-in-law, my husband's grandmother and my clients, but I wasn't taking care of myself. I didn't realize it, but I was burning my candle at both ends. On June 1, 2006 at 39 1/2 years old, my health took a wrong turn.

I developed heat exhaustion while mowing the lawn. What followed over the next weeks were a series of emergency room trips, doctor's visits, four days in the hospital, and appointments with specialists which included lots of blood work. Unfortunately for me, I didn't have any answers. I was told over and over "your blood work is normal." I'm thankful for doctors and their expertise and have many that are good friends. It was just difficult to figure out what was going on because I had so many symptoms. It wasn't something a pill could fix; I needed a lifestyle overhaul! The first clue into my diagnosis came from a retired family doctor friend that agreed to see me. Almost instantly he told my husband, "Del, I can see it in her eyes, she is exhausted, and her adrenals are exhausted."

I didn't know what he was talking about. I had never heard of adrenals. He pointed me in the direction of eating healthier and supplementing to support my adrenals.
Robin began going to the library and checking out several books at a time, reading, researching, taking notes on all she could find about adrenal exhaustion and hormonal imbalance. This crisis began a long, lonely two year journey of regaining my health. It didn't happen overnight, it was an hour by hour, day by day struggle for months.

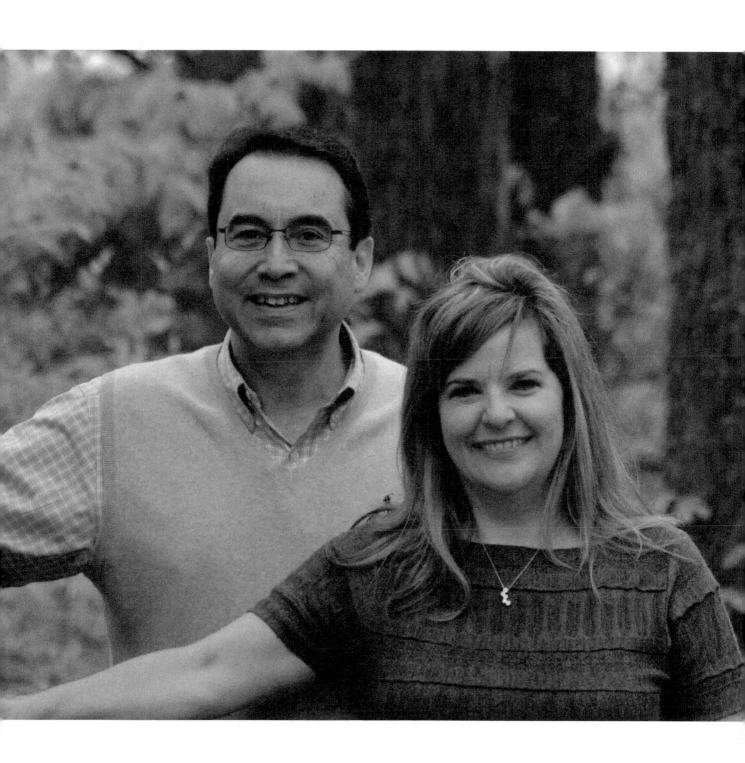

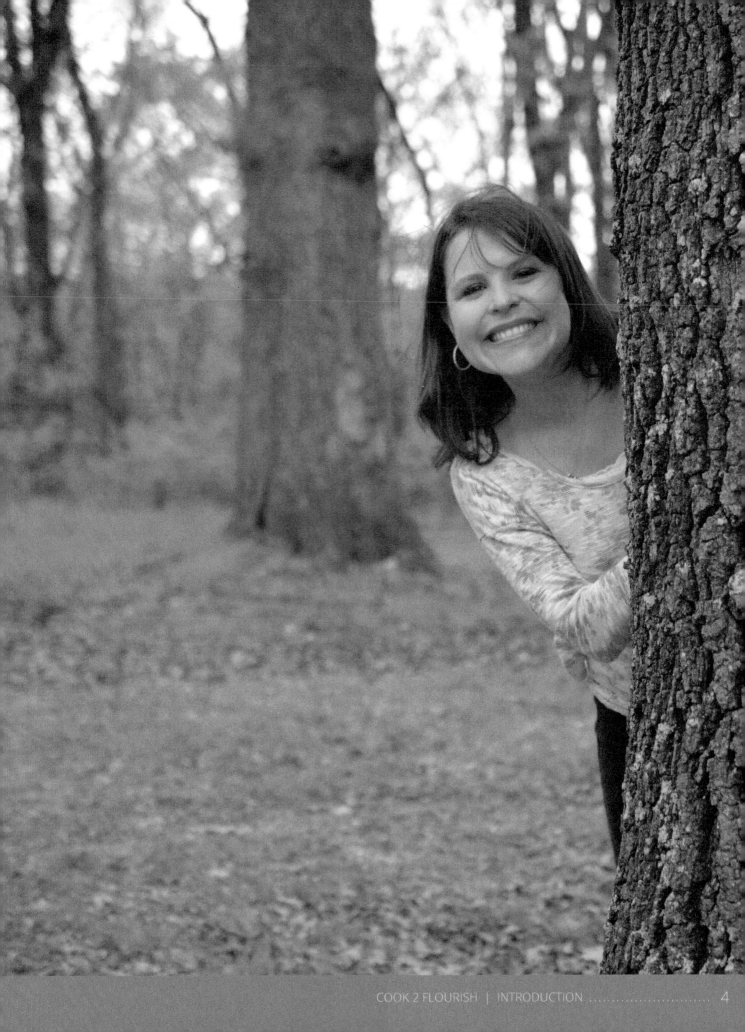

I had several symptoms I was dealing with besides the adrenal exhaustion and severe hormonal imbalance; extreme fatigue, sensitivity to heat, low thyroid, hair loss, weak and hoarse voice, constipation, irregular periods, heart racing and pounding, panic attacks, hypoglycemia, passing out while lying in bed and terrible insomnia, to name a few. I had 22 sleepless nights in 2 months. After that, I had to retrain myself to sleep by getting into a nightly routine of taking a shower and getting ready for bed, reading scripture and drinking hot herbal tea then turning the light out and saying a prayer. It took a few weeks, but finally I was sleeping again. Then there was fear and depression that came as a result of the imbalance and they became a battle in my mind. I was a sick young lady and I know I came close to dying twice.

I would not have made it without lots of prayers! I've known Jesus as my Savior all my life and this particular summer I was to really trust Him and get to know Him on a deeper level. I began to read my Bible and the scriptures came alive to me. It became like food, the more I read, the more I craved it; the passages were making sense like never before. This scripture meant so much to me, Jeremiah 17:8-9, "For he shall be like a tree planted by waters, which spreads out its roots by the river, and will not fear when heat comes; But her leaf will be green, and will not be anxious in the year of drought, nor will cease from yielding fruit." This gave me much hope!
He didn't choose to give me a quick fix and now, I'm thankful! I wouldn't have learned all I've learned, nor would I have changed my lifestyle and my pattern of eating. I went through a pruning process. I was cut off at the waist and only my roots went deep in the ground. (Psalms 1) It was just like remodeling a house from the inside out. My habits had to be pruned, my cravings and appetite had to be pruned, and my thinking had to be changed. All the processed foods in my kitchen had to be pruned if I was going to get my health back.

The Lord doesn't prune us because we're bad or in trouble, He prunes us just like a fruit tree is pruned, to bear more fruit, sweeter fruit, stronger limbs, more room to grow bigger; and then when future storms come, the tree can withstand the wind it brings. I emerged two years later 52 pounds lighter because of the foods I had been eating and with a stronger faith in Jesus and a strong prayer life. I really learned to pray during this journey and learned to listen after I prayed. I came to understand who God is and because of who He is, what He can do…
He is my Refuge and my Strong Tower,
I can trust Him and He protects me. He is my source, my strength for each new day comes from Him, He is my Healer, He is my Hope, and without Him there is no true hope or true peace. Dear friend, if you do not know Jesus as your Savior you can. If you are going through a struggle, He is right there waiting to help you, just ask Him to help you.

If you are sick in your body, He can help you. I encourage you to ask Jesus into your heart and life simply by saying, "Jesus, I need you! I need you in my life and in my heart. Please help me. Please change my situation, touch my health, heal my body, turn me around and point me in the right direction. Thank you for saving me and coming to my rescue."

If you just prayed this simple prayer, believe in your heart that you are saved and Jesus is with you. I encourage you to keep praying and find a Bible believing church to attend then get a Bible and begin reading the scriptures; they will guide you and give you peace. When my health took its turn, my husband was without my help at the store. The day by day anxiousness was very stressful for him and I want to thank him for his patience, tenderness, his continued love, encouragement and most of all for his prayers for me.

Robin stepped up to be the kitchen manager. At 13 years old, that was quite a task! PaPa would take her to the grocery store and she would prepare all of our meals for our family while maintaining her high grades in school and participating in the school theater plays. She continued this for years and became a great cook. Spiritually, this journey cultivated in her a deep faith and a strong prayer life. She is an amazing young woman now, wise and mature beyond her years. She has been a huge reason for my vitality today. I have learned so much from her, she is a wonderful teacher and I've been her hardest student. Change is hard. When this journey began, I felt like I was learning a new language. Reading labels, learning about healthier ingredients, giving up favorites, old ways of doing things and learning new things wasn't always delightfully accepted by me. I used to tell my husband, I don't like this, but I am eating it because I need it. Now, I have 15-20 new favorite super foods! My perspective on food changed; it was about eating vibrant greens and nutrients to really nourish my body instead of just eating whatever, which had included a lot of processed foods. I had thought food was food, but a whole new exciting world opened up to me with fresh whole foods. I studied what super foods did for me and began eating lots of them! My taste buds began to desire what I was feeding my body. Now the old things don't taste good to me or they make me sick when I eat them. So, thank you, Robin, for everything! I love you and appreciate you! Timo, you made me laugh when I didn't feel good. You've been a real trooper to walk this journey with me and to adjust to eating healthy when it's not cool for teens to eat that way. Actually, you didn't mind because your lunches were really good! One of your sandwiches was traded for a KC Chiefs ticket! Thanks for being a great taste tester. You too have changed your health by eating better and shedding 28 pounds!

Mom and Dad, thank you so much for all of your love and prayers and support during my journey. I so appreciate you! Thank you for the venison, it is so delicious and we enjoy cooking with it. Thank you for helping in the kitchen with preparing and keeping up with the dishes while proofing the recipes. We love you!

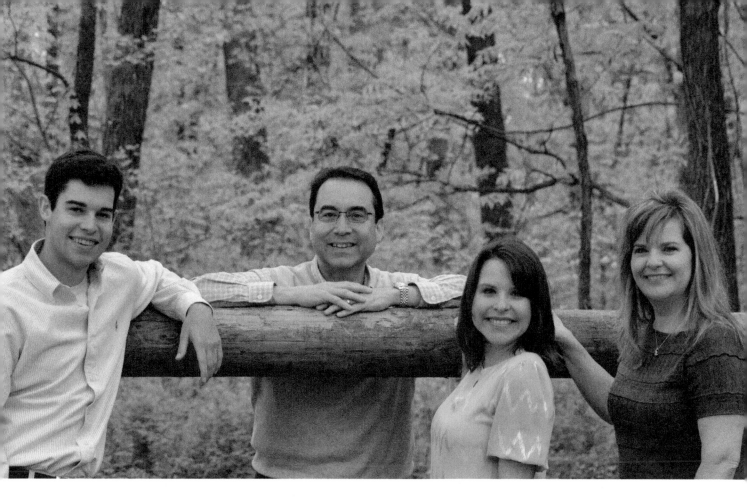

Although they are deceased now, Bill and TeTe were a huge blessing when I was sick. They cared for Robin and Timothy and prayed for me constantly. I'm so grateful! I miss them in our home and around our table. Thank you, Lord for the time we had with them and for bringing me through my journey, not leaving me in it. You are faithful! In May of 2012, I was frustrated that I wasn't completely over my fatigue and adrenal crashes when I over worked too much and I said "Lord, I'm done! I'm not taking another vitamin until you give me new direction!" I had tried so many different vitamins. I read about this, I heard about that one, I had been eating clean for six years, but I wasn't over it, I was done!

Two weeks later a lady from North Dakota who had been one of our very first customers back in 1998, came into our jewelry store and began talking with Robin about her college education. She asked, "What are you going to do to further your education? You should contact my doctor and see if you could be in a mentorship program under her." Then she looked directly at me and said "You need to know about Dr. Inge Wetzel and about Nature's Sunshine Supplements!" I replied, "Why?" "Because they work!" I took that as my new direction, so we got in touch with Dr. Inge and our whole family's health has been enhanced through Nature's Sunshine Products® and all the knowledge we have gained through Dr. Inge, for which we will always be so thankful! We have benefitted from the effectiveness and purity of these supplements. Robin continues to be mentored by her today.

Robin and I went on to become Nature's Sunshine® IN.FORMTM Burn Fat/ Be Fit/For Life coaches. We enjoy working together with our classes. People see us together now or meet us for the first time and think we are sisters; I've lost years off my face.

My top 21 out of over 500 Nature's Sunshine® Products are: Mineral Chi; it is a marvelous mineral drink for my adrenals! It ignites the energy in my cells!!! I put it in my smoothies in the morning and take a spoonful around 5PM. Love and Peas® and Nature's Harvest protein powder go in my smoothie! My other favorites are Flaxseed oil with Lignans, Adrenal Support, Thyroid Activator®/ Support, Master Gland® Formula, Super Trio®, JP-X, Lecithin, LBS II®, Lymph Gland Cleanse-HY, Women's X-Action®, Super Algae, MSM, Trigger Immune® TCM, Yeast & Fungal Detox, Breast Assured®, Target Endurance and Nervous Fatigue. If you would like to read more about these that I have mentioned, go to www.hope4health.mynsp.com

This cookbook is a vision that began over 3 years ago. Its timing is perfect and it is so needed in the kitchen of every home. My hope is that your health would be renewed and blessed as you eat these nutritious, delicious and colorful recipes. I want to encourage you that you can change your health and the health of your loved ones by cooking nutritious meals. You will feel better, have more energy, shed weight and look years younger.

Julie Cook
Ephesians 3:16-21

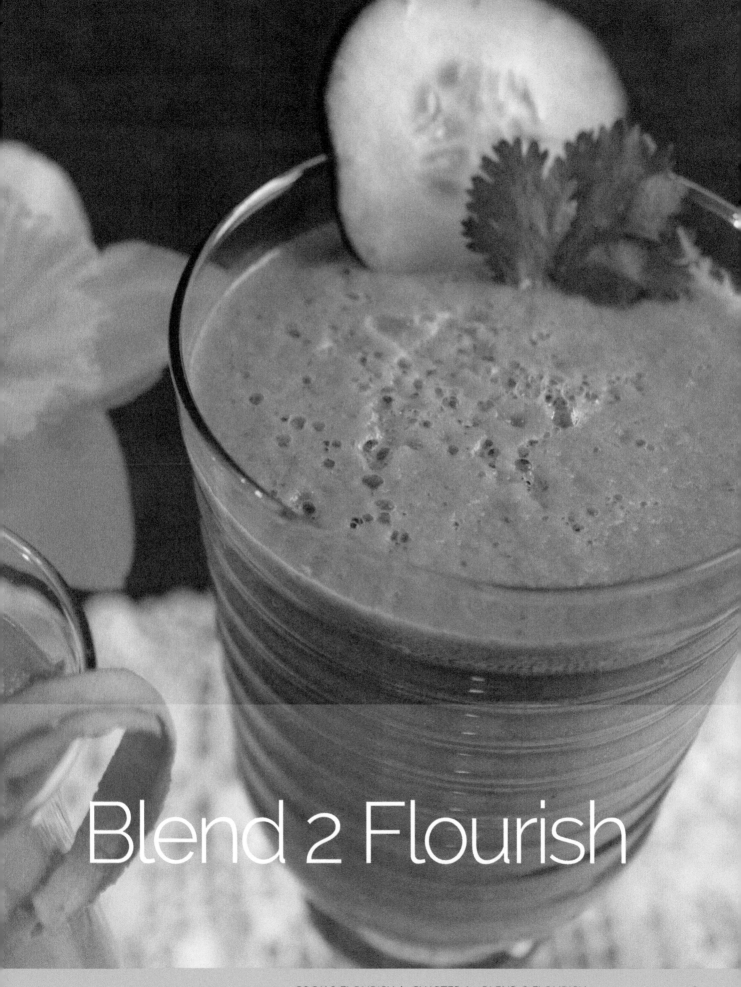

Blend 2 Flourish

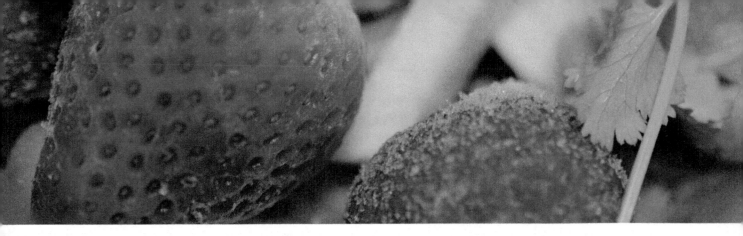

Nourish 2 Flourish Smoothie Formula

How to make 1 serving high speed blender with tight fitting lid

- **½ -1 cup Fresh or Frozen Fruit and Raw Sweet Vegetables:**

- organic carrot, with peeling	- organic strawberries	- banana	- blueberries
- organic peach, with peeling	- organic cherries	- kiwi	- pineapple
- organic red beet, with peeling	- organic apple, with peeling	- mango	- raspberries
- organic yellow beet, with peeling	- organic pear	- orange	- blackberries
			- sweet potato

- **½ -1 cup ice cubes**
- **1-1¼ cup (8-10 ounces) Fluid:**

- **1- 2 ½ cups total of Fresh Vegetables:**

- filtered water	- broccoli stems, peeled	- organic cucumber
- organic green or herbal tea	- organic parsley	- organic beet greens
- unsweetened almond milk	- organic cilantro	- organic dandelion greens
- unsweetened coconut milk	- organic celery ribs	- organic Swiss chard
	- organic kale, freeze the fresh	- organic spinach, freeze the fresh

---

Healthy Additions, choose as few or as many as you would like:

- ½ teaspoon Nature's Sunshine Stixated® powdered drink mix
- ½ Tablespoon Nature's Sunshine® flax seed oil with lignans
- 1-2 Tablespoons whole almonds, raw or soaked
- 1 Tablespoon Nature's Sunshine® Mineral Chi Tonic
- 1 Tablespoon cacao nibs
- ¼-1 teaspoon cinnamon
- ½ - 1 Tablespoon soaked flax seeds
- ¼ - ½ ripe avocado, pit removed and peeled, sliced

- ¼ - ½ inch slice fresh ginger
- 1 Tablespoon cocoa powder
- 1-2 Tablespoon walnuts
- 1-2 Tablespoon soaked chia seeds
- 5-10 drops liquid stevia, to taste
- 1 Tablespoon almond butter
- ½ Tablespoon unsweetened coconut flakes

Nature's Sunshine® Protein Powder, choose the equivalent of one serving:

- 1-2 scoops Love and Peas® protein powder (Sugar Free) (½-1 serving)
- 1-2 scoops Natures Harvest protein powder (½-1 serving)
- 1-2 scoops Nutri-Burn® protein powder, vanilla flavor (½-1 serving)

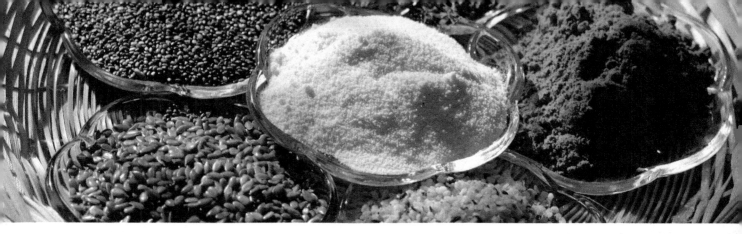

Directions:

1) Pour your choice of fluid into the high speed blender along with ice cubes.

2) Select your choice of fruit or sweet vegetable. If using carrot, scrub carrot to clean.

Cut the carrot into 6 or 7 pieces or grate it if your blender is not high powered. If using beets or sweet potato,

cut into small chunks so that you don't have big chunks at the bottom of your smoothie.

3) Select your choice of vegetables. If using celery ribs, cut into 6 or 7 pieces so it will blend up well.

Tip: purchase fresh greens such as kale, spinach or mixed greens and wash them then put them in a bag

in the freezer. They are then called "frozen fresh" and ready for your smoothies in the morning!

4) Select as few or as many of the additions as you would like. **Note: Although healthy, by combining the flax seed oil,**

avocado, cacao nibs, almond butter, walnuts and coconut flakes, the calorie content would be higher than necessary.

5) Protein in the morning within 20-50 minutes of waking up is essential for brain function, adrenal health, blood sugar

regulation and energy. Your body is in deficit without the protein. By using the Nature's Sunshine® protein powder, you

are receiving wholesome quality guaranteed nutrients to start your day that do not contain harmful additives, pesticide

residues or artificial sweeteners. Other protein powders may have heavy metal contaminants such as lead which can

disrupt hormones, artificial sweeteners that hinder brain function and are not tested for other pesticides or toxins.

6) Blend on high or on smoothie option.

> **Note:** For a smooth and creamy consistency, include avocado when using filtered water in your smoothie.
> Avocado is tasteless in the smoothie and really makes it creamy without the sugar content like a banana.
> Almond milk and coconut milk make a thicker and richer tasting smoothie, but has more calories and fat than
> filtered water. Be creative and be brave! Try more vegetables and less fruit! It's fun and satisfying!

Please note: We have labeled each recipe as either grain free, gluten free, dairy free or a combination of the three. Nature's Sunshine Stixated® powder drink mix sometimes does not agree with people with gluten intolerance, so we have not labeled recipes containing it "gluten free." As for the Love and Peas (Sugar Free)® protein powder, it is certainly gluten free, but since it has some protein derived from brown rice, we have not deemed it grain free.

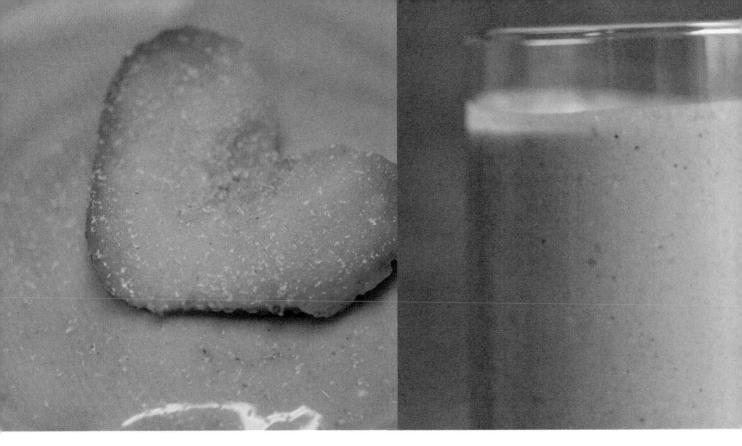

Berry Simple Smoothie

1 serving

- **8-10 ounces filtered water OR unsweetened almond milk**
- **1 cup frozen berries: strawberries, blueberries, mixed berries**
- **2 scoops Love and Peas® protein powder** *(Sugar Free)*

Directions:

1) Pour your choice of water or milk into the blender along with strawberries and protein powder.

2) Blend on high or on smoothie option until smooth and creamy.

Suggestion: add ½ cup ice if berries are not frozen. Super charge it with some spinach or organic celery. You could also do half water and half almond milk. For creamier consistency, add ¼ ripe avocado. Sweeten with stevia, to taste.

Apple Pie Smoothie

1 serving

- **½ cup unsweetened almond milk**
- **½ cup filtered water**
- **1 cup ice cubes**
- **½ an organic apple, Fuji or granny smith**
- **¼ ripe avocado, pit removed and peeled**
- **1 handful frozen fresh spinach leaves**
- **1 teaspoon cinnamon**
- **¼ teaspoon nutmeg**
- **Pinch pumpkin pie spice**
- **2 scoops Love and Peas® protein powder** *(Sugar Free)*

Directions:

1) Cut and core the apple.

2) Pour almond milk into blender along with water, ice cubes, apple, avocado, spinach, cinnamon, nutmeg, pumpkin pie spice, and protein powder.

3) Blend on high or on smoothie option until smooth and creamy.

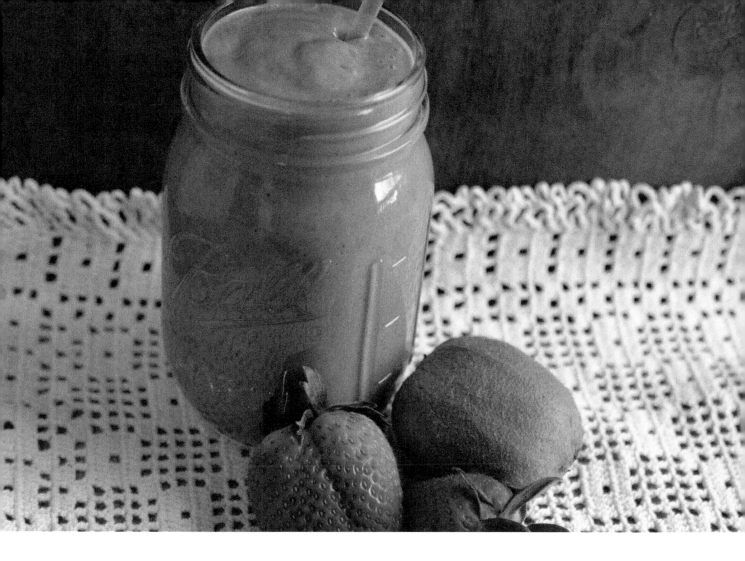

Strawberry Kiwi Smoothie

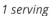

1 serving

- 8-10 ounces filtered water
- ½ cup ice cubes
- 1 kiwi
- ½-¾ cup strawberries, frozen
- 2 organic celery ribs
- ½ ripe avocado, pit removed and peeled
- ½ cup fresh organic cilantro

- ¼ inch slice fresh ginger root
- ½ teaspoon cinnamon
- ½ Tablespoon Nature's Sunshine® flax seed oil with lignans, optional
- 1 Tablespoon Nature's Sunshine® Mineral Chi Tonic, optional
- 2 scoops Love and Peas® protein powder *(Sugar Free)*

Directions:

1) Peel the kiwi. Cut the celery into 6 or 7 pieces.

2) Pour water into blender along with ice cubes, kiwi, strawberries, celery, avocado, cilantro, ginger root, cinnamon, flax seed oil (if desired), Mineral Chi Tonic (if desired) and protein powder.

3) Blend on high or on smoothie option until smooth and creamy.

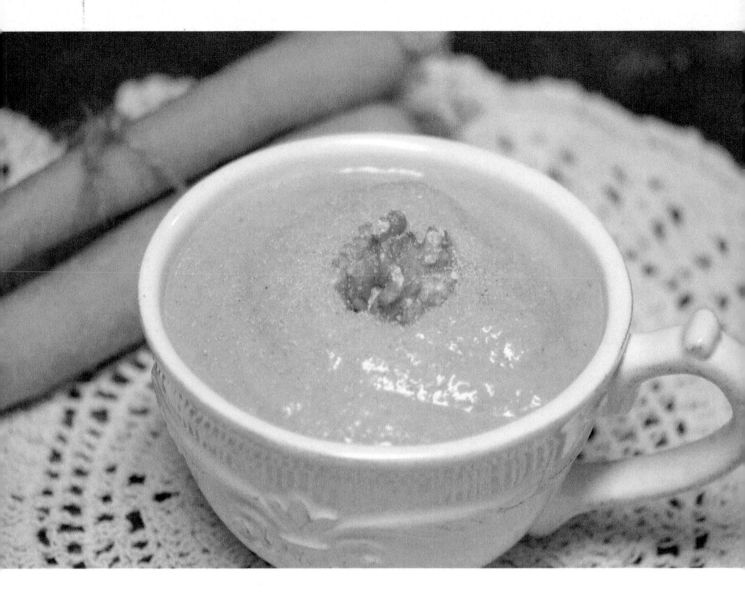

Carrot Cake Smoothie

1 serving

- 1 cup unsweetened almond milk
- 1 cup ice cubes
- 1 medium organic carrot
- ¼ ripe avocado, pit removed and peeled
- 1 Tablespoon walnuts
- 1 teaspoon cinnamon
- 2 scoops Love and Peas® protein powder
  (Sugar Free)

Directions:

1) Scrub carrot to clean. Cut the carrot into 6 or 7 pieces or grate it if your blender is not high powered.

2) Pour almond milk into blender along with water, ice cubes, carrot, avocado, walnuts, cinnamon and protein powder.

3) Blend on high or on smoothie option until smooth and creamy.

Now pretend that you are savoring a piece of carrot cake!

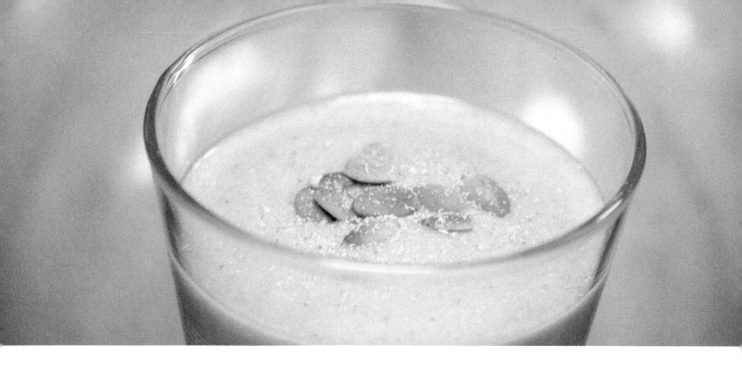

Pumpkin Spice Smoothie

1 serving

- **8 ounces unsweetened almond milk**
- **½ cup ice cubes**
- **½ cup unsweetened canned or fresh pumpkin puree**
- **1 cup frozen fresh spinach**
- **2 scoops Love and Peas® protein powder** *(Sugar Free)*
- **1 teaspoon cinnamon**
- **1 Tablespoons pumpkin seeds, optional**

Directions:

1) Pour milk into blender along with ice cubes, pumpkin, spinach, protein powder, cinnamon and pumpkin seeds (if desired). This is a green smoothie because of the spinach.

Pumpkin Patch Pudding Smoothie

1 serving

- **8 ounces unsweetened almond milk**
- **1 cup ice cubes**
- **¼ cup unsweetened canned or fresh pumpkin puree**
- **¼ avocado, pit removed and peeled**
- **2 scoops Love and Peas® protein powder** *(Sugar Free)*
- **¼ teaspoon cinnamon**
- **12 whole almonds**

Directions:

1) Pour milk into blender along with ice cubes, pumpkin, avocado, protein powder, cinnamon and almonds. This is an orange smoothie.

Tip: Make it a rich and delicious chocolate smoothie by adding 1 Tablespoon of carob powder.

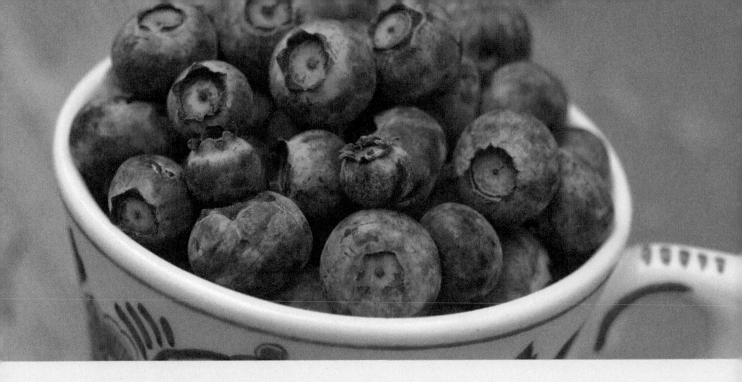

Spotlight : Blueberries

Whether you get to go pick your own blueberries and pop a few in your mouth or pick a bag up at the grocery store, blueberries are bursting with benefits!

Like walnuts, blueberries are beneficial for the brain, supporting memory and protecting the brain from accelerated decline. Blueberries are friendly to blood sugar since they are one of the lowest fruits on the glycemic index.

Not only do blueberries provide antioxidants for heart health, but also for the nervous system, digestive system, and structural system! In terms of heart health, cholesterol and triglycerides levels can be aided by blueberries and blood pressure levels can be positively affected. Continual stress wears on the nerves, but blueberries help to defend potential damage. Following a workout, muscles can be guarded from excessive breakdown by consuming blueberries; consider whirling them in a post workout smoothie with Nature's Sunshine® Love and Peas (Sugar Free)® or Nutri-Burn®.

Blueberries provide manganese, vitamin K, fiber, and vitamin C in addition to the benefits listed above.

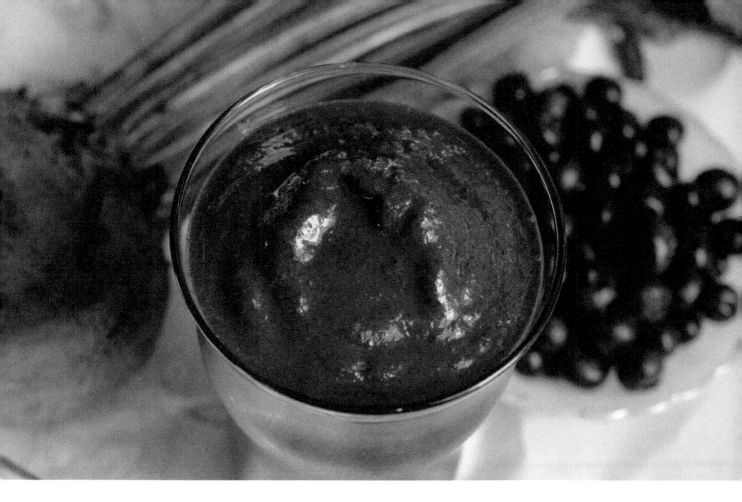

Julie's Morning Blueberry Smoothie

1 serving

- 8-10 ounces filtered water
- 1 cup ice cubes
- ½ cup blueberries, frozen
- 2 organic celery ribs
- ½ inch slice red beet
- ¼ inch slice fresh ginger
- 1 cup frozen fresh kale OR spinach

- 1 scoop Love and Peas® protein powder *(Sugar Free)*
- 1 scoop Natures Harvest protein powder (½ serving)
- ½ teaspoon cinnamon
- ¼ ripe avocado, pit removed and peeled
- 1 Tablespoon Nature's Sunshine® flax seed oil with lignans, optional
- 1 Tablespoon Nature's Sunshine® Mineral Chi Tonic, optional

Directions:

1) Cut each celery rib into 6 or 7 pieces.

2) Pour water into blender along with ice cubes, blueberries, celery, beet, avocado, your choice of kale or spinach, protein powder, cinnamon, ginger, flax seed oil (if desired), Mineral Chi Tonic

3) Blend on high or on smoothie option until smooth and creamy.

Note: Mom packs a lot of nutrition into her smoothie in the morning.

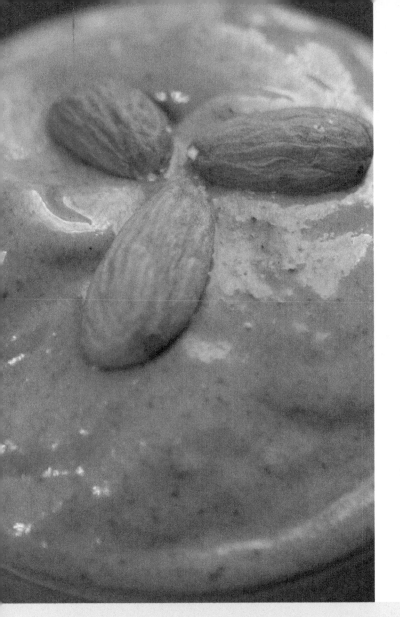

Carob Almond Smoothie

1 serving

Gluten Free
Dairy Free

- **8 ounces filtered water
  OR unsweetened almond milk**
- **1 cup ice cubes**
- **2 scoops Love & Peas® protein powder** *(Sugar Free)*
- **1 ½ cups frozen fresh kale**
- **1 Tablespoon unsweetened carob powder**
- **1 Tablespoon almond butter OR 10 whole almonds**

Directions:

1) Pour your choice of water or milk into blender along with ice cubes, protein powder, kale, carob powder, and almond butter.

2) Blend on high or on smoothie option until smooth and creamy.

> **Suggestion:** Substitutions are possible. Use spinach instead of kale, cocoa powder instead of carob powder. Half of a frozen banana is also good in this smoothie.

Cordyceps Concoction...

When I was interning with Dr. Inge Wetzel, she introduced me to a vast assortment of herbs. On occasion, I would get to make her breakfast shake in between appointments, and I asked her what she wanted in it. To my amazement, she requested that I include the Nature's Sunshine® Cordyceps in her health shake concoction. Curious what this tasted like, I included Cordyceps in my Nature's Sunshine® order and gave it a whirl.

To me, it gives the shake an earthy mocha note with benefits. Cordyceps is a Chinese herb that encourages vitality, supports the respiratory system, encourages the immune system, aids the endocrine system, provides energy for exercise, and has been shown to support heart health.

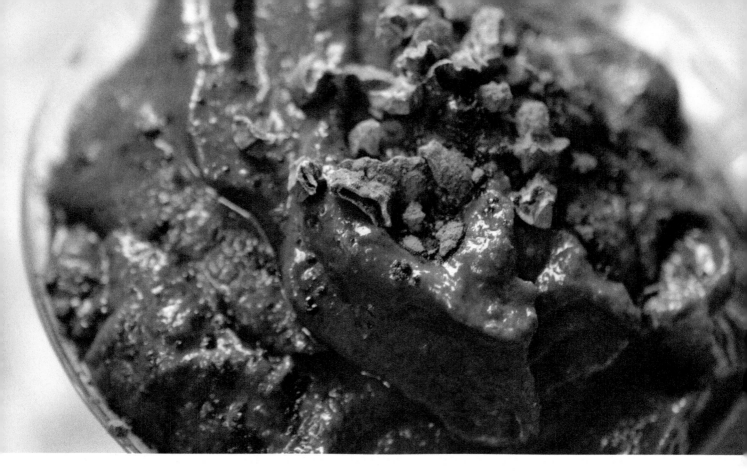

Robin's Power Smoothie

1 serving

- 8-10 ounces filtered water
- 1 cup ice cubes
- ½ cup slice fresh red beet
- 1 cup frozen fresh kale
- ½ ripe avocado, pit removed and peeled

- 2 Tablespoons carob powder
- 2 scoops Love and Peas® protein powder *(Sugar Free)*
- 2 capsules of Nature's Sunshine® Cordyceps
- Dash stevia, to taste
- ½ Tablespoon cacao nibs, optional

Directions:

1) Scrub beet to clean. Cut the beet into 6 or 7 pieces or grate it if your blender is not high powered.

2) Pour water into blender along with ice cubes, beet, kale, avocado, carob powder, cacao nibs (if desired) and protein powder. Open the Cordyceps capsules and empty the contents into the blender.

3) Blend on high or on smoothie option until smooth and creamy. Add stevia to taste and top with cacao nibs (if desired).

Detox smoothie idea:

Omit Kale, cacao nibs and carob powder and replace with:
- ½ cup fresh organic cilantro
- ¼ inch slice fresh ginger root
- 1 teaspoon cinnamon
- ¼ inch slice fresh turmeric root OR 1 Nature's Sunshine® CurcuminBP™ capsule

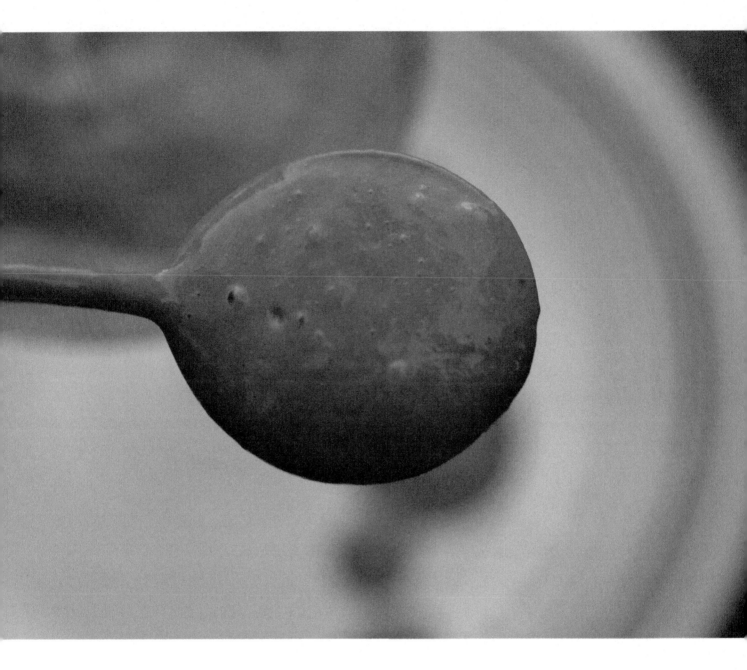

Chocolate Fudgesicle Smoothie

Gluten Free
Dairy Free

1 serving

- **8 ounces unsweetened almond milk**
- **1 ½ Tablespoons cocoa powder OR carob powder**
- **¼ ripe avocado, pit removed and peeled**
- **1 cup ice cubes**
- **2 scoops Love and Peas® protein powder** *(Sugar Free)*

Directions:

1) Pour almond milk into blender along with your choice of cocoa powder or carob powder, protein powder, avocado and ice.

2) Blend on high or on smoothie option until smooth and creamy.

Pour into Popsicle containers and freeze to make Fudgesicles.

Simple Chocolate Shake

1 serving

- **8-10 ounces filtered water**
  OR unsweetened almond milk
- **½ Tablespoon cocoa powder OR carob powder**
- **½ cup ice cubes**
- **2 scoops Love and Peas® protein powder**
  (Sugar Free)

Directions:

1) Pour your choice of water or milk into a sealed drink cup along with your choice of cocoa powder or carob powder, protein powder and ice.

2) Shake until mixed well.

Suggestion: You could do half water and half almond milk if you would like to.

We call this chapter Blend 2 Flourish because making smoothies is a simple, quick and delicious way to get both protein and essential nutrients to start your day. Why is protein so vital you ask, well let me tell you! Sipping on protein within 20 to 50 minutes of waking will set the tone for your: metabolism, satiety, blood sugar balance, adrenal health, brain power, and more! We like using the Nature's Sunshine® Love and Peas (Sugar Free)® protein because it provides 20 grams of protein per serving to begin our day!

Cocoa Mocha Almond Smoothie

1 serving

- **1 cup unsweetened almond milk**
- **½ cup filtered water**
- **1 cup ice cubes**
- **½ banana, frozen**
- **1 cup frozen fresh spinach**
- **1 Tablespoon cacao nibs**
- **1 Tablespoon carob powder**
- **½ teaspoon cinnamon**
- **1 Tablespoon almond butter OR 10 whole almonds**
- **2 capsules Nature's Sunshine® Cordyceps**
- **1 capsule Nature's Sunshine® Maca**
- **2 scoops Love & Peas® protein powder (Sugar Free)**

Directions:

1) Pour milk and water into blender along with ice cubes, protein powder, banana, spinach, cacao nibs, carob powder, cinnamon and almond butter.

2) Open the Cordyceps capsules and the Maca capsule and empty the contents into the blender.

3) Blend on high or on smoothie option until smooth and creamy.

Tip: Substitute ½ cup ice cubes for the ½ cup water for a thicker ice cream like consistency.

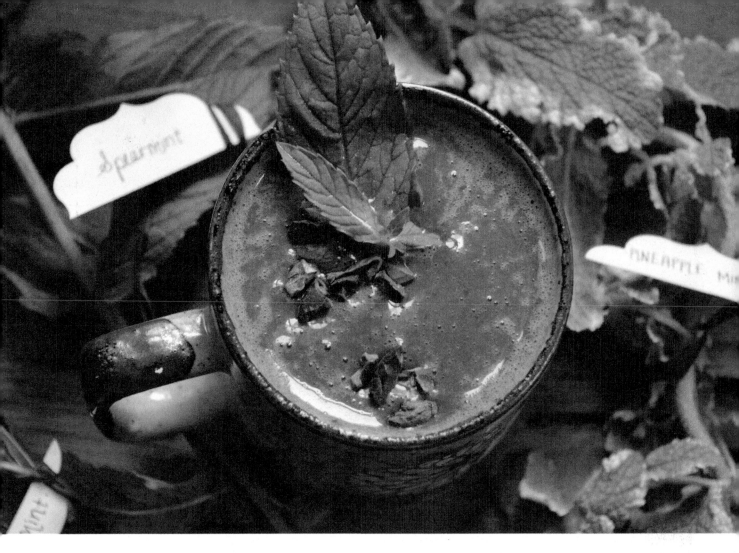

Fresh Mint Morning Smoothie

Although this smoothie can be enjoyed any time of day, drink it to help sip the morning grogginess away.

1 serving

- **2-4 fresh mint leaves, to taste**
- **10-12 ounces filtered water or unsweetened almond milk**
- **2 scoops Love & Peas® protein powder** *(Sugar Free)*
- **1 cup ice cubes**
- **1 cup frozen fresh kale**
- **¼ ripe avocado, pit removed and peeled**
- **2 Tablespoons carob powder**
- **½ Tablespoon Liquid Chlorophyll ES™**
- **8-10 drops liquid stevia, to taste, optional**
- **½ Tablespoon cacao nibs, optional**

Directions:

1) Pour water into blender along with ice cubes, mint leaves, kale, avocado, carob powder, chlorophyll and protein powder. If desired, add stevia to taste and cacao nibs.

2) Blend on high or on smoothie option until smooth and creamy.

Tip: If you want a thicker, spoon-able consistency, use 8 ounces of liquid. For a regular smoothie, use 10 ounces of liquid.

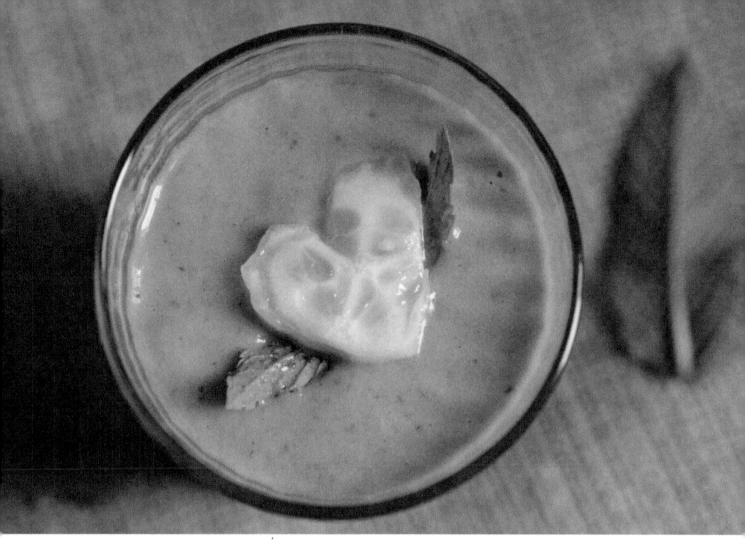

Cucumber Mint Smoothie

Gluten Free
Dairy Free

1 serving

- **6-8 ounces filtered water
  or unsweetened almond milk**
- **1 cup ice cubes**
- **1 cup organic cucumber**
- **¼ ripe avocado, pit removed and peeled**
- **1 teaspoon Liquid Chlorophyll ES™**
- **2 scoops Love & Peas® protein powder** *(Sugar Free)*
- **8-10 drops liquid stevia, to taste, optional**
- **8 fresh mint leaves, optional**
- **1 cup frozen fresh kale, optional**

Directions:

1) Pour water into blender along with ice cubes, cucumber, avocado, chlorophyll and protein powder. If desired, add stevia, mint leaves and kale.

2) Blend on high or on smoothie option until smooth and creamy.

Tip: If you want a thicker, spoon-able consistency, use 6 ounces of liquid. For a regular smoothie, use 8 ounces of liquid.

Soak 2 Flourish

When a seed goes into the ground, it does not sprout until it has come in contact with water. It is at this time that all of its stored nutrients begin to be mobilized and available for the growing seed. When you soak your seeds, nuts, and grains in your kitchen, you realize a similar effect.

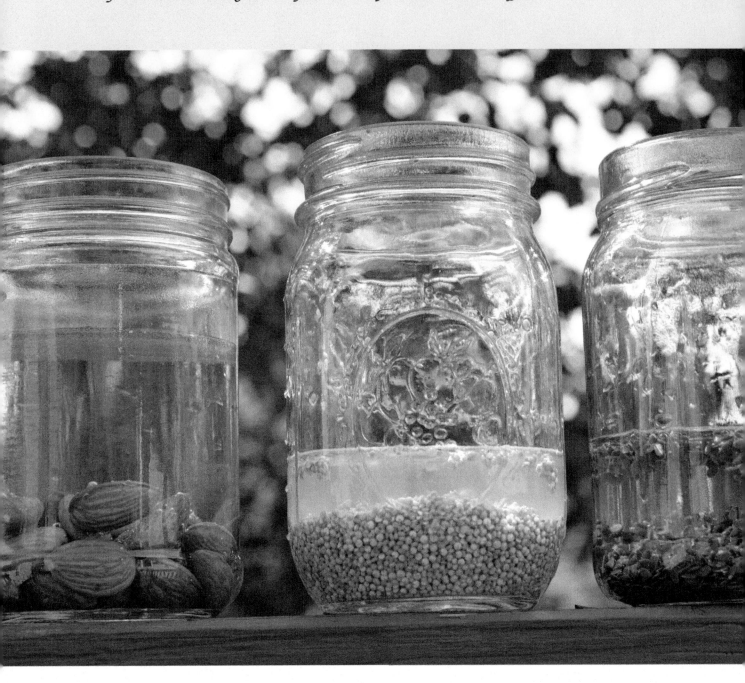

When soaked, the pH is more alkaline, there are fewer enzyme inhibitors which improves digestion, their nutrients are easier are more readily absorbable, and much more. Yes, it does take some planning ahead, but your digestive system and wallet will thank you since you will be efficiently accessing the nutrients and getting more for your money.

Soaking varies based on what seed, nut, or grain that you are soaking. For highly absorbable seeds like chia seeds, you may need 6 parts water to 1 part chia seeds. Flaxseeds are closer to a 4 to 1 ratio of water to seeds. The spelt berries, brown rice, quinoa, and almonds that are used in this book are simply placed in a glass jar with approximately 3 times the amount of water to grain/ nut and soaked 8 hours or overnight. For optimal digestion, add Nature's Sunshine® sea salt to the water, stir to dissolve and add almonds or other nuts you may wish to soak. For spelt berries, brown rice, and quinoa, add 1 teaspoon of lemon juice to the soaking water to diminish the negative effects of phytic acid.

Simply drain the seeds, nuts, or grains after soaking and rinse well before using or sprouting, and enjoy the soaked benefits!

	Chia seeds	Flaxseeds	Almonds	Brown rice	Quinoa	Spelt berries
Water ratio*	6 : 1	4 : 1	3 : 1	3 : 1	2 : 1	3 : 1
Sea salt**	None	None	1 teaspoon	None	None	None
Lemon juice**	None	None	None	1 teaspoon	1 teaspoon	1 teaspoon
Time	10 minutes - overnight	30 minutes - overnight	8 hours - overnight	8 hours - overnight	4 hours - overnight	8 hours - overnight

*water to seed/nut/grain ratio
**use accordingly; 1 teaspoon per 2 cups water

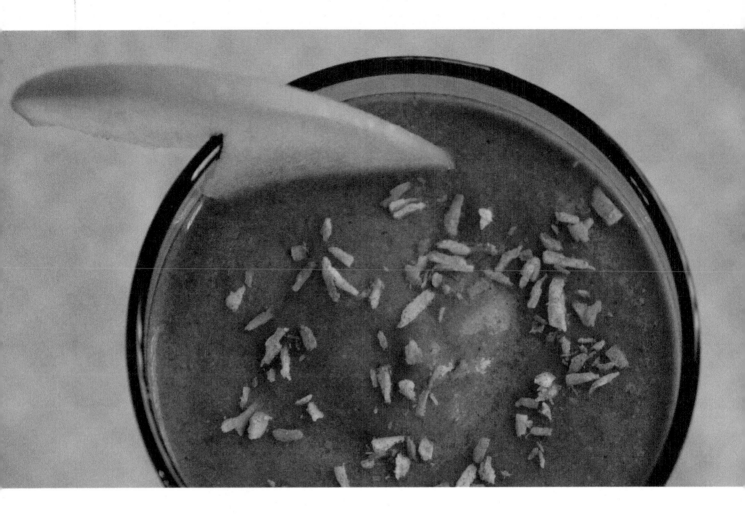

Morning Joy Smoothie

1 serving

- ½ cup filtered water
- 1 cup ice cubes
- ½ an organic carrot
- ½ an organic apple, Fuji or granny smith
- ¼ ripe avocado, pit removed and peeled
- 1 cup frozen fresh kale or spinach
- 1 teaspoon cinnamon
- 1 Tablespoon soaked flax seeds
- 1 Tablespoon unsweetened coconut flakes
- 1 scoop Love and Peas® protein powder
  (Sugar Free) (½ **serving**)
- Stevia, to taste
- 1 scoop Nature's Harvest protein powder
  (½ serving)

Directions:

1) Scrub carrot to clean. Cut the carrot into 6 or 7 pieces or grate it if your blender is not high powered.

2) Cut and core the apple.

3) Pour water into blender along with ice cubes, carrot, apple, avocado, your choice of kale or spinach, cinnamon, flax seeds, coconut, protein powder and stevia.

4) Blend on high or on smoothie option until smooth and creamy.

> ***Psalms 30:5b NLT***
> *"Weeping may last through the night,*
> *but joy comes with the morning."*

Morning Joy

· · · · · · · · · · · · · · ·

Psalms 30: 4-5 ESV

"Sing praises to the Lord, O you his saints,

    and give thanks to his holy name.

5 For his anger is but for a moment,

    and his favor is for a lifetime.

Weeping may tarry for the night,

    but joy comes with the morning."

Yesterday may have been rough, but God promises to bring joy.

Through His great grace and redemption, even the most painful of times can be used for good.

Romans 8:28 assures

"And we know that God causes everything to work together for the good of those who love God and are

called according to his purpose for them."

Resting in this truth gives hope for the day ahead and the days to come.

Romans 8:28 NLT

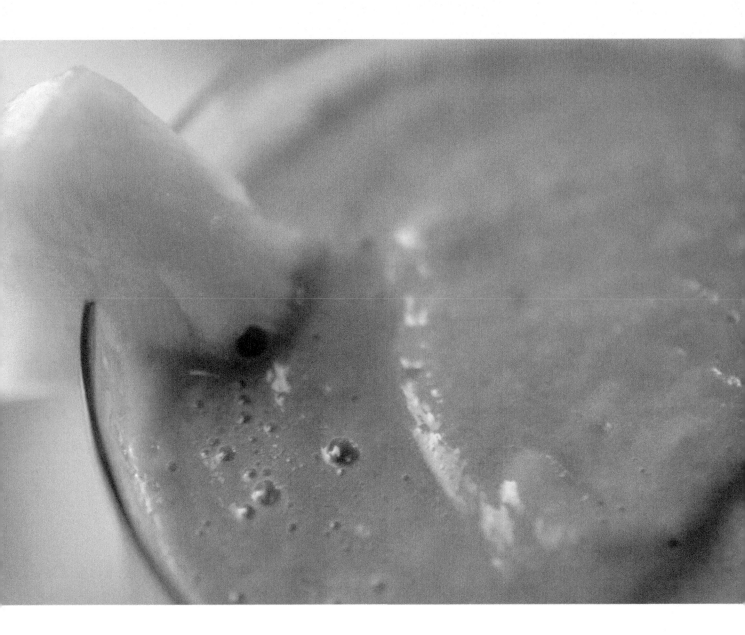

Pina-Kalada Smoothie

1 serving

- 1 cup filtered water OR unsweetened almond milk
- 1 cup ice cubes
- ¼ ripe avocado, pit removed and peeled
- 1 cup fresh frozen kale
- 1 cup fresh pineapple
- 2 scoops Love and Peas® protein powder *(Sugar Free)*
- 5-10 drops liquid stevia, to taste, optional

Directions:

1) Pour your choice of water or almond milk into blender along with ice cubes, avocado, kale and pineapple.

2) Add protein powder. Blend on high or on smoothie option until thick and creamy.

3) Add stevia (if desired).

Simple Chocolate Chai Shake

1 serving

- **8-10 ounces filtered water**
OR unsweetened almond milk
- **½ Tablespoon cocoa powder OR carob powder**
- **1 teaspoon cinnamon**
- **2 scoops Love and Peas® protein powder** *(Sugar Free)*
- **½ cup ice cubes**

Directions:

1) Pour your choice of water or milk into a sealed drink cup along with your choice of cocoa powder or carob powder, cinnamon, protein powder and ice.

2) Shake until mixed well.

> **Suggestion:** *You could do half water and half almond milk if you would like to.*

Carob Mint Smoothie

1 serving

- **8-10 ounces filtered water**
  or unsweetened almond milk
- **1 cup ice cubes**
- **1 cup frozen fresh kale**
- **¼ ripe avocado, pit removed and peeled**
- **1 Tablespoon carob powder**

- **2 Tablespoons soaked flax seeds**
- **1 teaspoon Liquid Chlorophyll ES™**
- **2 scoops Love & Peas® protein powder** *(Sugar Free)*
- **8-10 drops liquid stevia, to taste**
- **2 Nature's Sunshine® peppermint mints**
- **½ Tablespoon cacao nibs, optional**

Directions:

1) Pour your choice of water or almond milk into blender along with ice cubes, kale, avocado, carob powder, soaked flax seeds, liquid chlorophyll, protein powder, stevia, and peppermints.

2) Blend on high or on smoothie option until smooth and creamy. Garnish with cacao nibs (if desired).

Simple Cinnamon Shake

1 serving

- **8-10 ounces filtered water**
  OR unsweetened almond milk
- **1 teaspoon cinnamon**
- **½ cup ice cubes**
- **2 scoops Love and Peas® protein powder** *(Sugar Free)*

Directions:

1) Pour your choice of water or milk into a sealed drink cup along with the cinnamon, protein powder and ice.

2) Shake until mixed well.

> **Suggestion:** *You could do half water and half almond milk if you would like to.*

Refreshing Kiwi Smoothie

1 serving

- **8 ounces filtered water**
- **1 cup ice cubes**
- **1 kiwi**
- **2 organic celery ribs**

- **Stevia, to taste**
- **¼ ripe avocado, pit removed and peeled**
- **1 scoop Love and Peas® protein powder** *(sugar free)* **(½ serving)**
- **1 scoop Nature's Harvest (½ serving)**
- **1 Tablespoon unsweetened coconut flakes OR soaked flax/chia seeds**

Directions:

1) Peel the kiwi. Cut the celery into 6 or 7 pieces.

2) Pour water into blender along with ice cubes, kiwi, celery, avocado, protein powder and coconut.

3) Blend on high or on smoothie option until smooth and creamy. Add stevia to taste.

How to cut open a ripe Avocado

Directions:

1) Wash the ripe avocado. Using a sharp knife, cut into it lengthwise while turning the avocado and cutting all the way around. With your hands, twist the avocado in opposite directions to open it up. Remove the stem at the top. Whack the seed with your knife and twist your knife clockwise and the seed will come out. (Caution: Never put the seed into your mouth to clean the goodie off of it! The seed is so slick and it could cause you to choke!)

Cut the avocado in half again and peel back the skin and release the fruit. By peeling back the skin instead of spooning it out, you get the maximum health benefits of the antioxidants just under the thick outer shell. If you do use a spoon to scoop it out, scrape the shell to get these health benefits.

2) A potato masher or a fork will easily mash an avocado.

3) To keep the open avocado from turning brown, keep the seed in it.

4) To keep guacamole from turning brown, squeeze lime juice in the recipe or place the seed in the middle of the guacamole. Cover the guacamole with BPA free plastic wrap by placing the plastic wrap directly on the avocado mixture so no air is in the bowl.

5) Eat avocados by themselves, on toast with an egg, stuffed with tuna salad, guacamole, put them in smoothies, put them in soup, in a salad, in seaweed chips or put them in salad dressings.

They are so good! Enjoy!

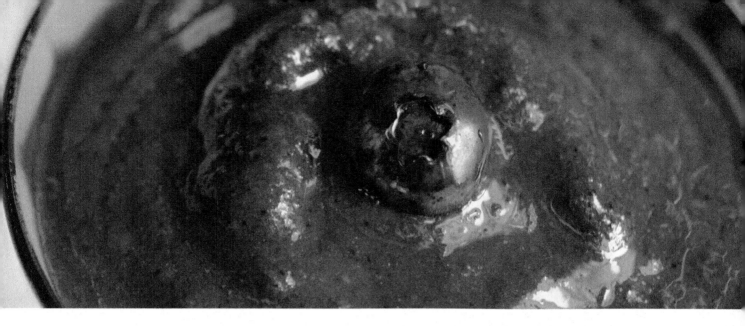

Blueberry Smoothie

Gluten Free
Dairy Free

1 serving

- 8 ounces unsweetened almond milk
- 1 cup ice cubes
- 1 cup blueberries, frozen
- 1 big handful spinach leaves
- 3-5 drops liquid stevia, to taste, optional
- 2 scoops Love and Peas® protein powder *(Sugar Free)*
- ¼ ripe avocado, pit removed and peeled, optional
- ½ teaspoon cinnamon OR 1 Tablespoon carob powder, optional

Directions:

1) Pour milk into blender along with ice cubes, blueberries, spinach, protein powder, avocado and your choice of cinnamon or carob powder (if using).

2) Blend on high or on smoothie option until smooth and creamy. Sweeten with stevia (if desired).

Suggestion: You could replace the avocado with ½ of a frozen banana to thicken and sweeten the smoothie (if so, use ½ cup blueberries and omit the stevia). Cocoa powder may be substituted for the carob powder. Filtered water may be substituted for the milk. Add in a slice or two of fresh red beet for added nutrients and a sweet taste.

Simple Stixated Smoothie

Dairy Free

1 serving

- ½ cup ice cubes
- 2 scoops Love and Peas® protein powder *(Sugar Free)*
- 8-10 ounces filtered water OR unsweetened almond milk
- ½ packet Nature's Sunshine Stixated® powdered drink mix

Directions:

1) Pour your choice of water or milk into a sealed drink cup along with the Stixated® powdered drink mix, protein powder and ice.

2) Shake until mixed well.

Suggestion: *You could do half water and half almond milk if you would like to.*

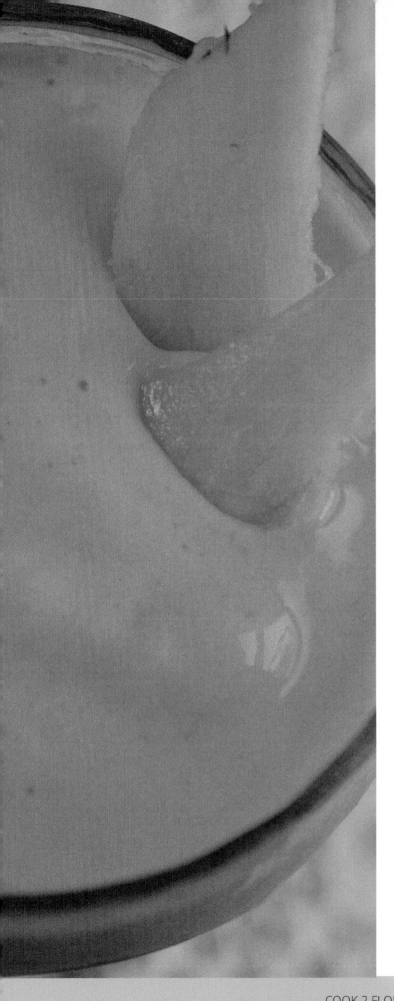

Tropical Tango Smoothie

1 serving

Gluten Free
Dairy Free

- 1 cup unsweetened almond milk
- 1 cup ice cubes
- 1 cup fresh mango   OR   pineapple
- 1 organic carrot   OR   2 organic celery ribs
- ¼ ripe avocado, pit removed and peeled
- 2 scoops Love and Peas® protein powder *(Sugar Free)*
- 1 Tablespoon soaked flax seeds
  OR 2 teaspoons soaked chia seeds

Directions:

1) Cut the fruit and the vegetable into pieces.

2) Pour milk into blender along with ice cubes, your choice of mango or pineapple, your choice of carrot or celery, avocado, protein powder and your choice of flax seeds or chia seeds.

3) Blend on high or on smoothie option until smooth and creamy.

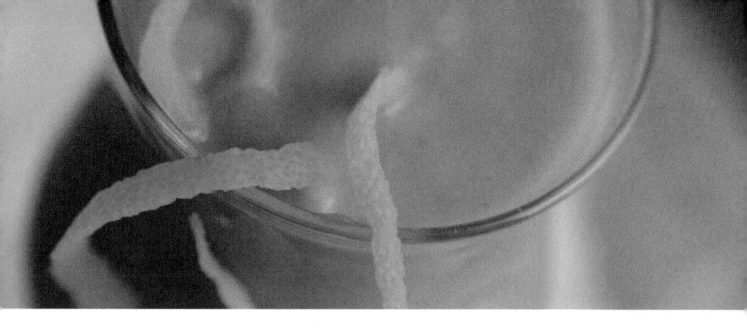

Refreshing Cucumber Lemonade Smoothie

1 serving

- ¾ cup filtered water
- 1 cup ice cubes
- ½ ripe avocado, pit removed and peeled
- 1 cup organic cucumber, sliced, with peeling
- 1 small lemon
- 2 scoops Love and Peas® protein powder *(Sugar Free)*
- 5-10 drops liquid stevia, to taste, optional

Directions:

1) Pour water into blender along with ice cubes, avocado and cucumber.

2) Peel the lemon. Cut it in slices and remove the seeds. Place in the blender.

3) Add protein powder. Blend on high or on smoothie option until thick and creamy.

4) Add stevia (if desired).

Substitution: Spinach for the cucumber.

Cucumber Pineapple Cilantro Smoothie

1 serving

- 8 ounces filtered water, chilled
- 1 cup ice cubes
- ½ ripe avocado, pit removed and peeled
- 1 ½ cups organic cucumber, sliced
- 1 cup fresh pineapple
- 1 cup frozen fresh spinach
- ½ cup fresh organic cilantro
- 2 scoops Love and Peas® protein powder *(Sugar Free)*
- 1 Tablespoon soaked flax seeds

Directions:

1) Pour water into blender along with ice cubes, avocado, cucumber, pineapple, spinach, cilantro, protein powder and flax seeds.

2) Blend on high or on smoothie option until thick and creamy.

Substitutions can be made: Substitute organic celery for the cucumber, any fruit can be substituted for the pineapple, kale can be substituted for the spinach and if you want, you can substitute 1 teaspoon chia seeds for the flax seeds.
Be creative!

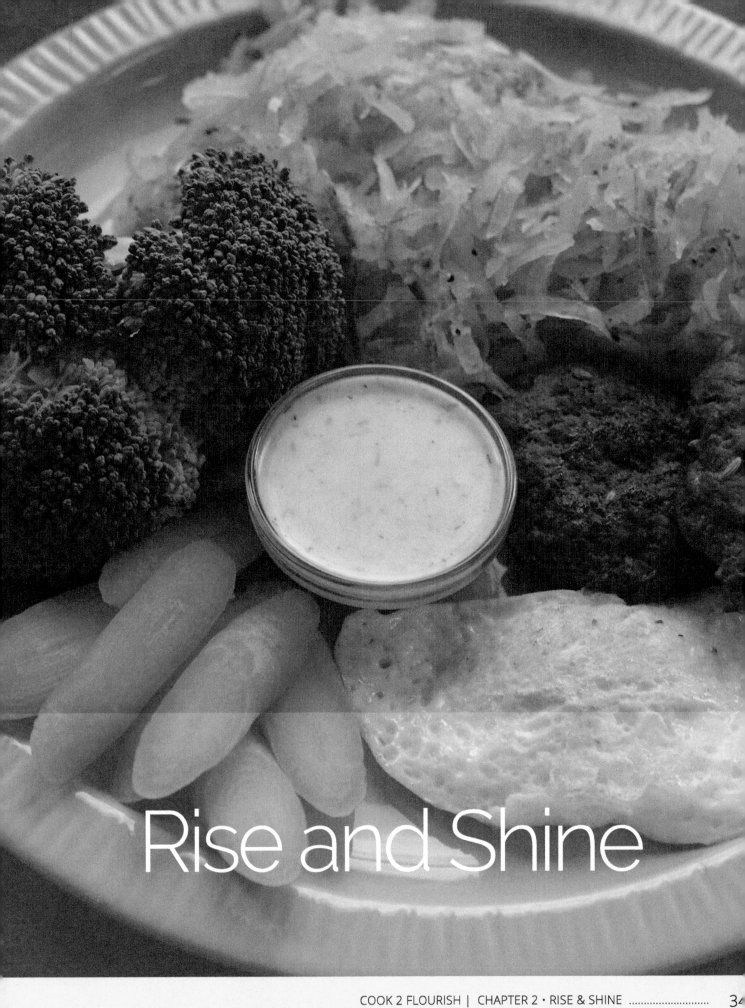

Rise and Shine

Breakfast Sausage

Gluten Free
Grain Free
Dairy Free

4 sausage patties

- ½ pound organic grass fed ground beef
- 2 ½ teaspoons breakfast sausage seasoning (page 238)

Directions:

1) Add the spices to the ground beef and mix well. Form into patties and fry in a stainless steel skillet turning often to keep from sticking. Serve immediately.

Remember to eat some fresh veggies with your breakfast. Raw broccoli and carrots are easy and you can dip them in Homemade Ranch Style Dressing (page 112).

Hash Browns

Gluten Free
Grain Free
Dairy Free

4 servings

- 3 small-medium organic russet potatoes, with skin
- 1 Tablespoon avocado oil OR grapeseed oil
- Nature's Sunshine® sea salt, to taste
- Ground black pepper, to taste

Directions:

1) Wash and dry the potatoes. Shred the potatoes then quickly place them in a colander and rinse them thoroughly under running water. Drain well.

2) Pour oil in a stainless steel skillet over medium heat and place the potatoes in the skillet while making sure the potatoes do not drip water into the skillet, as it will pop when the oil is hot. Spread out the potatoes evenly in the skillet.

3) Cook uncovered for 15-18 minutes, turning only once during cooking time. Serve hot.

Hen Berries

In the early days of getting our jewelry business started, Bernie would come over and help my dad while he worked in the "The Little Repair Shop" in our basement. I was three years old. Now, Bernie frequents our jewelry store to bring us fresh eggs, which he calls hen berries.

Every morning we are thankful for his generosity and for the unparalleled flavor of the golden yolks.

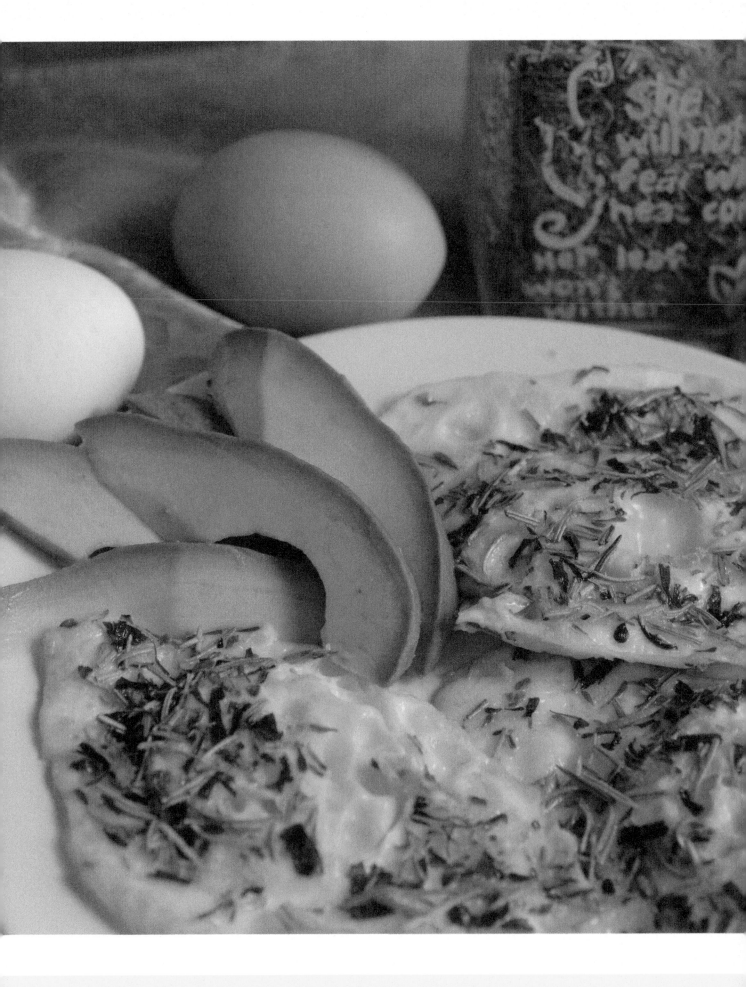

Green Eggs NO Ham

1 serving

Gluten Free
Grain Free
Dairy Free

- 2 organic eggs
- Dash cayenne pepper
- Dash ground black pepper
- ½ teaspoon extra-virgin coconut oil
- Dash Nature's Sunshine® sea salt
- ½ Tablespoon Her Leaf Won't Wither seasoning

Directions:

1) Place the coconut oil in a stainless steel skillet on medium-low heat.

2) Drop the eggs into the skillet and season the eggs with seasonings.

3) Cook the eggs on medium-low until thoroughly done (or to your preference) flipping over once during cooking time. Remove from heat and serve immediately.

Her Leaf Won't Wither

Makes < ½ cup

- 2 Tablespoons dried whole rosemary
- 2 Tablespoons dried oregano
- 1 Tablespoon dried tarragon leaf
- 1 Tablespoon dried thyme
- 1 Tablespoon dried parsley

Directions:

1) Combine all the herbs together in a bowl and stir well. Pour into a spice container.

Note: Please use organic herbs, if possible, to get the most nutritional benefit.

Her Leaf Won't Wither

It is amazing what God has put into herbs to benefit our bodies! In my quest to find any food to help my mom regain her strength, I came across an article on tarragon recounting how travelers would stuff their shoes with the herb to bolster their stamina. Taking this nugget of information, we began putting tarragon on our morning eggs and added other green herbs.

In honor of Dr. Seuss we laughed and said we were eating green eggs with no ham. We call this blend of herbs "Her Leaf Won't Wither" to commemorate this journey and the hope we clung to in Jeremiah 17:8 that my mom's life was not going to fade, but flourish! It has been a journey, but God has been faithful through it all! May your leaf be green, too!

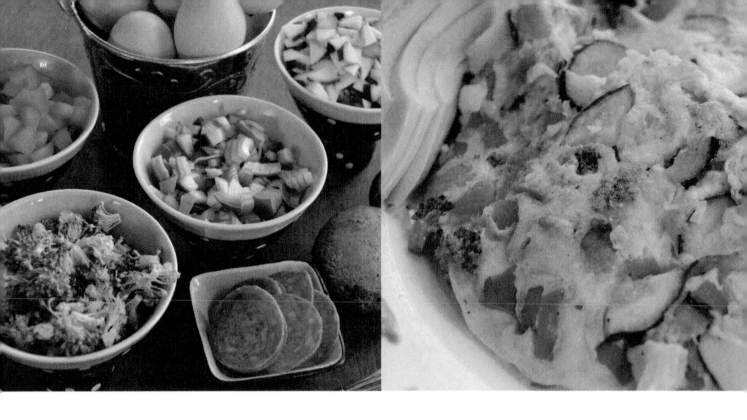

O'mazing Omelet

How to make 1 serving

- **½ teaspoon grapeseed oil**
- **2 organic eggs**
- **1-1 ½ cups total of fresh vegetables:**

    - bell pepper   - broccoli

    - black olives   - mushrooms

    - garlic   - onion

    - tomatoes   - zucchini

- **¼ cup unsweetened milk:**

    - almond   - coconut

- **Seasoning:**

    - cayenne pepper   - dried oregano

    - dried whole rosemary   - dried thyme

    - Nature's Sunshine® sea salt

    - ground black pepper

- **Toppings:**

    - ½ ripe avocado, pit removed and peeled, sliced

    - 1 Tablespoon white cheese

    - 1 Tablespoon organic cilantro

    - 1 Tablespoon dried parsley

    - 2 Tablespoons salsa

Directions:

1) Pour the grapeseed oil in a stainless steel skillet on medium heat. Sprinkle in the fresh vegetables of your choice and the amount you desire. Sauté for 3 or 4 minutes so that the vegetables get a head start of the eggs. Lower the temperature to medium-low.

2) Beat the eggs and your choice of milk together then pour over the vegetables.

3) Season the eggs with your choice of seasonings and the amount you desire.

4) Cook the eggs until thoroughly done, flipping over once during cooking time. Approximately 3-5 minutes.

5) Remove from heat and plate. Garnish with any toppings (if desired). Serve immediately.

Tip: Do not allow the oil to get too hot and smoke! It becomes a trans-fat and is rancid. If this happens, let the pan cool, wash it and start over. It is best to wash the pan between each omelet you make.

Egg Omelet Muffins

Gluten Free
Grain Free
Dairy Free

Makes 6 muffins

- **6 organic eggs, beaten**
- **¼ cup bell pepper, chopped**
- **½ cup zucchini, diced**
- **½ cup onion, chopped**
- **1 Tablespoon fresh basil, minced**
- **½ teaspoon garlic granules**
- **¼ teaspoon Nature's Sunshine® sea salt**
- **⅛ teaspoon ground black pepper**
- **Dash cayenne pepper**
- **¼ cup sundried tomatoes in extra-virgin olive oil, chopped**

Directions:

1) In a mixing bowl, mix together the eggs, tomatoes, bell pepper, zucchini, onion, basil, garlic, sea salt, black pepper and cayenne pepper until combined.

2) Pour the egg mixture into unbleached muffin liners in a stainless steel muffin pan or use a stoneware muffin pan only! Bake in preheated 350 degree oven for 25-30 minutes. Serve immediately and refrigerate any leftovers.

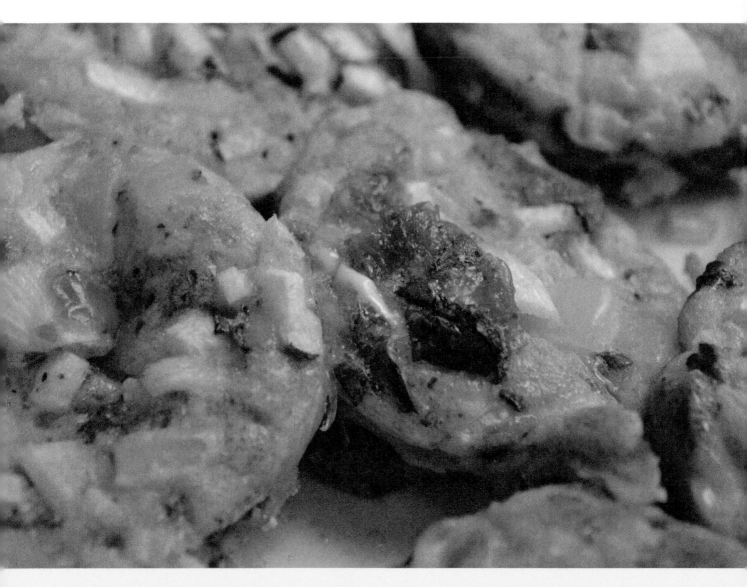

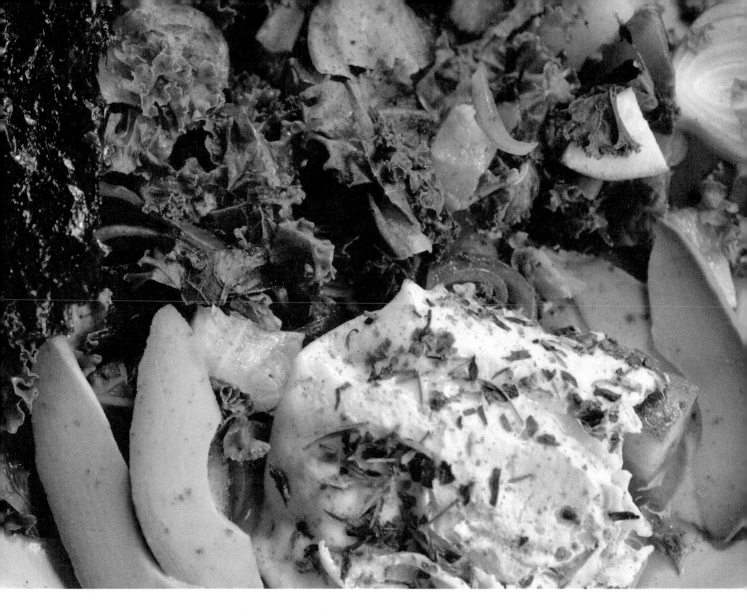

Egg Superfood Sauté

Gluten Free
Grain Free
Dairy Free

1 serving

- **2 organic eggs, cooked, seasoned with dash cayenne pepper**
- **⅓ cup chicken broth**
- **Dash Nature's Sunshine® sea salt**
- **Dash ground black pepper**
- **4 cups total your choice of veggies:**
  - Kale, Swiss chard, beet greens, onion slices, mushroom slices

Directions:

1) Place the chicken broth in a stainless steel skillet and bring to a boil over medium heat. Add the veggies, sea salt and pepper. Cover with a lid and steam sauté for 5-8 minutes to desired al dente' doneness.

2) Plate your veggies and top with the cooked eggs.

This is also really good served with seasoned salmon instead of the egg! Serve with seaweed chips or toast.

Spotlight : Kale

Kale... I can remember the awestruck moment in the grocery store when my mom and I discovered kale. What drew me in was its impressive line-up of nutrients, the longest list of vitamins and minerals I had ever seen on a food, everything from folic acid to omega 3! This was a stark contrast to the processed food with the laundry list of unpronounceable ingredients that had contributed to my mom's health crisis. I felt as if I had struck gold, finding a new power tool for my healing super food tool box. I encourage you to try kale if you haven't already in kale chips or one of our delicious salads- your body's cells will be glad you did!

Believe it or not, kale is not a new health food find at all; its cultivation dates back to 600 years before Christ and many a peasant thrived off this leafy wonder in the Middle Ages. Kale made it to America in the 1600's and is becoming increasingly renowned for its nutrient density and versatility in smoothies, salads, soups, and other delicious dishes!

Each fork-full has its benefits:

• kale's contributions include calcium, carotenoids and chlorophyll

• as a plant source of omega 3 (ALA), kale may provide anti-inflammatory action

• especially when steamed, kale may help lower cholesterol

• kale aids in ridding the body of toxins

A note about antioxidants:

Like a thief, free radicals (oxidants) are out of control trying to regain their lost electron, and to do so, steal the electron from a healthy cell. Meet antioxidants. A deficiency of antioxidants ("against the robber") can make our bodies more vulnerable to "oxidative stress" or cell stress. If our cells are stressed, no wonder we are stressed! Antioxidant rich foods like kale to the rescue!

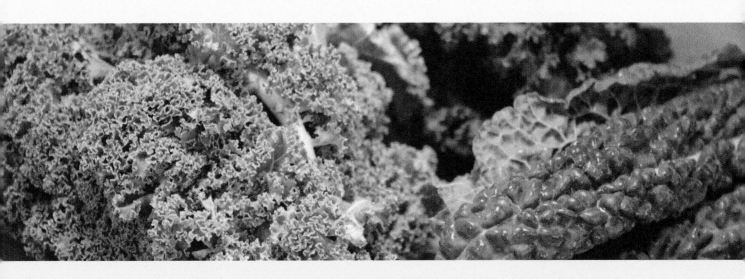

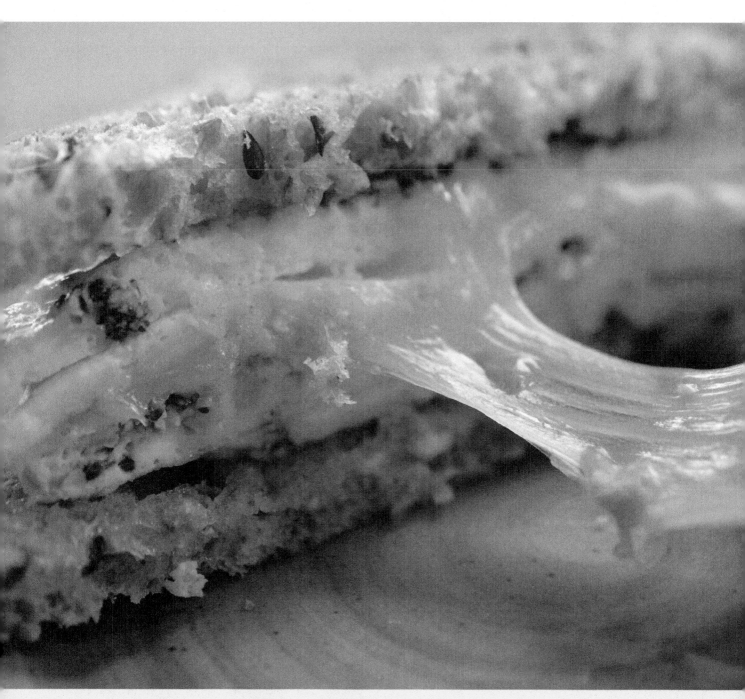

Egg Man-wich

Egg Man-wich

Eat in Moderation

1 serving

- ½ teaspoon extra-virgin coconut oil
- 2 organic eggs
- Dash Nature's Sunshine® sea salt
- Dash cayenne pepper
- 2-3 Tablespoons broccoli floret, tips only
- 2 slices Alvarado ST.® essential flax seed bread OR Ezekiel® 100% sprouted whole grain bread
- 1 Tablespoon organic butter
- ½ ounce slice of pepper jack cheese

Directions:

1) Place the coconut oil in a stainless steel skillet on medium-low heat.

2) Lightly beat the eggs and pour into the skillet.

3) Season the eggs with sea salt and cayenne pepper.

4) Slice the broccoli floret tips into the egg mixture.

5) Let the eggs cook on medium-low for about 4 or 5 minutes then flip over and continue cooking until thoroughly done.

6) Toast and butter the bread. Cut the eggs in half. Fold one piece of egg onto each slice of toast. Top one egg with the cheese and bring the two slices of toast together to make a sandwich. Serve immediately.

Tip: This is a breakfast sandwich you can eat on the go. Just wrap a paper towel around the bottom of the sandwich and enjoy!

Breakfast in a Baggie

Gluten Free
Grain Free
Dairy Free

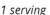

1 serving

- 2 organic eggs, boiled and shelled
- 4 broccoli florets
- 6 organic baby carrots
- 8 walnut halves

Directions:

1) Place the above ingredients in a sandwich baggie and eat on your way to work.

Tip:
This is a quick and nourishing breakfast you can eat on the go.

Scrambled Eggs

Gluten Free
Grain Free
Dairy Free

1 serving

- ½ teaspoon extra-virgin coconut oil
- 2 organic eggs
- 3 Tablespoons unsweetened almond milk
- Dash Nature's Sunshine® sea salt
- Dash ground black pepper

Directions:

1) Place the coconut oil in a stainless steel skillet on medium-low heat.

2) Whisk the eggs and milk together with a fork until combined then pour into the skillet.

3) Season the eggs with sea salt and pepper.

4) Let the eggs cook on medium-low for about 3 minutes then take a spatula and lightly scrape the edges of the skillet. Then fold the eggs over in small amounts. Let cook another minute and repeat folding until the eggs are thoroughly done. Eggs are considered done when all the runny liquid is cooked and the eggs are light and fluffy.

Cook by Name

My PaPa was a cook by name, not by deed. He was a wonderful man, and what a gift it was to have him live in our home growing up.

He couldn't cook a lick... except one dish, scrambled eggs. Before one particular Saturday tee time, the two of us [I was 10 years old] hovered over the stove, PaPa recalling his scrambled egg duty in the army.

After a few cracks, stirs and a dash of patience, we had a plate of fluffy scrambled eggs. Despite his limited kitchen aptitude, his loving, Godly legacy lives on.

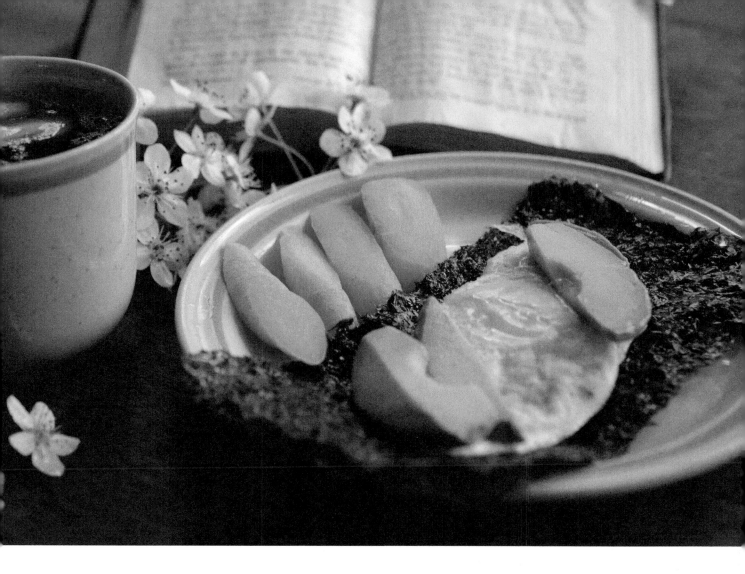

Early Bird Egg Wrap

1 serving

- ½ teaspoon extra-virgin coconut oil
- 2 organic eggs
- Dash Nature's Sunshine® sea salt
- Dash cayenne pepper
- **Choose Wrap – seaweed, lettuce, kale or cauliflower flat bread**
- **Choose Garnish – avocado, spinach leaves, shredded carrots or sundried tomatoes**
- **Fresh herbs, if desired**

Directions:

1) Place the coconut oil in a stainless steel skillet on medium-low heat.

2) Drop the eggs into the skillet. Season the eggs with sea salt and cayenne pepper.

3) Cook the eggs on medium-low until thoroughly done or to your preference, flipping over once during cooking time. Less time for sunny side up (liquid yolk) or a few minutes more for firm yolk.

4) Place the eggs on your choice of wrap. Top with your choice of garnishes.

5) Sprinkle with fresh herbs (if using).

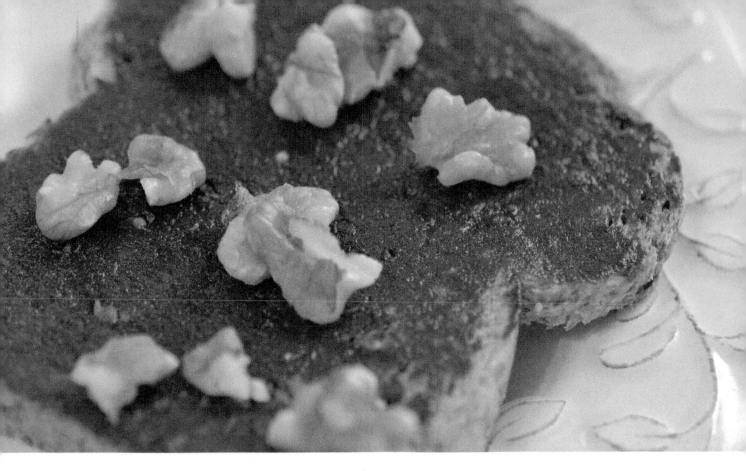

Cinnamon Breakfast Toast

Dairy Free

1 serving

- **½ teaspoon ground ginger**
- **1 teaspoon cinnamon**
- **1 teaspoon extra-virgin olive oil**
- **1 teaspoon raw honey**
- **1 slice Ezekiel® bread**
- **2 Tablespoons English walnuts, chopped**

Directions:

1) In a ¼ cup measuring cup or ¼ cup small rounded bowl, combine ginger, cinnamon, olive oil and honey. Stir with a butter knife.

2) Toast the slice of bread. Remove from toaster and spread all of the cinnamon mixture on the bread. Top with walnuts.

Benefits:

Supports metabolism and circulatory system as well as helps your body to detox. This recipe has healthy fats and fiber. It reminds me of eating a cinnamon roll!

Timo's Morning Oatmeal

Dairy Free

1 serving

- ½ cup filtered water
- ½ cup unsweetened almond milk
- ½ cup organic gluten free old fashioned rolled oats
- 1 teaspoon raw honey OR 2-4 drops liquid stevia
- 1 teaspoon cinnamon
- ½ Tablespoon organic oat bran
- 1 teaspoon extra-virgin coconut oil
- ½ scoop Love and Peas® protein powder (Sugar Free)
- 8 pecans, for serving

Directions:

1) In a small sauce pan, heat the water and milk for 2-3 minutes.

2) Add in the oats, your choice of sweetener, cinnamon, and oat bran.

3) Simmer over medium heat for 7-8 minutes, stirring often, until oats are cooked and the consistency is thick and bubbly.

4) Remove from heat and stir in the protein powder and coconut oil.

5) Pour into a cereal bowl and top with the pecans. Serve immediately.

Tip:
For gluten free, omit the organic oat bran.

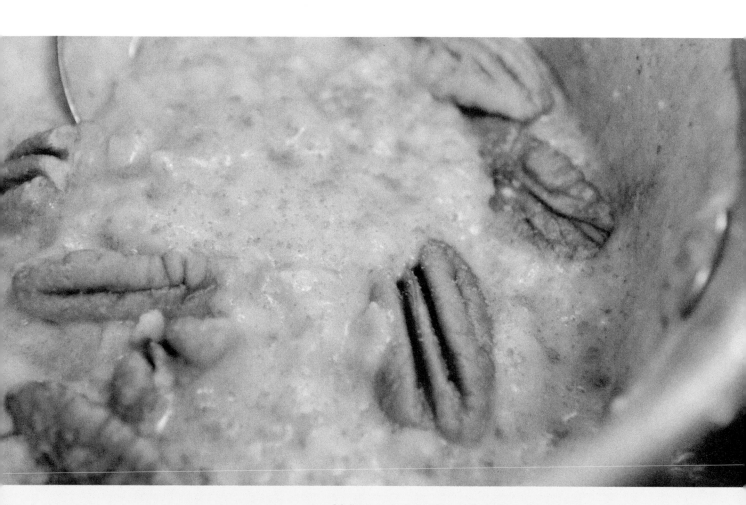

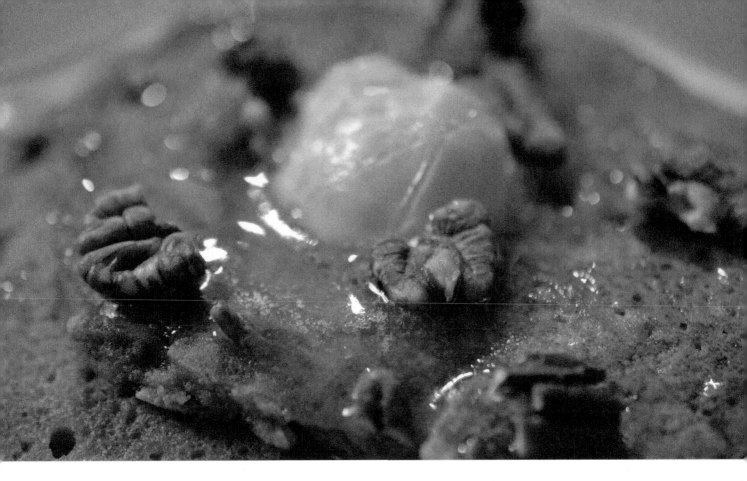

Pumpkin Protein Pancakes

Makes 6-8 pancakes

- ½ cup unsweetened canned pumpkin puree
- 3 organic eggs
- 2 Tablespoons extra-virgin coconut oil, melted
- ½ cup unsweetened almond milk
- ½ teaspoon organic pure vanilla extract
- 2 scoops Love & Peas® protein powder *(Sugar Free)*
- ½ teaspoon baking powder
- ½ Tablespoon cinnamon
- ¼ cup coconut flour
- 2 Tablespoons raw honey OR coconut sugar

Directions:

1) Beat the eggs and pumpkin together in a small bowl. Stir in 2 Tablespoons coconut oil, almond milk and vanilla extract.

2) In a separate bowl mix together the protein powder, baking powder, cinnamon, coconut flour and your choice of honey or coconut sugar.

3) Combine the dry ingredients into the wet ingredients and stir to thoroughly combine.

4) Line a stainless steel baking sheet with unbleached parchment paper. Spray the parchment paper lightly with non-stick grapeseed oil spray or better yet, bake on stoneware. Pour ¼ cup of batter onto stoneware per serving.

5) Bake in preheated 320 degree oven for 15-20 minutes.

6) Serve immediately with organic butter (omit for dairy free), raw honey, pure maple syrup grade B, pecans or fresh fruit.

Tip: If you have leftovers, you could use as a wrap with almond butter and apple slices or along side of a salad with a chicken breast.

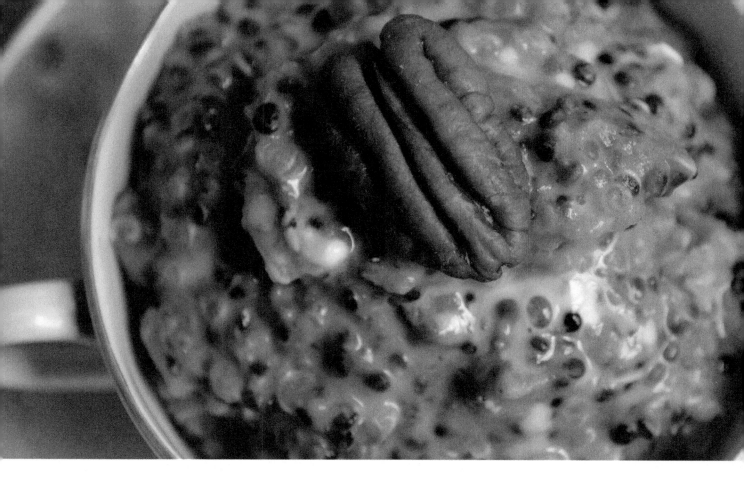

Pumpkin Pecan Quinoa

1 serving

- ¼ cup quinoa, soaked overnight
- ½ cup unsweetened almond milk
- ¼ cup canned pumpkin puree
- 2 Tablespoons canned full fat coconut milk
- ½ -1 teaspoon cinnamon, to taste
- 5 drops liquid stevia, to taste
- 2 Tablespoons pecans, chopped

Directions:

1) Place the dry quinoa in a glass jar and fill with enough water to cover by one inch and allow to soak overnight.

2) In the morning, drain and rinse the quinoa.

3) Bring the almond milk to a boil in a small saucepan.

4) Add the soaked quinoa to the almond milk and cook approximately 8 minutes or until the quinoa is cooked and most, if not all, of the almond milk is absorbed. Reduce the heat to low and drain off any excess almond milk (if desired).

5) Stir in the pumpkin, coconut milk, cinnamon, stevia, and pecans. Serve as soon as the quinoa mixture is thoroughly heated.

Note: This recipe easily doubles and will keep 1-2 days in the fridge. It would be tasty hot or cold. Substitutions: Omit the pumpkin and add in blueberries or mashed banana. To bolster the protein content, add raw shelled hemp hearts.

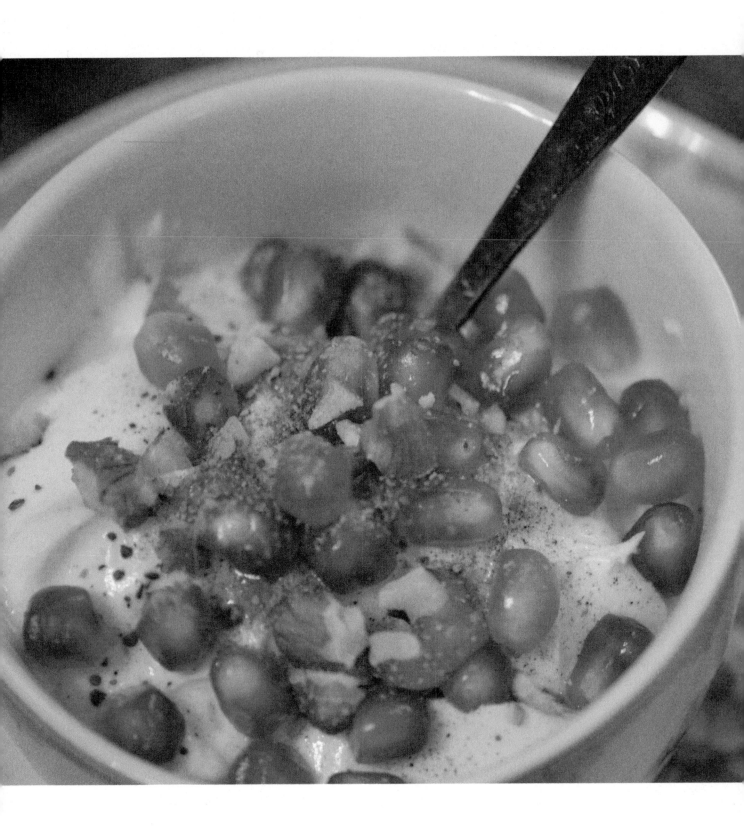

Flaxy-Pomegranate Yummiest Yogurt

1 serving

- **1 cup organic Greek yogurt, plain whole milk**
- **½ teaspoon Nature's Sunshine Stixated® powdered drink mix**
- **½ - 1 teaspoon Nature's Sunshine® flax seed oil with lignans**
- **⅓ cup pomegranate arils**
- **2 Tablespoons walnuts, chopped**
- **½ teaspoon cinnamon**

Directions:

1) In a small serving bowl mix together the yogurt, Stixated® powder, and flaxseed oil.

2) Wash the pomegranate then cut it in half. Over a bowl, peel back the peeling while breaking the half in half. This will cause the little arils to fall into the bowl. Remove any pith or peeling. Add pomegranate arils to the yogurt.

3) Top with walnuts and sprinkle on the cinnamon.

This is such a tasty yogurt to eat!
The pomegranate arils burst in your mouth with a touch of cinnamon and the crunch of the walnut!

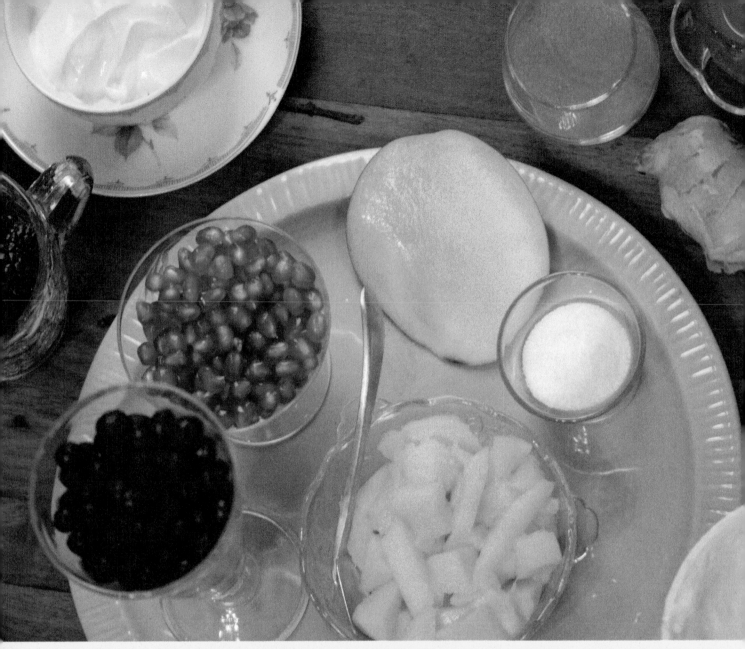

Yogurt Sundae Buffet

Blueberry Yogurt

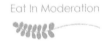

1 serving

- 1 cup organic Greek yogurt, plain whole milk
- ½ teaspoon cinnamon
- ¼ cup blueberries, fresh or frozen
- 2 Tablespoons black walnuts

Directions:

1) Place the yogurt in a small serving bowl. Sprinkle the cinnamon on top, add the blueberries and black walnuts.

Yogurt Sundae Buffet

How to make 1 serving

- **½ -1 cup yogurt:**
    - Wallaby® organic Greek yogurt, plain whole milk
    - goat's milk yogurt, plain whole milk
    - coconut milk yogurt, plain unsweetened
    - almond milk yogurt, plain unsweetened

- **½ teaspoon flavoring:**
    - cinnamon   **-** carob powder
    - fresh ginger, grated
    - Nature's Sunshine® flax seed oil with lignans
    - Nature's Sunshine Stixated® powdered drink mix

- **Crunchy toppings:**
    - ½ teaspoon chia seeds
    - ½ teaspoon flax seeds
    - 1 Tablespoon unsweetened coconut flakes
    - 1 Tablespoon pumpkin seeds
    - 1 Tablespoon raw wheat germ
    - 2 Tablespoons soaked almonds
    - 2 Tablespoons pecans OR walnuts

- **Sweetness:**
    - ½-1 teaspoon raw honey
    - ½-1 teaspoon pure maple syrup grade B
    - 3-5 drops stevia, to taste

- **½ cup fresh fruit:**

- banana	- blue berries	- organic apple
- kiwi	- black berries	- organic cherries
- mango	- raspberries	- organic peaches
- pineapple	- pomegranate	- organic strawberries

Directions:

1) Spoon your choice of yogurt and the amount you desire in a small serving bowl.
2) Mix in one flavoring of your choice.
3) Stir in one serving of your choice of sweetness, to taste (if desired).
4) Add in your choice of fresh fruit.
5) Sprinkle with one or two crunchy toppings of your choice.

Strawberry Yogurt

Eat In Moderation

1 serving

- **5 strawberries, divided**
- **1 cup organic Greek yogurt, plain whole milk**
- **½ - 1 teaspoon Nature's Sunshine® flax seed oil with lignans**
- **½ - 1 teaspoon raw honey OR 2-4 drops liquid stevia**
- **1 capsule Nature's Sunshine Probiotic 11®**
- **½ teaspoon Nature's Sunshine Stixated®**
  powdered drink mix

Directions:

1) In a small serving bowl mix together the yogurt, Stixated® powder, flaxseed oil, your choice of honey or stevia, and only the contents of the Probiotic capsule.
2) Mash 3 strawberries and stir into the yogurt. Slice the remaining 2 strawberries and garnish on top of the yogurt.

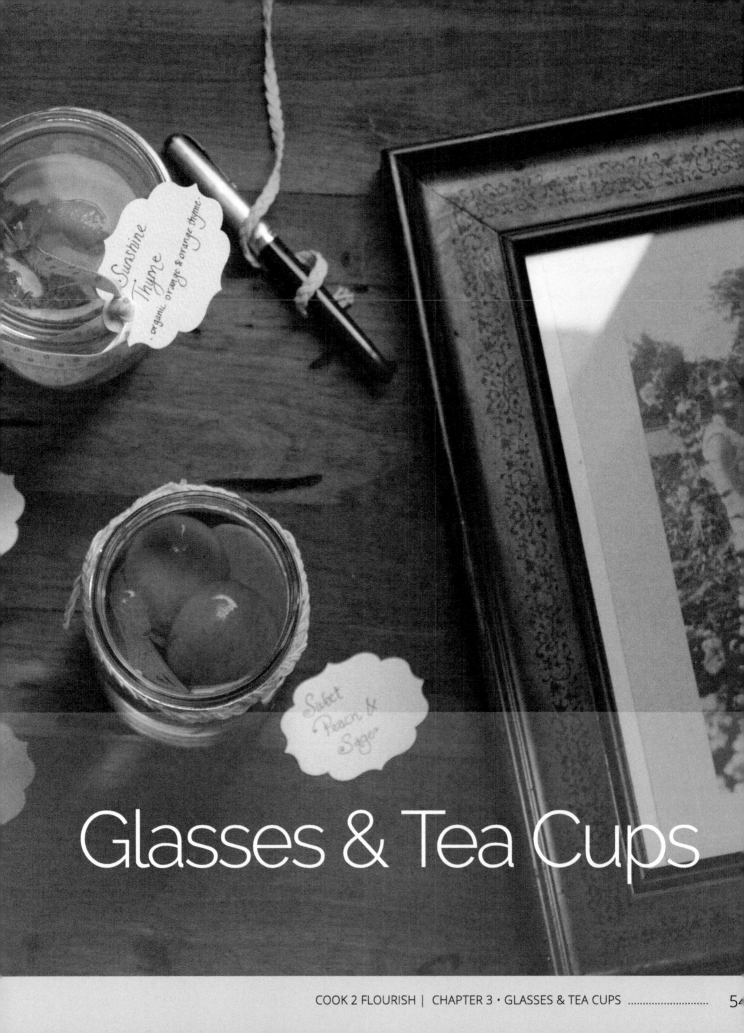

Sunshine
Thyme
· organic orange & orange thyme.

Sweet
· Peach &
Sage·

Glasses & Tea Cups

Hydrate 2 Flourish

• *Mint 2 Enjoy - Organic Cucumber and mint*

• *Sunshine Thyme - Organic orange and orange thyme*
• *Sweet Peach and Sage - Organic Peach and sage*

• *Immune H2O - Organic lemon and lemon thyme*
• *Berry Basil - Organic Strawberry and basil*

• *The above suggested combinations are pictured in the photo.*

Select your choice of organic fruits or vegetables and pair them with fresh herbs, if desired. Dice or slice the fruits and vegetables and crush or bruise the herbs to release their essence. This is a tasty, healthy way to drink more water each day. Simply place your flavorful selections into a glass jar and begin sipping or cover and place in the refrigerator up to 8 hours. It is important to drink half your body weight in ounces up to 100 ounces of water each day. Your body requires water to function optimally for joint health, mental clarity, energy, metabolism/weight management, detoxification and elimination, as well as preventing headaches and much more! So, hydrate your thirsty cells and sip 2 flourish!

Please note, that although these delightful water additions do help hydrate your body, some sources insist that there is no replacement for pure water. Pure water helps to flush the kidneys and does not have to be filtered by the liver first, so just make sure you get ample pure water each day, enjoying these flavored waters as a bonus!

Chai a Latte'

1 serving

• **1 ½ cups almond milk, divided**

• **1 Chai flavor tea bag**

• **2 Tablespoons** *Love and Peas® protein powder (Sugar Free)*, **fluffed**

• **7 drops liquid stevia, to taste**

Directions:

1) Bring 1 cup almond milk up to a boil and remove from burner. Remove half of the unsweetened almond milk from the saucepan and pour into a small mixing bowl. Place tea bag into the saucepan of milk and steep for 5 minutes, covered with a lid.

2) Meanwhile, beat the protein powder into the warm almond milk with an electric mixer for 30 seconds. Pour back into the saucepan to keep warm.

3) Beat the remaining cold almond milk for 40 seconds until foamy.

4) Remove tea bag and press between 2 spoons to extract as much tea as possible. Add in the stevia to taste.

5) Pour the warm milk from saucepan into a mug then pour the foamy milk on top.

Try a Latte':

Madagascar Vanilla with1/8 teaspoon cinnamon (added in Step 3).

Moroccan Mint with ½ -1 teaspoon carob powder (added in Step 3).

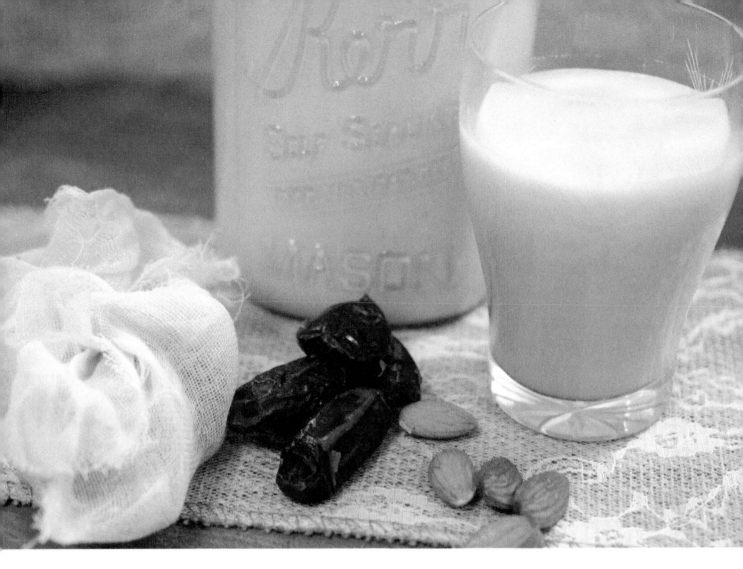

Warm Me Up Hot Chocolate

Gluten Free
Dairy Free

1 serving

- 1 cup unsweetened almond milk
- 1 Tablespoon carob powder
- ½ Tablespoon *Love and Peas®* protein powder
  (Sugar Free)
- 1 teaspoon raw honey OR coconut sugar
- 10 drops liquid stevia, to taste

Directions:

1) Warm almond milk over medium heat for 3-5 minutes.

2) Sift the carob powder into a mug then add the protein powder and your choice of honey or coconut sugar and stir.

3) Pour the hot almond milk into the mug then stir well.

4) Add stevia to taste.

Cold Chocolate Milk: *Pour almond milk, carob powder, protein powder and your choice of honey or coconut sugar in a blender and blend on high for 15 seconds. Add stevia to taste and ice cubes.*

How to make Almond Milk

Makes 5 ½ cups

- **1 cup raw almonds**
- **5 Medjool dates, pitted**
- **3 cups high alkaline water or filtered water**
- **5 cups high alkaline water or filtered water, divided**
- **½ teaspoon cinnamon**
- **½ teaspoon organic pure vanilla extract, optional**

Tools:

1 quart glass jar, a glass pitcher, high speed blender, cheese cloth or nut milk bag, wire mesh strainer and a sturdy glass bowl to fit strainer across.

Directions:

1) Place the almonds in the 1 quart glass jar and fill with the 3 cups of water. Place the dates in a small cup and fill with enough water to cover by one inch. Soak the almonds and dates overnight or for 8 to 12 hours.

2) Drain and rinse the almonds to wash away nutrient inhibitors. This way your body gets the nutrients more easily in the soaked almonds. Drain the dates.

3) Place the cheese cloth in the wire mesh strainer over the sturdy bowl. Place the almonds, 3 dates and cinnamon in the blender with 3 cups of water. Blend for one minute on high.

4) Pour the almond milk into the cheese cloth. Gather the four corners of the cheese cloth and gently twist and continue twisting the almond pulp to release the milk. Twist and squeeze as much milk out as possible.

5) Place the almond pulp back into the blender with the remaining 2 dates and 2 cups of water. Blend for one minute on high. Pour the almond milk back into the cheese cloth. Gather the four corners of the cheese cloth and gently twist and continue twisting to release as much milk as possible. Keep the almond pulp to be used in other recipes listed below (if desired).

6) Pour the almond milk into a glass pitcher and add the vanilla extract (if desired). Refrigerate and seal almond milk in a glass pitcher or large jar. Stir or shake well before serving. Homemade almond milk must be refrigerated and used within 3 or 4 days.

7) Rinse the cheese cloth and the residue from the almond pulp will wash off. Add dish soap and wash in a small bowl and rinse well. Hang to dry.

Suggestions: Almond pulp can be mixed into tuna salad, a smoothie, or meatless taco filling. If you prefer to use stevia, omit the dates, and add 5 drops liquid stevia, to taste.

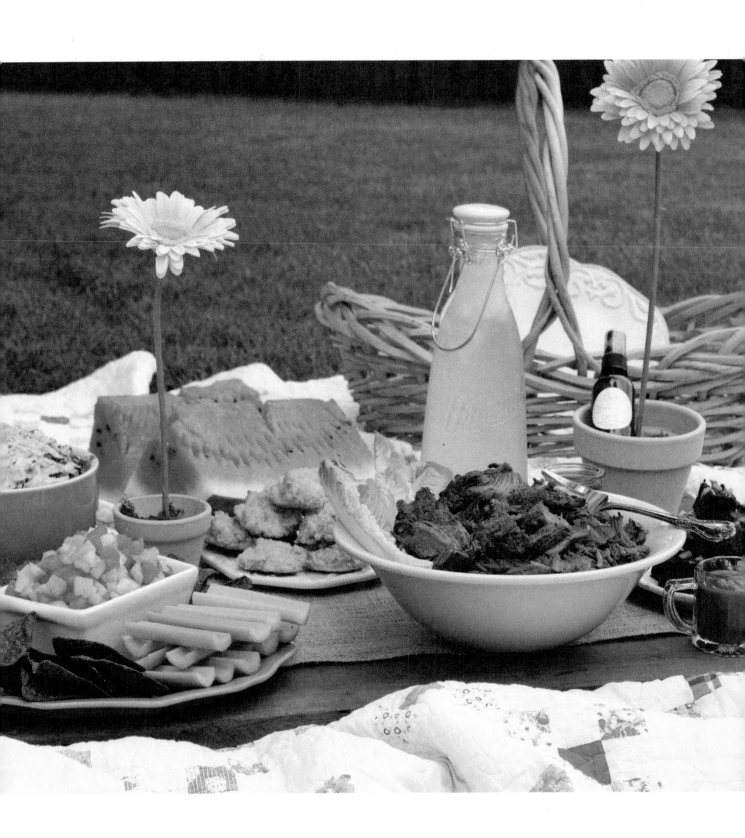

Licious' Lemonade

How to make 1 serving

- ½ cup fresh squeezed lemon juice
- ¾ teaspoon liquid stevia, to taste
- 9 cups cold filtered water
- 4 cups ice, for serving

Directions:

1) Combine the fresh squeezed lemon juice, liquid stevia and cold water then stir well.

2) Taste to see if you need more stevia.

3) Pour over ice in individual glasses. Serve immediately.

Lemon Cold Remedy

1 serving

- 1 cup filtered water
- Juice of 1 fresh lemon
- 1 Tablespoon raw honey
- ½ teaspoon organic butter
- Big pinch of nutmeg
- Pinch of ground ginger
- Dash cayenne pepper

Directions:

1) Bring filtered water to a boil.

2) In a mug combine juice from the lemon, honey, butter, nutmeg, ginger and cayenne.

3) Pour the hot water into the mug then stir to combine. Drink this as hot as you can take it. Then go to bed.

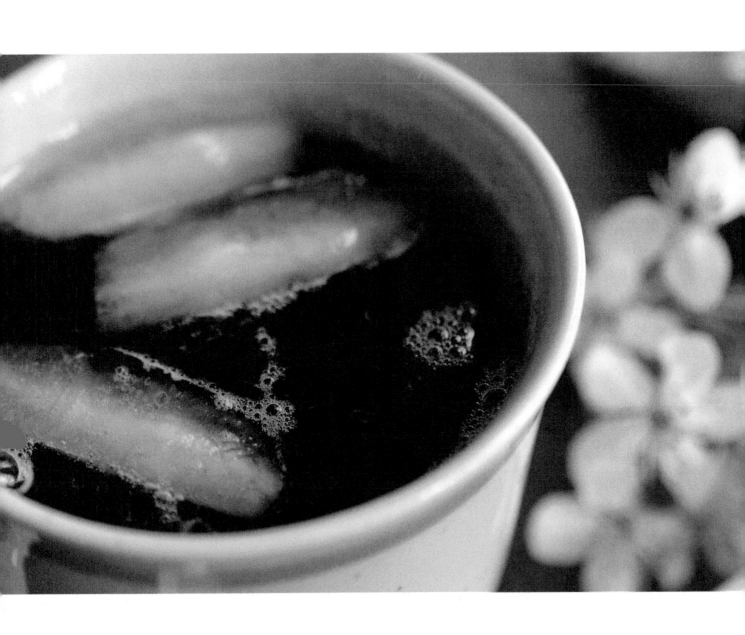

Mint 2 Flourish

· · · · · · · · · · · · · · · · · · · ·

One of my favorite drinks is Liquid Chlorophyll ES™ from Nature's Sunshine®.

Chlorophyll is the green pigment that gives green leafy vegetables their vibrant hue.

With such a refreshing mint taste, chlorophyll is cooling to the body and offers wonderful

benefits: gently detoxifying, may promote regularity, promotes a balanced pH in the

body, deodorizes the body, and it has antioxidant properties.

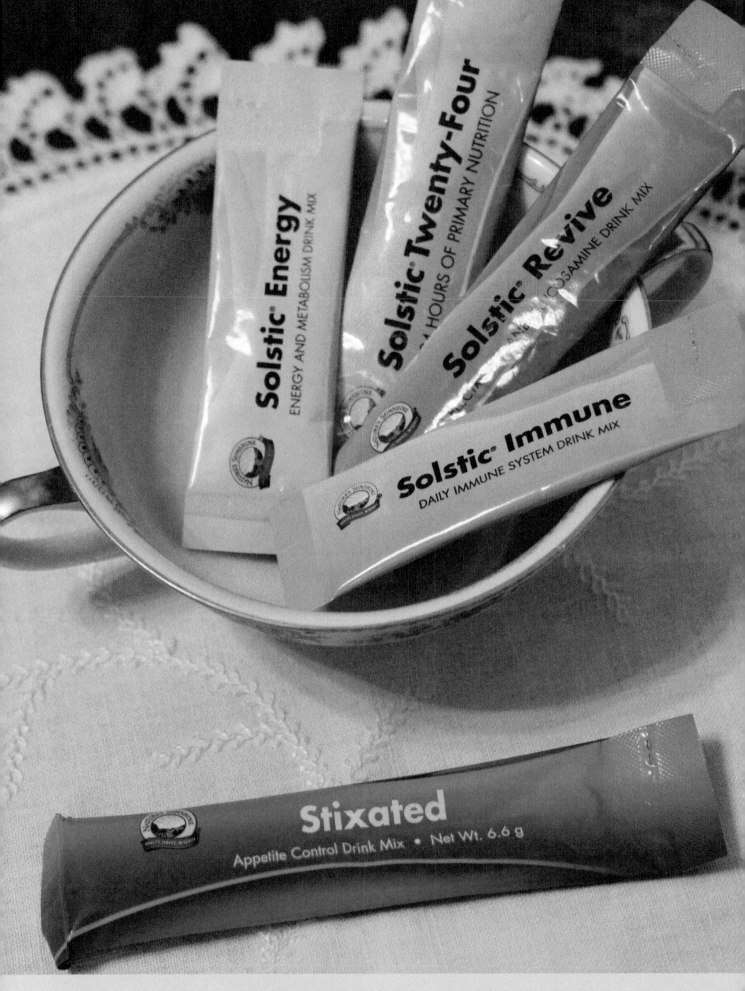

Sip 2 Flourish with Flavor

In addition to drinking pure water, the Solstic® drink packets from Nature's Sunshine® provide a fun, tasty way to get more nutrients in your day! There are 6 flavors that have a specific health benefit. All of these delicious drinks are available in boxes with 30 packets each from Nature's Sunshine® (www.n2flourish.mynsp.com):

The citrus pineapple flavor Solstic® Energy is great for a coffee replacement without the jitters while enhancing metabolism and mental clarity with caffeine from the herb guarana.

The pink lemonade flavor Solstic® Revive is wonderful for replenishing electrolytes and for a post workout recovery and supporting joint health (no caffeine). It also has antioxidants and helps with stamina.

The berry flavored Stixated™ can help with appetite control and cravings and supplies chromium.

The tart berry flavor of Solstic® Immune is wonderful for boosting the body's natural defense mechanisms. It features vitamin C, vitamin D, and elderberry.

The berry flavor Solstic® Twenty-Four is a multi vitamin in a drink- vitamins A-E plus minerals.

The strawberry lemon flavor Solstic® Cardio is for supporting heart health and improving workout endurance.

These statements have not been evaluated by the FDA. These products are not intended to diagnose, treat, prevent or cure disease.

Time 2 Flourish - Organic Teas

Make time for yourself, it's important. Sipping a cup of tea can do the body a lot of good. It's relaxing and simple. Whether you read a book or your Bible or have quality time with a friend, enjoy your tea time and reap the benefits!

• Chamomile (Roman) - soothing to the digestive tract, calming, promotes sleep, may lessen premenstrual bloating and cramping.

• Peppermint - has been noted for its decongestant effects, eases stomach spasming and nausea.

• Lavender - has been known to support mood, promote relaxation, ease stress, and promote digestion and sleep.

• Echinacea - may improve immune function and has been used to fight colds and flu's. (Caution for auto-immune concerns.)

• Jasmine - calming and may ease premenstrual tension. (Do not use during pregnancy.)

• Green - rich in antioxidants, has less caffeine than coffee, contains the amino acid L-theanine that can support brain health, may improve metabolism, may provide anti-inflammatory benefits, may improve oral health, may aid blood sugar, and may support cardiovascular health. (Organic is highly recommended)

• Ginger - may decrease intestinal gas and combat nausea, has a warming effect and can boost the immune system.

• Pau D'Arco - has been used to support immune function and has shown anti-fungal, anti-viral, anti-parasitic and anti-inflammatory effects. (Do not use during pregnancy.)

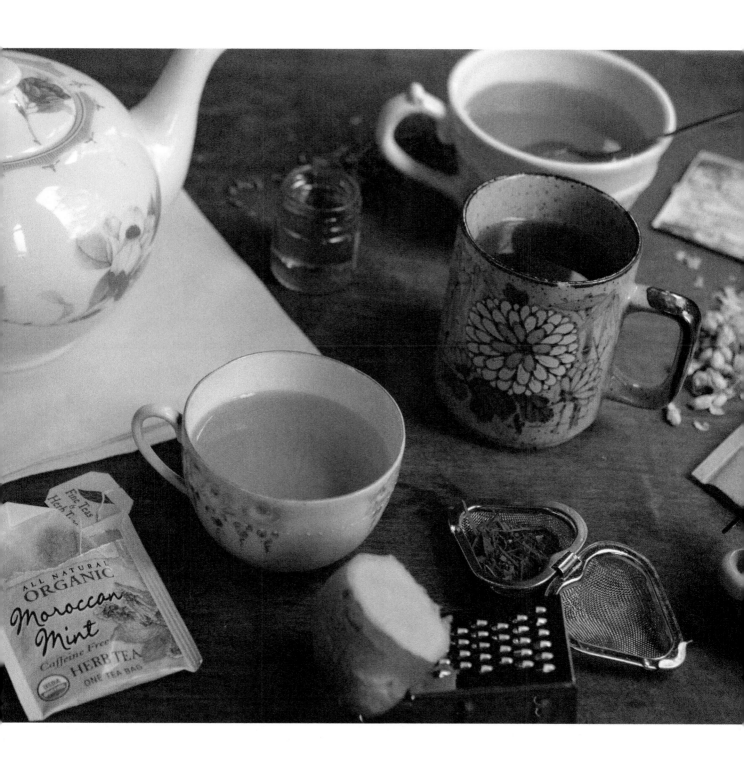

These statements have not been evaluated by the FDA. The reader assumes full responsibility for his/her health; this information is not intended to diagnose, treat, prevent or cure disease.

Fruity Frosty

. . . .

Gluten Free
Grain Free
Dairy Free

2 servings

- 2 cups ice
- Liquid stevia, to taste
- ¼ ripe avocado, pit removed and peeled (for creaminess and blood sugar stability)
- 2 cups your choice fresh fruits
- Optional additions: cinnamon, ginger, mint
- Fresh Fruits: blueberries, blackberries, cherries, kiwi, lemon, lime, mango, melons, peach, pineapple, raspberries and strawberries.

FRESH: Melon Fruity Frosty
- ¼ ripe avocado,
  pit removed and peeled
- 1 cup watermelon
- 1 cup cantaloupe
- 2 cups ice
- 3-5 drops liquid stevia, to taste

FROZEN: Strawberry Fruity Frosty
- ¼ ripe avocado, pit removed and peeled
- 2 cups strawberries, frozen
- 2 cups ice
- 10 drops liquid stevia, to taste
- 1 ½ cups filtered water

Directions:

1) Combine the avocado, your choice of fresh fruit or a combination of fruits, ice and liquid stevia to taste. Blend in a high speed blender on high or smoothie option until smooth.

2) Taste to see if you need more stevia. Serve immediately with a straw or a spoon

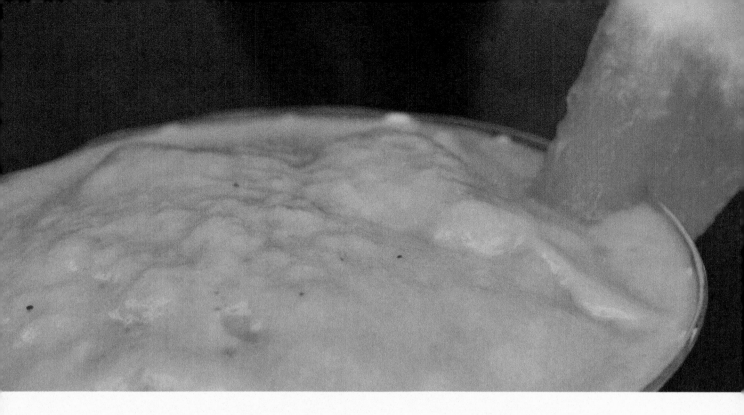

Encourage 2 Flourish : Raspberry Story

Usually my market acquisitions include tomatoes, various squashes, kale, and other health gems. One particular day raspberries were available, which is a rarity at my market. I just couldn't resist their ruby hue. Eager to pop one into my mouth I just knew they would be sweet... my taste buds said otherwise; they were sour!

Disappointed, I thought, "Lord, I just spent $4 on these berries, and they're sour!" Almost immediately I felt Him say, "They weren't in the sun long enough."

These $4 berries had just turned into a goldmine revelation. When we as people do not take the time to soak in the Son of God, our fruit can be sour. Sour fruit may look different for each of us, but when we are in the Son- receiving His grace, talking with Him in prayer, desiring to be increasingly more like Him, listening to His voice and reading His Word daily, we can produce the fruit of the Holy Spirit: love, joy, peace, patience, kindness, goodness, faithfulness, gentleness, and self control. That sounds like sweet fruit to me!

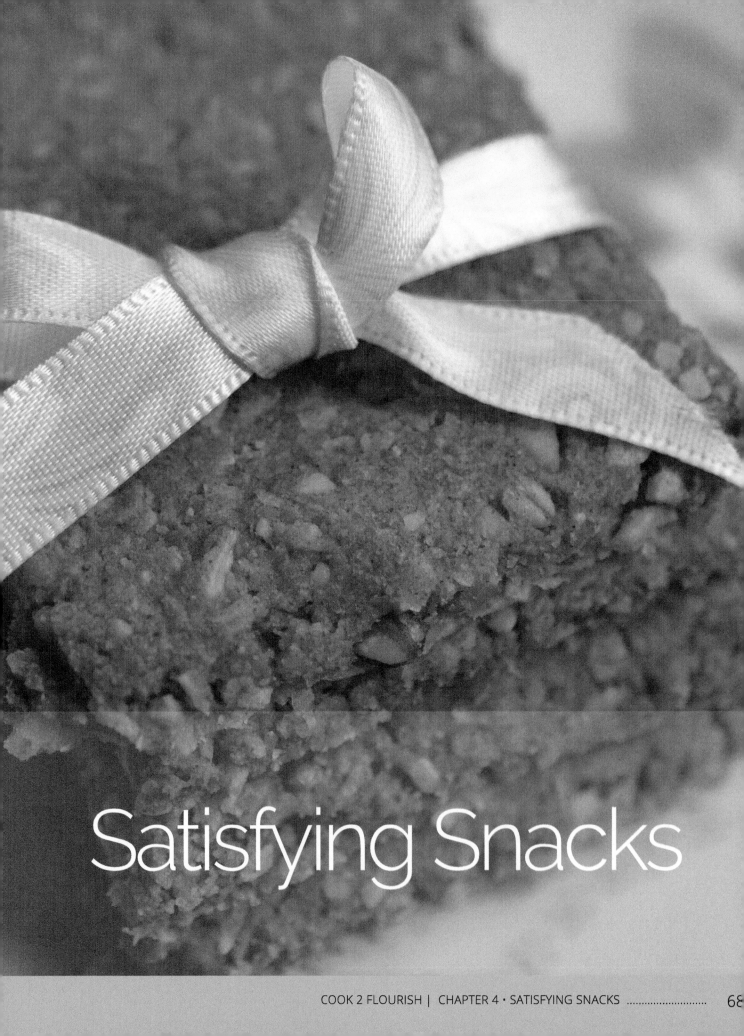

Satisfying Snacks

Soaked Oats Granola Bars

Makes 12-15 bars

- ¼ cup gluten free oat bran
- ¾ cup organic gluten free old fashioned rolled oats
- ¼ cup almond butter
- ¼ cup raw honey
- ¼ teaspoon stevia
- ¼ teaspoon Nature's Sunshine® sea salt
- 1 teaspoon organic pure vanilla extract
- 2 Tablespoons extra-virgin coconut oil

- ½ cup unsweetened coconut flakes
- ¼ cup coconut flour
- ¼ cup Love and Peas® protein powder *(Sugar Free)*
- 1 Tablespoon cinnamon
- ¼ cup pumpkin seeds

Directions:

1) In a 2 cup measuring cup place the oat bran and oats then fill with enough water to cover by one inch. Let soak for 2 hours. Drain and lightly rinse in mesh strainer. Shake to release as much excess liquid as possible then set aside and continue to drain.

2) In a large mixing bowl, add the almond butter, honey, stevia, sea salt, vanilla and coconut oil and mix until smooth and creamy.

3) Add in the coconut flakes, coconut flour, protein powder, cinnamon and pumpkin seeds. Stir to combine thoroughly.

4) Add the soaked oats and stir until well combined.

5) Coat a 15x10x1 inch stoneware bar baking pan with non-stick grapeseed oil spray or line a stainless steel baking sheet with unbleached parchment paper and pour the batter onto the pan. The batter should be a stiff, cohesive dough. Oil your fingers with coconut oil first then spread evenly to about ¼ inch. Cut into desired square pieces with a pizza cutter.

6) Bake in preheated 350 degree oven for 28-30 minutes. Remove from oven and place on a cooling rack to cool completely. Store uncovered for 24 hours or place in the oven overnight in the OFF position. It is dry and there is no dampness in there.

> ***Tip:*** *If your granola bars are thicker than ¼ inch, you will need to bake them just a little longer than 30 minutes. Watch them carefully so they don't burn.*

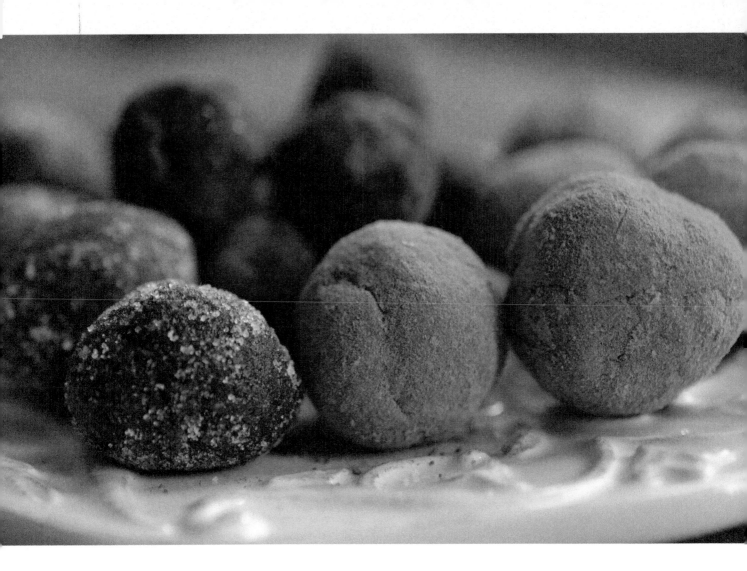

Energy Balls

Makes 1 ½ - 2 dozen

- ⅓ cup unsweetened canned pumpkin puree
- 1 teaspoon cinnamon
- 1 scoop Love and Peas® protein powder *(Sugar Free)*

- ⅓ cup almond butter
- 2 Tablespoons coconut flour

Directions:

1) Place the pumpkin, cinnamon, protein powder, almond butter and coconut flour in a food processor and process until a soft, moldable dough is formed. You may need to scrape down the sides in between processing.

2) Pinch off a small amount of dough and roll between your hands to make large gumball size balls.

3) Place a few of them in a sandwich baggie and shake to coat with your favorite coating:

Ground cinnamon / Coconut flakes / Chia seeds / Finely chopped nuts or pumpkin seeds

4) Store in the refrigerator or freezer.

Energy Balls - Goji Berry

Makes 1 ½ - 2 dozen

Dairy Free

- 3 Tablespoons almond butter
- 3 Tablespoons Goji berries, dried
- 2 Tablespoons beet powder
- 2 Tablespoons unsweetened canned pumpkin puree
- ½ teaspoon Nature's Sunshine® Stixated powdered drink mix
- 1 scoop Love and Peas® protein powder *(Sugar Free)*

Directions:

1) Place the almond butter, Goji berries, beet powder, pumpkin, Stixated® and protein powder in a food processor and process until a soft, moldable dough is formed. You may need to scrape down the sides in between processing.

2) Pinch off a small amount of dough and roll between your hands to make large gumball size balls.

3) These are good without a coating, but if you would like to coat them with something that is optional. If coating, place a few of them in a sandwich baggie and shake to coat with your favorite coating:

Cocoa powder / Coconut flakes / Chia seeds / Finely chopped nuts

4) Store in the refrigerator or freezer.

Energy Balls - Chocolate Mint

Makes 1 ½ - 2 dozen

Gluten Free
Dairy Free

- ⅓ cup cocoa almond butter (page 73)
- 1 Tablespoon cocoa powder
- 1 Tablespoon cacao nibs
- 1 Tablespoon raw honey OR 6-8 drops liquid stevia
- 1 Tablespoon unsweetened coconut flakes
- 2 Tablespoons Nature's Harvest protein powder
- 2 Tablespoons unsweetened canned pumpkin puree
- 1 teaspoon Nature's Sunshine® Liquid Chlorophyll ES™
- 5 Nature's Sunshine® Xylitol Peppermints

Directions:

1) Place the cocoa almond butter, cocoa powder, cacao nibs, your choice of honey or stevia, coconut, protein powder, pumpkin, chlorophyll and mints in a food processor and blend until finely ground and smooth. You may need to scrape down the sides in between processing.

2) Pinch off a small amount of dough and roll between your hands to make large gumball size balls.

3) These are good without a coating, but if you would like to coat them with something that is optional. If coating, place a few of them in a sandwich baggie and shake to coat with your favorite coating:

Cocoa powder / Coconut flakes / Chia seeds / Sesame seeds / Finely chopped nuts

4) Store in the refrigerator or freezer.

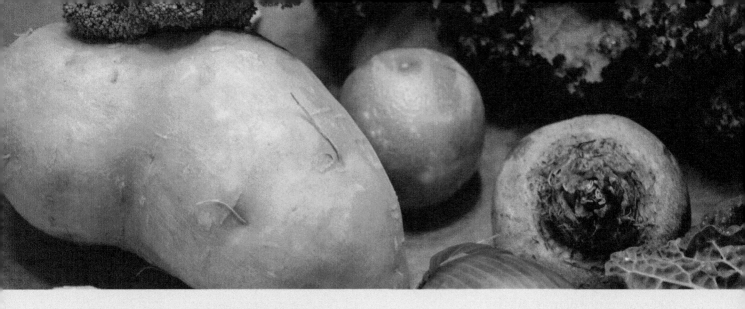

Spotlight : Sweet Potatoes:

Sweet potatoes, one of my favorite sweet treats...with vegetable benefits! Did you know that sweet potatoes come in more colors besides orange, such as purple, and that they are not in the same family as yams?

However you slice them, sweet potatoes have been known to:

• offer a generous amount of beta carotene, benefitting both the eyes and the skin

• lessen the effects of toxic heavy metals in the body

• supply fiber thereby being one of the best starches for blood sugar

• support energy levels and adrenal health because of their B vitamin content

Take a family classic sugary sweet potato casserole and transform it by preparing from fresh sweet potatoes and topped with pecans and blood sugar balancing cinnamon!

Perhaps the most unique attribute of sweet potatoes involves the role of "storage proteins." God designed sweet potatoes that in the event that the tuber gets damaged, it develops these compounds useful for antioxidant benefit in our bodies that it wouldn't have possessed otherwise.

How amazing is that?

Let's take it beyond sweet potatoes, and see the parallel in our lives. When we experience pain, we have the opportunity to use it as a catalyst for growth- a maturing agent in our lives. Through the fruit of that pain, we can be used by the Lord to encourage others who encounter similar situations. Romans 8:28 NIV "And we know that in all things God works for the good of those who love him, who have been called according to his purpose."

Though the enemy meant it for harm, God meant it for good! When trials come, we can be sure that when we are walking with Christ, He will never leave us nor forsake us!

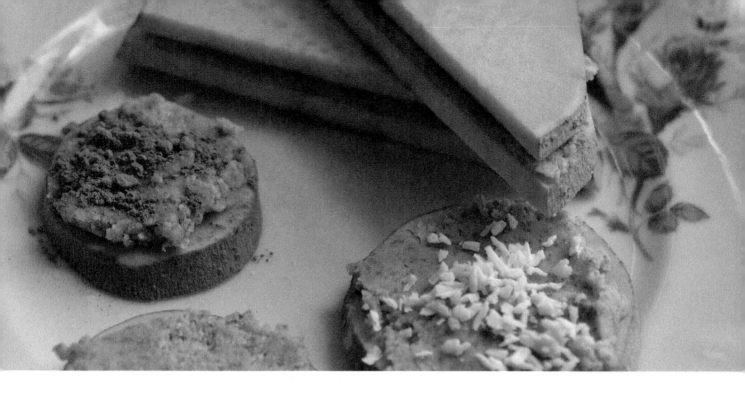

Sweet Potato Sandwich Snack

1 serving

- **1 small sweet potato**
- **Almond butter**

Directions:

1) Slice the raw sweet potato into ¼ inch thick slices or round discs.

2) Top one slice with 1 Tablespoon of almond butter.

3) Place another slice of sweet potato on top to make a sandwich.

4) Repeat for additional little sandwiches.

Almond Butter

Makes 1 2/3 – 2 cups

- **3 cups raw whole almonds**
- **¼ teaspoon Nature's Sunshine® sea salt**
- **¼ teaspoon cinnamon**
- **2 Tablespoon extra-virgin coconut oil, melted**

Directions:

1) Place the almonds in a food processor along with sea salt, cinnamon and melted coconut oil. Blend until finely ground or paste.

Make Your Own Nutella® Spread by adding the following ingredients to the above almond butter and process 30 seconds until thoroughly combined:

Cocoa Almond Butter
- *1-2 Tablespoons cocoa powder*   - *½ teaspoon cinnamon*   - *2 teaspoons raw honey*   - *½ teaspoon stevia*

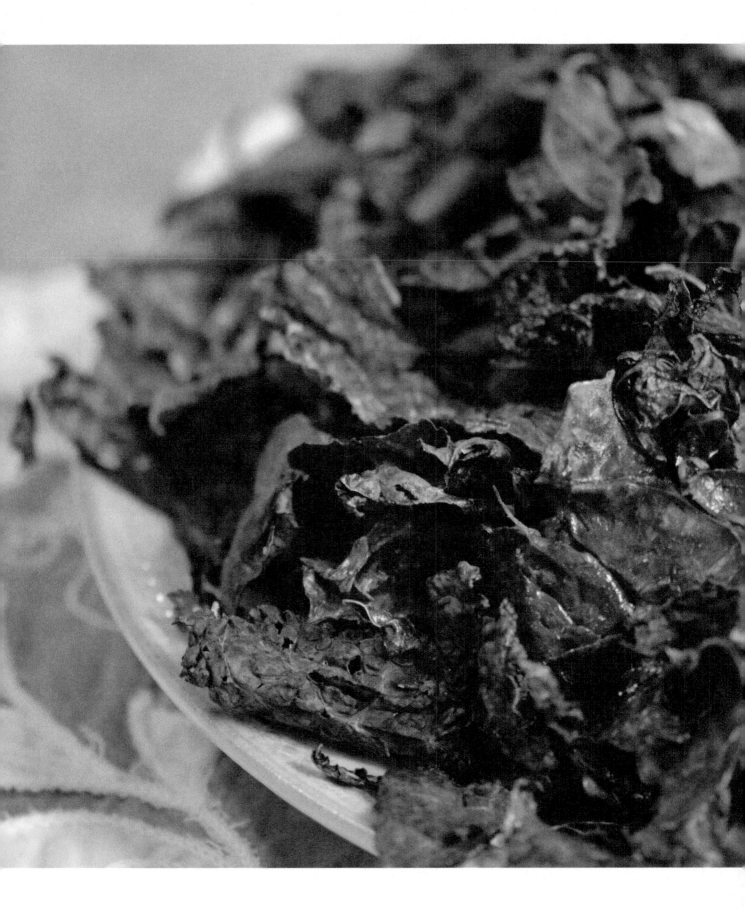

Kale Chips

2-4 servings

- **8 cups fresh Kale, washed and drained well**
- **1 teaspoon grapeseed oil**
- **¾ teaspoon garlic powder**
- **½ teaspoon Nature's Sunshine® sea salt**
- **Dash or more cayenne pepper**

Directions:

1) Preheat oven to 350 degrees and line a large stainless steel baking sheet with unbleached parchment paper.

2) In a large bowl, tear the kale into pieces and strip the kale off of the large part of the stem.

3) Pour the oil over the kale and toss to coat.

4) Sprinkle with garlic powder, sea salt and cayenne pepper. Toss to coat.

5) Spread out the kale on the parchment paper and bake for 15 minutes.

6) Remove from the oven and fluff the kale chips around with a fork. Place back in the oven for 5 to 10 more minutes.

7) Remove from oven and fluff one more time. If they are crunchy, they are done. If they are still wet, bake 3-5 more minutes.

8) Pour them into a bowl or serve them directly off of the parchment paper.

Kid approved kale chips

After coming home with nearly a trunk load of kale, kale chips were definitely on the menu! Having plenty to share, we decided to make a batch for our little neighbor friends next door. The chips had come out of the oven, so we called to have the four children pick up their bowl of crispy [green] goodness.

The look on their faces was priceless- excitement veiled in hesitance. Our phone rang soon after and the little voice said "them tastes weird, but we kept on eating them... we like them!" Sure enough, the kale chips have now become one of their go-to snacks.

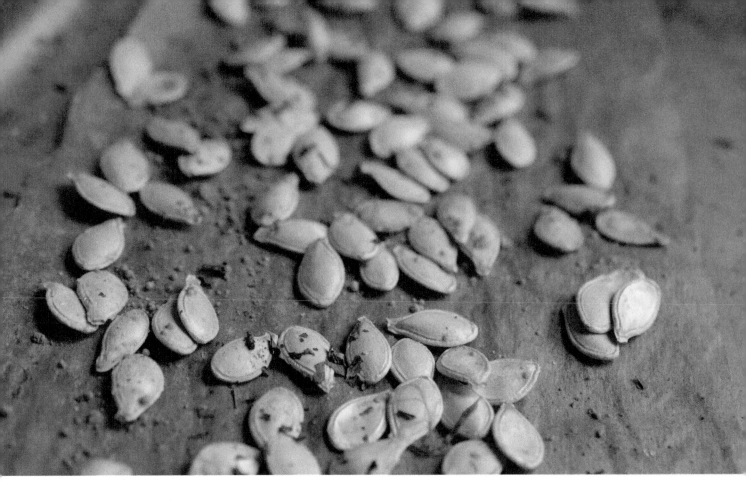

Savory Seeds

1 or 2 servings

- Nature's Sunshine® sea salt, to taste
- Dash cayenne pepper
- Dash dried parsley
- ½ teaspoon garlic powder

These are a tasty treat right out of the oven or on top of a salad!

Directions:

1) Scoop out the seeds from your pumpkin, spaghetti squash or butternut squash then rinse the seeds in a colander, removing any stringing flesh.

2) Place the damp seeds on an unbleached parchment paper lined stainless steel baking sheet. Season with sea salt and a dash of cayenne pepper OR sea salt, parsley flakes and garlic powder. Whatever you desire!

3) Bake in a preheated 350 degree oven for 18-20 minutes until just turning golden brown. Don't let them turn dark golden brown, they may taste burnt.

Sweet Seeds: Coat seeds with ½ Tablespoon of raw honey and ¼ teaspoon of cinnamon.

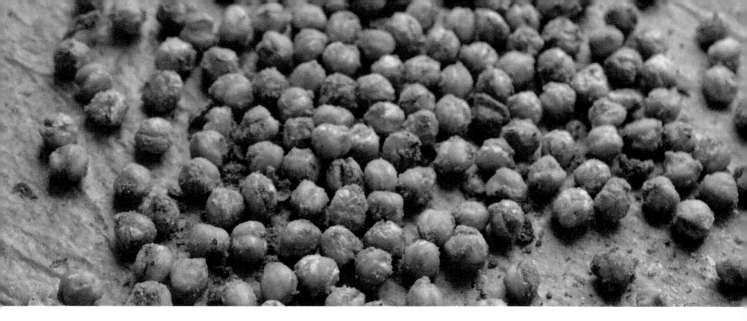

Katie's Chickpeas

. . . .

Makes 2 cups

Gluten Free
Grain Free
Dairy Free

- 2 cups garbanzo beans
- 2 teaspoons ground cumin
- 1 ½ teaspoons garlic powder
- 1 Tablespoon avocado oil OR grapeseed oil
- ¼ teaspoon ground black pepper
- ½ teaspoon Nature's Sunshine® sea salt

Directions:

1) Use canned or cooked garbanzo beans for this recipe. Drain, rinse and pat dry then pour into a small mixing bowl along with the oil, pepper, sea salt, cumin and garlic powder. Mix well.

2) Spread the garbanzo beans out on an unbleached parchment paper lined stainless steel baking sheet.

3) Bake in preheated 375 degree oven for:
- 45-50   Minutes for hard shell and soft inside
- 55-65   Minutes for very crunchy

4) Stir every 15-20 minutes to make sure they do not burn. Keep special watch over them after they have been cooking for 30 minutes.

Katie's Chickpeas
. . . .

Friends since freshman year of high school, Katie and I met with the common ground of kitchen fever—we both really enjoyed cooking. Nearly every time we cook together, Brussels sprouts are on the menu. I cherish our times in Bible study together, our excursions to Whole Foods®, and creating new recipes with our favorite foods...this is one of them.

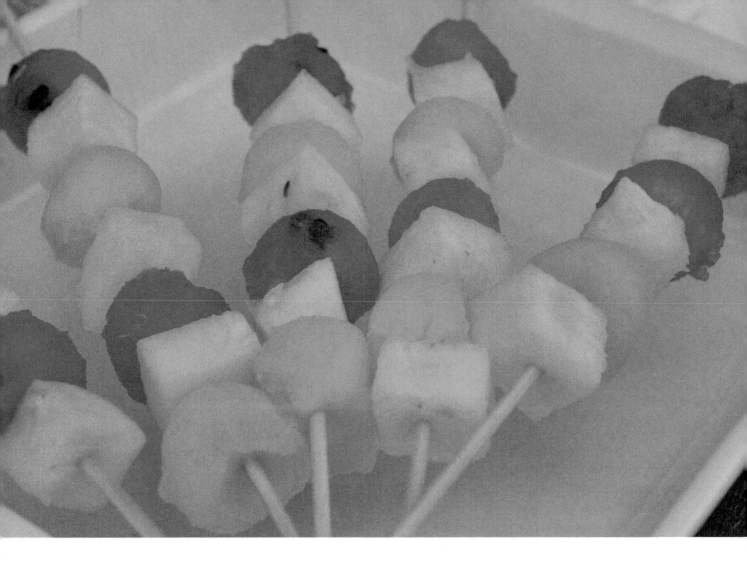

Fruity Spinach Smoothie

. . . .

2 servings

- 1 cup unsweetened almond milk
- ½-1 cup ice cubes
- 1 cup frozen fresh spinach leaves
- ½ ripe avocado, peeled and pit removed
- ½ cup strawberries
- 1 cup pineapple
- 10-15 drops liquid stevia, to taste

Directions:

1) Pour milk into blender along with ice cubes, spinach, avocado, strawberries, pineapple and stevia.

2) Blend on high or on smoothie option until thick and creamy.

Soft Serve Creamy Ice – Carob Almond

2-4 servings

- **6 ounces unsweetened almond milk**
- **2 cups ice cubes**
- **2 scoops Love & Peas® protein powder** *(Sugar Free)*
- **1 ½ cups frozen fresh kale**
- **½ banana, frozen**
- **1 ½ Tablespoon unsweetened carob powder**
- **1 ½ Tablespoon almond butter OR 28 whole almonds**

Directions:

1) Pour milk into high speed blender along with ice cubes, protein powder, kale, banana, carob powder and your choice of almond butter or almonds.

2) Blend on high for 50 seconds until smooth and creamy. Serve immediately in chilled bowls!

Soft Serve Creamy Ice - Fruit

1 serving

- **4 ounces unsweetened almond milk**
- **1 cup ice cubes**
- **⅓ cup frozen berries OR pineapple**
- **⅓ banana, frozen**
- **⅔ cup frozen fresh kale (only if using blueberries)**
- **¼-½ ripe avocado, pit removed and peeled**
- **3-5 drops liquid stevia, to taste**
- **½ packet Nature's Sunshine Stixated® powdered drink mix**
- **1 scoop Love and Peas® protein powder** *(Sugar Free)* **(½ serving)**

Directions:

1) Pour milk into high speed blender along with ice cubes, your choice of fruit, banana, kale (if desired), avocado, stevia, Stixated® powder and protein powder. Blend on high until smooth and creamy. Serve immediately in chilled bowls!

Creamy Stuffed Eggs

Makes 12 halves

- 6 organic eggs, hard cooked and shelled
- 3 Tablespoons Vegenaise®
- 2 Tablespoons organic Greek yogurt, plain whole milk
- 1 ½ teaspoons prepared mustard

- ¼ teaspoon garlic powder
- ¼ teaspoon onion granules
- ¼ teaspoon Nature's Sunshine® sea salt
- Smoked paprika, for serving

Directions:

1) Cook eggs according to directions below.

2) Slice eggs in half and place each egg yolk into a small mixing bowl. Mash the yolks with a fork or potato masher.

3) Add in the Vegenaise®, yogurt, mustard, garlic powder, onion powder and sea salt.
Mash and stir until well combined and smooth.

4) Arrange the halved egg whites on a dish and scoop one spoonful of the yolk mixture into the hole in the egg white.
Garnish with a sprinkle of paprika, if desired.

5) Lightly cover the eggs and refrigerate until ready to serve.

> **Tip:**
> To keep the stuffed eggs from falling over on each other, slice off a small piece from the bottom of each egg white shell before filling with the yolk mixture.

How to make Boiled Eggs

Makes 6 eggs

- 6 organic eggs

- Water
- 1 teaspoon sea salt

Directions:

1) Place the eggs in a single layer in a medium-large saucepan and fill with enough water to cover by one inch.
Cover the saucepan with a lid. Bring eggs to a boil over medium heat.

2) When you hear the eggs boiling and bouncing in the pan, wait one minute then turn off the heat and remove
from the burner. Let eggs stand in the hot water for 12 minutes for medium size eggs,
15 minutes for large size eggs and 18 minutes for extra large eggs.

3) Drain and rinse under cold water until thoroughly cooled to prevent darkening around the yolks
and this will make shelling easier too.

4) To shell: Tap large end of egg to break the shell, roll on the counter to loosen the shell.
Peel egg under running cold water.

Stuffed Avocado

Gluten Free
Grain Free
Dairy Free

Makes 2 halves

- 1 ripe avocado, pit removed and peeled
- ½ cup garbanzo beans, drained and rinsed
- ½ Tablespoon Vegenaise®
- 1 teaspoon sundried tomato olive oil
- ¼ teaspoon garlic powder
- ⅛ teaspoon onion granules
- ⅛ teaspoon Nature's Sunshine® sea salt
- ⅛ teaspoon smoked paprika
- Sesame seeds, for serving

Directions:

1) Place peeled avocado halves on a plate. Slice off a small piece from the bottom to keep them from falling over.

2) Mash the garbanzo beans with a fork or a potato masher. Add in the Vegenaise®, oil, garlic powder, onion powder, sea salt and paprika. Mash and stir until well combined and smooth. Scoop half of the mixture into each hole in the avocado halves.

3) Garnish with sesame seeds. Lightly cover the avocadoes and chill before serving.

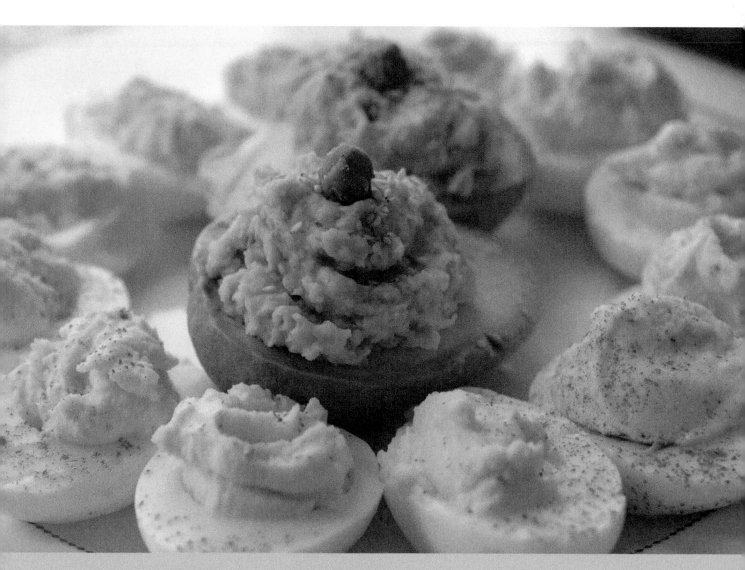

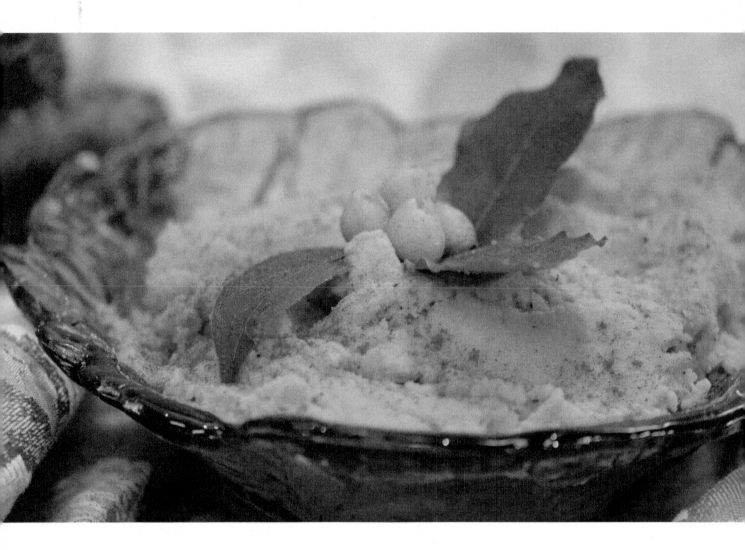

Gluten Free
Grain Free
Dairy Free

Hunger Hampering Hummus

Makes 1 ½ - 2 cups

- 1 (15.5 ounces) can garbanzo beans, drained and rinsed
- 1 ½ Tablespoons lemon juice
- 2 ½ Tablespoons extra-virgin olive oil
- 2 Tablespoon filtered water
- ½ teaspoon smoked paprika
- 1 teaspoon ground cumin
- ½ teaspoon Nature's Sunshine® sea salt
- ½ teaspoon ground black pepper to taste
- Dash cayenne pepper
- 1 garlic clove OR 2 Tablespoons roasted garlic

Directions:

1) Place all ingredients into a high speed blender and blend until smooth and creamy!

Enjoy with veggies! For a deeper, sweeter flavor, add in ½ cup roasted onions and ½ cup roasted red bell peppers.

Tomato Basil Hummus

Makes 2 cups

- 1 (15.5 ounces) can garbanzo beans, drained and rinsed
- ¼ cup sundried tomatoes in extra-virgin olive oil, drained
- 2 ½ Tablespoons oil from sundried tomatoes
- 1 Tablespoon fresh basil
- 1 ½ Tablespoons lemon juice

- 2 Tablespoons filtered water
- ½ teaspoon garlic powder or 1 garlic clove
- ½ teaspoon ground cumin
- ½ teaspoon Nature's Sunshine® sea salt
- ½ teaspoon ground black pepper, to taste

Directions:

1) Place all ingredients into a high speed blender and blend until smooth and creamy!

Airport Hummus

Although traveling can pose a threat to healthy eating, passion and planning can override its attempts. Researching the destination and the nearby grocers can help immensely, as can taking a lunch or snack of your own on board the plane. When my friend Jennifer and I traveled to the Nature's Sunshine® Convention, we took a container of this hummus, baby carrots, and Mary's Gone Crackers® to give us fuel to flourish for the remainder of our travel time.

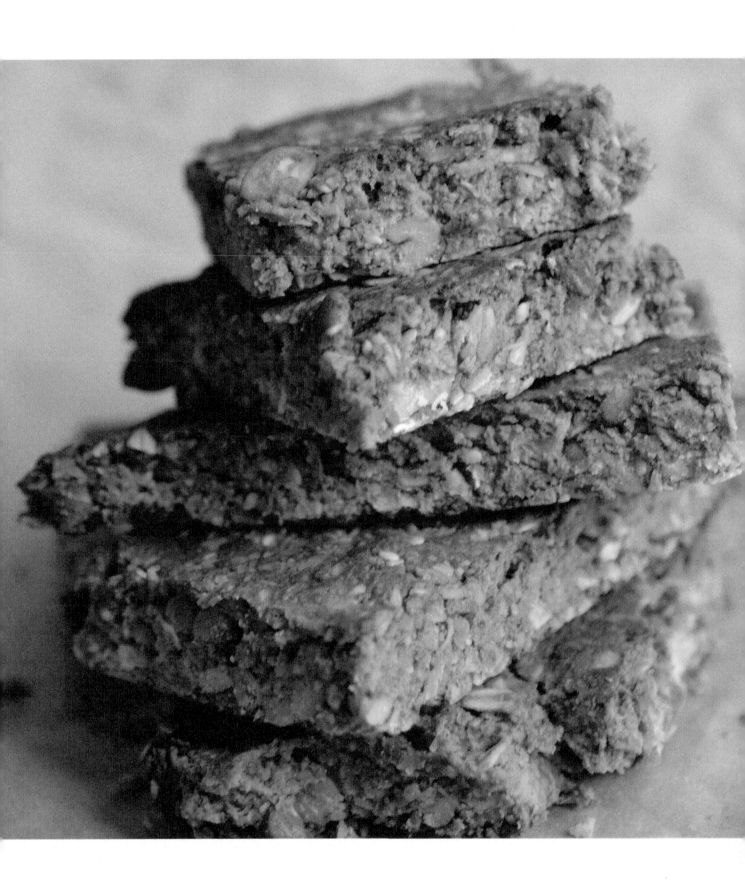

Easy Granola Bars

Makes 12 bars

- ¼ cup almond butter
- ⅓ cup raw honey
- ¼ teaspoon stevia
- ¼ teaspoon Nature's Sunshine® sea salt
- 1 teaspoon organic pure vanilla extract
- 2 Tablespoons extra-virgin coconut oil
- 1 Tablespoon coconut flour
- 1 Tablespoon cinnamon
- ¼ cup almond flour
- ¼ cup Love and Peas® protein powder *(Sugar Free)*
- ¼ cup gluten free oat bran
- ¾ cup organic gluten free old fashioned rolled oats
- ¾ cup add-ins

Directions:

1) In a food processor or mixing bowl, mix the almond butter, honey, stevia, sea salt, vanilla and coconut oil until smooth and creamy.

2) In a large mixing bowl stir together the coconut flour, cinnamon, almond flour, protein powder, oat bran, oats and your choice of add-ins, see below for ideas.

3) Add the creamy almond butter mixture to the large mixing bowl and stir well with a durable spatula.

4) Place a piece of unbleached parchment paper in a 9x13x2 inch glass baking dish then press the granola into the dish with a durable spatula or with your hand. (Oil your fingers with coconut oil first).

5) Bake in preheated 350 degree oven for 18 minutes.

6) Remove from oven and cut into 12 squares with a pizza cutter or sharp knife. Put back into the oven for 3–5 minutes. Watch that it doesn't burn. Then remove the granola and parchment paper from the baking dish and let completely cool on a cooling rack. Once completely cool, store in tightly closed container for about 7-10 days.

Add-ins: coconut flakes, almonds, cashews, pecans, walnuts, pumpkin seeds, sesame seeds, sunflower seeds, 70% or higher chocolate chunks, unsulfured apricots, figs or raisins.

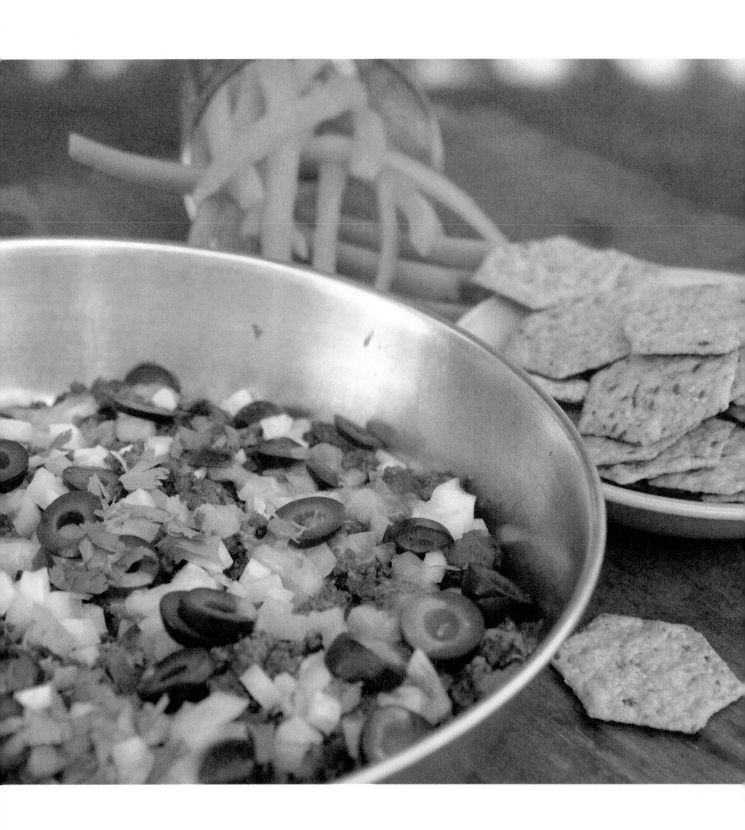

Marvelous Mexican Dip (serve warm)

4-5 servings

• 1 (29 ounce can) refried pinto beans
• 1 cup leftover seasoned taco meat
• ½ cup red or yellow bell pepper, diced
• 2 Tablespoons onion, chopped
• 1 teaspoon garlic powder
• 12 black olives, drained well and sliced, optional
• ¼ cup shredded white cheese, optional (Monterey Jack or Colby Jack cheese)
• 1 teaspoon fresh cilantro leaves

Directions:

1) In a stainless steel skillet, coated with grapeseed oil spray, spread out the beans evenly.
Turn burner on to medium-low.

2) Spread the seasoned taco meat over the beans followed by the bell pepper and onion.
Season with garlic powder then cover with a lid and heat for 5 minutes.

3) Add the black olives (if desired) and the cheese (if using). Cover with the lid until the cheese melts.
Garnish with the cilantro leaves.

This is a quick snack for after school or when a group of kids arrive unexpectedly. Serve with sliced carrots, bell pepper slices, Crunchmaster® Multi-Grain crackers or organic blue corn chips. If you do not have leftover taco meat, season the beans with 1 teaspoon taco seasoning and ½ teaspoon cumin. Serve right in the skillet to keep it warm.

Tip: Many refried beans contain hydrogenated oils so read the label to avoid them!

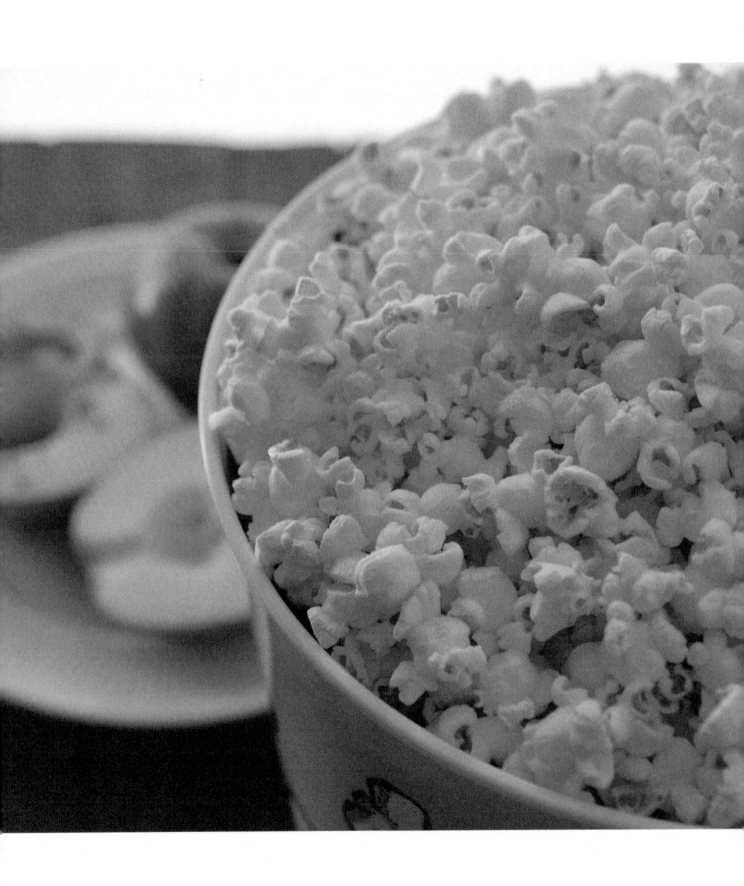

Microwave & Movie Popcorn Alternative

Makes 14 cups

• ½ cup organic, non-GMO popcorn kernels
• 1-2 Tablespoons extra-virgin olive oil
• ½ teaspoon Nature's Sunshine® sea salt, to taste
• Apple slices, for serving
• Cinnamon, for serving

Directions:

1) Place the ½ cup organic, non-GMO popcorn kernels in an air popper popcorn machine. Plug in machine and follow manufacturer's directions for popping the kernels. Place a large bowl under the funnel of the air popper.

2) When the popcorn is finished popping, unplug the air popper and drizzle the olive oil over the popped corn.

3) Season with Nature's Sunshine® sea salt.

4) Wash, core and slice apples then sprinkle them with cinnamon.

Note:

½ cup of popcorn kernels pops approximately 14 cups of popcorn.

One serving is approximately 3 cups of popped popcorn. Why Nature's Sunshine Sea Salt? Sea salt is supposed to have minerals in it to balance out the natural sodium; Nature's Sunshine® sea salt contains at least 50 minerals in it and tastes wonderful! Why an air popper? This way, you do not have to heat the oil while cooking that could turn to a trans-fat.

Do not shy away from the extra-virgin olive oil on top because the healthy fats in it will help to balance the rise in blood sugar from the popcorn. Why apples and cinnamon?

Apples will provide fiber and the cinnamon will help to maintain a healthy blood sugar level. Have the children sit at the table to eat this and they won't eat as much as they would in front of the TV.

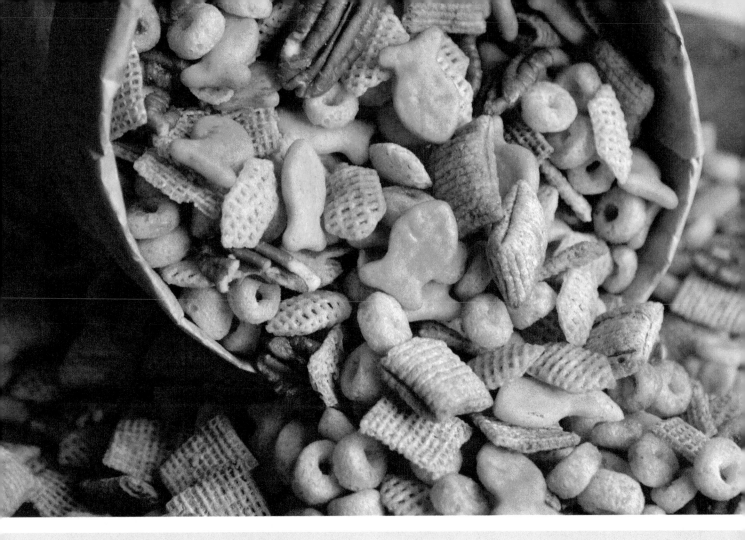

Timo's Snack Mix

Some of you reading this may have a life or death situation where you are trying to change your eating radically and rapidly, like my mom did. One thing about changing to a healthy eating lifestyle is that often it involves the whole family. In our case, this involved my brother in his teenage years. The store brand mix was his very favorite and we had to come up with a healthier version of it to help with the transition of change. Recipes such as this one are a splurge and offer a healthier alternative to their conventional counterparts so that feelings of deprivation and rebellion are minimized. We don't make it very often, but when we do, we make it last. Always remember that no matter where you are in your health journey, there is hope and every day is a new day... let's make it a healthy one.

Timo's Snack Mix

Makes 14 cups

• 14 cups total your choice of the following:
- Love Grown® Foods Power O's original
- Cascadian Farm® Organic Purely O's
- Pepperidge Farm® Wholegrain Goldfish brand snack crackers
- Cascadian Farm® Organic multi grain squares
- Nature's Path Organic™ Oaty Bites®
- Crunchmaster® Multi-Grain Crackers
- Mary's Gone Crackers™ sea salt pretzels
- Pecans OR almonds

• Sauce:
- 7 Tablespoons organic butter, no substitutes
- 1 teaspoon Bragg® liquid aminos
- 1 Tablespoon white wine vinegar
- 2 Tablespoons filtered water
- 2 Tablespoons molasses
- 1 ½ teaspoons garlic powder

Directions:
1) In a small saucepan over low heat, combine the butter, liquid aminos, vinegar, water, molasses and garlic powder. Stir well until the butter is melted.
2) Pour the 14 cups of your choice dry ingredients into a large roasting pan or glass baking dish.
Using a large spoon or spatula to stir the cereal, pour the butter mixture over the cereal and mix well.
3) Place the roasting pan in a preheated 250 degree oven and bake for 1 hour, stirring the cereal mixture every 15 minutes. Let cool completely and store in a tightly sealed container for up to 3 weeks.

Tip: If you want this more salty, add ½-1 teaspoon more of Bragg® liquid aminos.

Note: These cereal brands may change ingredients or certain grocers may not carry them. The goal is to purchase the cereal made with the most whole food ingredients (organic whole grains), the most amount of fiber, and the least amount of sugar.

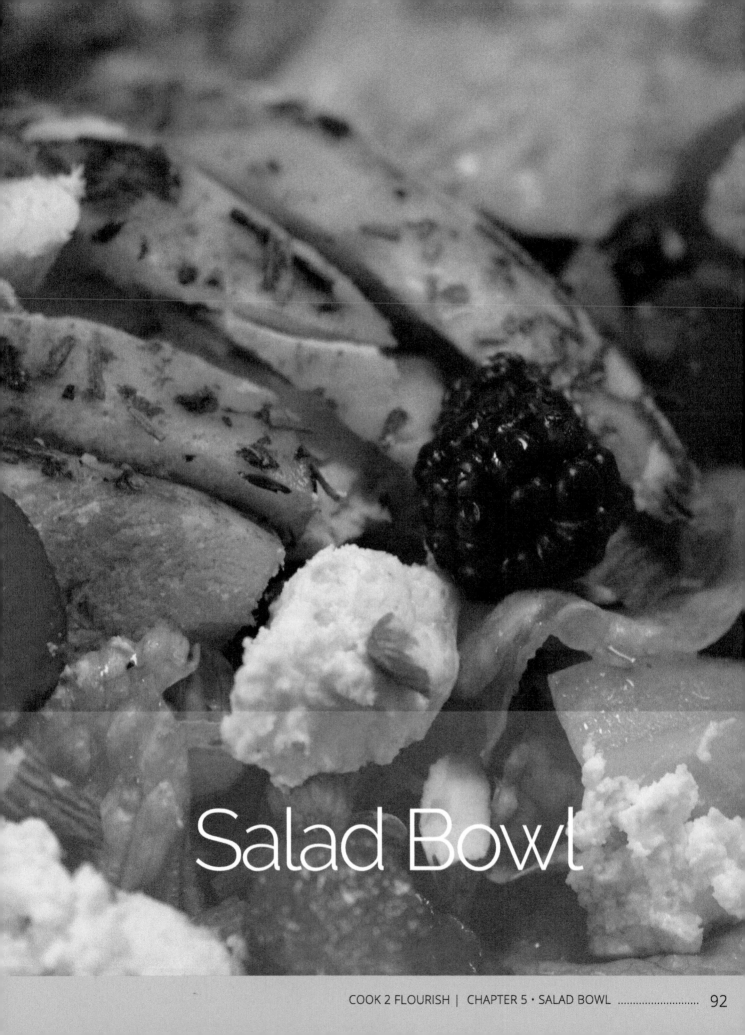

Salad Bowl

Berry Delicious Salad

4 servings

Antioxidant Dressing:

Makes ⅔ cup

- **¼ cup extra-virgin olive oil**
- **⅓ cup Nature's Sunshine® Nature's Noni® juice OR Thai-Go®**
- **2 Tablespoons filtered water**
- **½ teaspoon garlic, minced**
- **¼ teaspoon Nature's Sunshine® sea salt**
- **¼ teaspoon ground black pepper**
- **⅛ teaspoon stevia, to taste**

Salad:
- **8 cups fresh greens, including Romaine and spinach**
- **1 small organic red beet, vegetable peeler ribbons**
- **1 large carrot, vegetable peeler ribbons**
- **1 medium red onion, sliced**
- **½ cup red cabbage, thinly sliced, optional**
- **8 organic strawberries, sliced, optional**
- **¾ cup organic blackberries**
- **½ cup almonds (toasted or soaked), chopped**
- **¼ cup feta OR goat cheese, crumbled**
- **2 fully cooked and seasoned chicken breasts, sliced**

Directions:

1) Combine all ingredients for the dressing in a blender and blend on high speed until mixed well.
Stir again before serving as the dressing tends to separate.

2) In a large salad bowl place the salad greens, beet, carrot, onion and red cabbage (if using).
Pour in half of the dressing and toss well to coat.

3) Plate your individual salad servings and arrange the strawberries and blackberries. Sprinkle with almonds and your choice of crumbled cheese. Position the sliced chicken on top and if desired, add more dressing.

Robin's Recipe for a Loaded Salad

Who said "salad means boring lettuce?"

I understand that plain lettuce salad is not something to beam with excitement about like the aroma of baked chicken and cinnamon sweet potatoes filling the room, but accenting with a few delectable, not extravagant, but delicious toppings can make your salad a hit! Yes, a raving report is not solely for the main dish- make your salad delish!

The toppings that will please like the plethora of combinations at a salad bar- with the quality and comfort of your own home and creativity...

Salad Greens:
- Romaine lettuce
- Napa cabbage
- spinach
- spring mix salad greens
- baby kale
- arugula

Fresh Vegetables:
- broccoli florets
- cauliflower florets
- carrot ribbons or shredded
- beet ribbons or shredded

Accent Vegetables:
- bell pepper- red, yellow, orange, green
- onion
- tomatoes
- radish
- cucumbers
- cabbage- red or green

Fresh Fruit:
- organic apple
- black berries
- raspberries
- orange
- pear
- kiwi
- mango
- organic peaches
- organic strawberries
- pomegranate arils

Toppings:
- sundried tomatoes
- kalamata olives
- avocado
- boiled egg
- mushrooms
- black olives
- artichoke hearts
- garbanzo beans
- frozen peas

• Crunchy toppings:
- pecans
- raw almonds
- walnuts
- raw sunflower seeds
- raw pumpkin seeds
- pecans

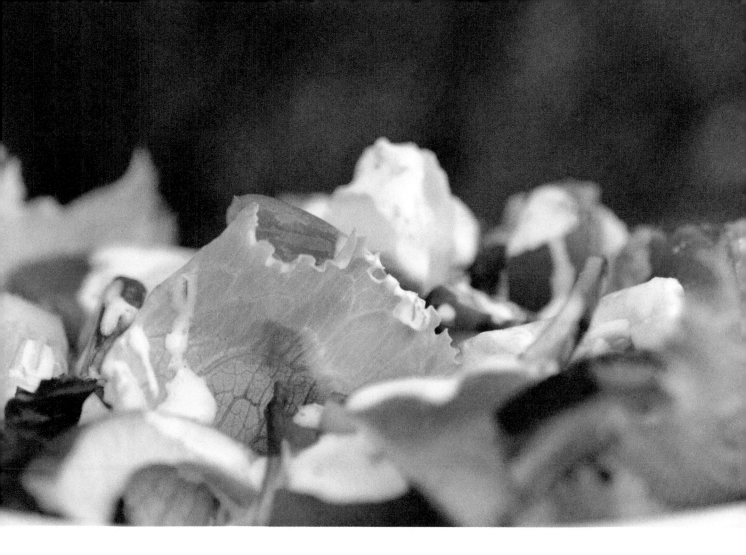

Dressing:

Prepare either our Ranch style dressing or one of the many delicious vinaigrettes here in Cook 2 Flourish. They are quick and easy to make! Save money by making your own flavorful dressings and enjoy the benefits of antioxidants without the empty calories, hydrogenated oil and refined sugars!

Directions:

1) Choose a large salad bowl or a single serving bowl to make your salad in.

2) Choose the salad greens you want for the base of your salad. Then choose the fresh vegetables you would like to add to the salad. If desired, add a small amount of any desired accent vegetables to your salad bowl. You can toss the salad or layer the salad.

3) Would you like to add some fruit? A salad with fruit is really good with a vinaigrette dressing with avocado or chicken breast on top. Make your selection from the list. Leave strawberries whole or slice them. Slice or dice the apple, peach, kiwi or pear. Sprinkle on the pomegranate arils and small berries.

4) Maybe you would rather an Italian flair! Toss chopped sundried tomatoes, olives, artichoke hearts and garbanzo beans into mixed greens. Then make our Italian vinaigrette dressing and garnish with feta cheese. Whatever the salad, add a few toppings and enjoy!

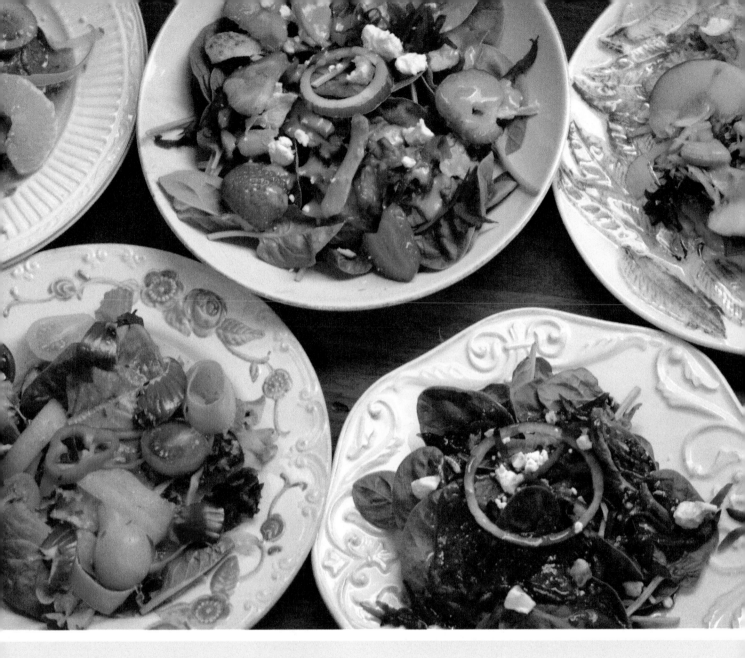

Salad Party

. . . .

Among the wonderful taste testers for the cookbook, our friend Joyce was our "salad girl" because she loves vinaigrette salads! In an effort to proof five of the salads for this book, we made a project into a party. One afternoon we three ladies tossed and tasted five vibrant salads, and each one we tasted we decided it was our new favorite. We hope you really enjoy them, too!

Citrus Thyme Sublime Dressing

Makes ½ cup

- 2 Tablespoons extra-virgin olive oil
- ¼ cup fresh squeezed blood orange juice
- 2 Tablespoons Persian lime flavor olive oil
- 1 Tablespoon peach flavor balsamic vinegar
- ¼ teaspoon ground black pepper
- ¼ teaspoon Nature's Sunshine® sea salt
- 6-9 drops liquid stevia, to taste
- ½ teaspoon fresh orange thyme

Salad:
- 8 cups fresh organic spring mix greens
- 1 small organic yellow beet, vegetable peeler ribbons
- 1 large carrot, shredded
- 1 medium red onion, sliced
- Assorted organic edible flowers, baby pansies

Directions:

1) Blend the dressing in a blender until all the ingredients are mixed well.

2) Place the salad greens, beet, carrot and onion in a large salad bowl. Pour in half of the dressing and toss well to coat. Position the edible flowers on top. Plate your individual salad servings and if desired, add more dressing.

Berry Kissed Quinoa Salad

4-6 servings

Dressing:
- 12-18 drops liquid stevia, to taste
- ⅛ teaspoon organic pure vanilla extract
- 1 teaspoon cinnamon
- Pinch of ground nutmeg, optional

Salad:
- 8 cups fresh spinach
- ½ cup cooked quinoa, chilled

- 2 Tablespoons toasted sesame oil
  OR Nature's Sunshine® flax seed oil with lignans
- 3 Tablespoons Nature's Sunshine® Nature's Noni® juice
  OR Thai-Go®
- ¼ cup unsweetened almond milk OR prepared organic green tea

- ½ cup soaked almonds OR toasted almonds
- ½ cup fresh berries (strawberries, blackberries, blueberries)

Directions:

1) In a measuring cup combine your choice of oil, your choice of Noni juice or Thai-Go, your choice of almond milk or green tea, stevia, vanilla, cinnamon and nutmeg (if desired) then stir well. Pour over the spinach and the chilled quinoa then toss to coat.

2) Plate the salad and top each salad plate with almonds and your choice of fresh berries.
Refrigerate until ready to serve or serve immediately.

Substitutions for the Nature's Noni® and Thai-Go®: (Choose one)

3 Tablespoons Cinnamon Pear balsamic vinegar

2 Tablespoons Cinnamon Pear balsamic vinegar with 1 Tablespoon Chocolate balsamic vinegar

---

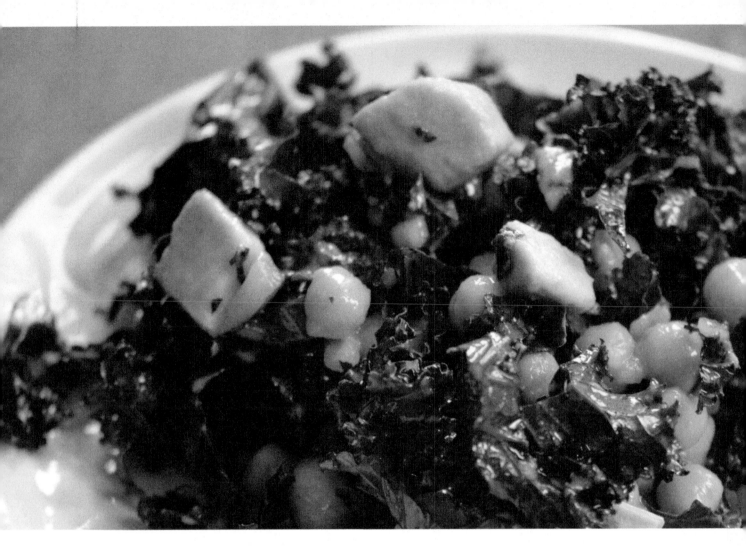

Kraving Kale Salad

2-4 servings

- 3 cups baby Kale OR curly Kale, thinly sliced
- 1 (15 ounce) can garbanzo beans, drained and rinsed
- 1 small avocado, pit removed and peeled, diced
- ½ cup red onion, chopped
- 2 Tablespoons fresh squeezed lemon juice
- 2 Tablespoons extra-virgin olive oil
- ½ teaspoon garlic, minced
- ½ teaspoon Bragg® liquid aminos
- 3-6 drops liquid stevia, to taste

Directions:

1) Combine the Kale, garbanzo beans, avocado and red onion in a large salad bowl.

2) In a measuring cup, combine the lemon juice, oil, garlic, liquid aminos and stevia to taste. Mix well with a fork. Pour the dressing on the salad and toss well.

Tip: Use roasted garlic if you want a milder taste. Roasted garlic is not as noticeable.

Italian Flair: Omit avocado. Add sundried tomatoes in extra-virgin olive oil, drained and chopped and feta cheese.

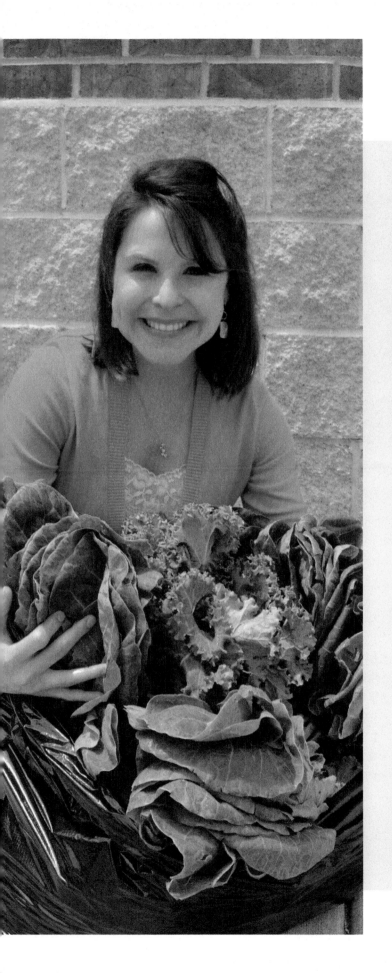

Perfect Provision
························

To all who have supported me through the writing of this book, thank you! Your prayers and encouragements mean so much! I must also share that all along this journey God has been so faithful. We have seen His gracious hand of provision time after time- from the choosing of the publisher to discounted purple cauliflower and 20 pounds of free Farmer's Market kale. I stand in awe of all the perfect provision- no request is too small nor, need too great; be encouraged to trust God and wait for His provision.

Philippians 4:19

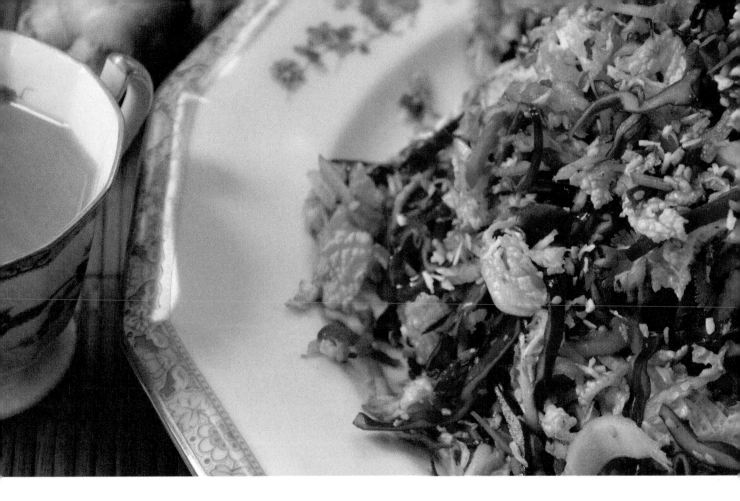

Sesame Cashew Crunch Coleslaw

4-6 Servings

- 4 cups Napa cabbage, finely sliced
- 1 cup red cabbage, finely sliced
- 1 cup organic carrots, shredded
- ½ cup beet, shredded
- ½ cup fresh organic cilantro, minced
- 1 garlic clove, pressed
- 2 Tablespoons sesame oil
- 1 Tablespoon filtered water

- 1 Tablespoon Bragg® liquid aminos
- 1 teaspoon raw honey OR 2-4 drops liquid stevia
- ½ teaspoon ground ginger
- ¼ cup raw cashews, chopped
- 1 Tablespoon sesame seeds
- 1 Tablespoon unsweetened shredded coconut, for garnish
- ½ Tablespoon Nature's Sunshine® flax seed oil with lignans
- 1 Tablespoon coconut aminos

Directions:

1) Slice the cabbage into a large mixing bowl then add the shredded carrots, beets and cilantro. Toss to combine.

2) In a measuring cup combine the garlic, sesame oil, flax seed oil, coconut aminos, liquid aminos, water, your choice honey or stevia and ginger. Stir well and pour over the cabbage mixture. Toss to combine.

3) Add in the cashews and sesame seeds then sprinkle the coconut on top as a garnish.

Cherry on the Top Kale Salad

2-4 servings

Dressing:
- 2 Tablespoons extra-virgin olive oil
- 2 Tablespoons Napa Valley Naturals® Cherry Wood Aged Organic Balsamic Vinegar
- ¼ cup sweet cherries, frozen
- 1 Tablespoon water
- 1 small garlic clove, minced
- Dash Nature's Sunshine® sea salt
- Dash ground black pepper
- ¼ teaspoon Dijon mustard
- ⅛ teaspoon stevia, to taste

Salad:
- 8 cups total: curly kale, Tuscan kale
- ½ medium red onion, spiralized
- ½ medium red beet, spiralized
- ⅓ - ½ cup frozen sweet cherries OR fresh Bing cherries, pitted
- ⅓ cup walnuts, chopped
- ¼ cup feta OR goat cheese, crumbled, optional

Directions:

1) Combine all dressing ingredients into a blender and blend on high speed for 20 to 30 seconds until all the ingredients are mixed well.

2) Slice the kale thinly and massage it with the dressing for 5 minutes until it wilts and is half the size. (Salad pictured has both varieties of kale in it).

3) Spiralize the onion and the beet then slice through the spirals four times to make them smaller pieces. Add to the kale.

4) Slice the cherries in half or fourths and add to the kale salad. Toss to combine then plate the kale salad onto individual plates.

5) Garnish with walnuts and cheese (if desired)...and a cherry on top!

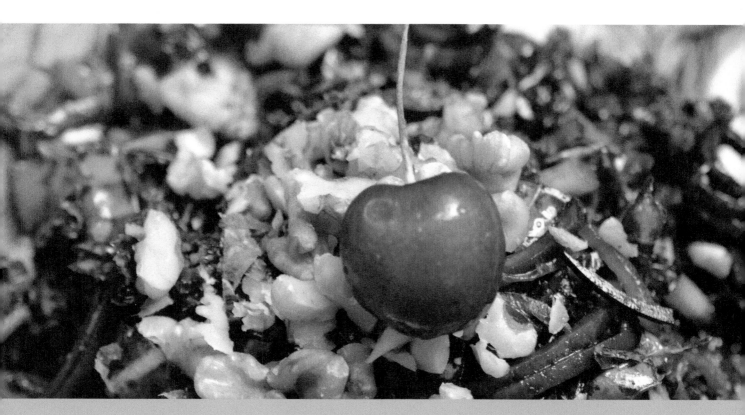

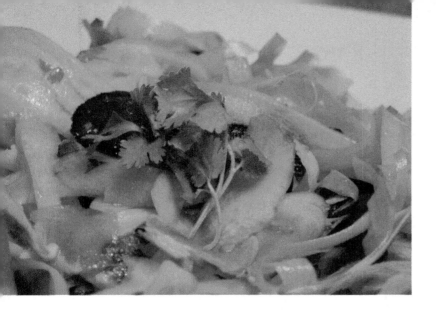

Happy Salad

4 servings

Dressing:
- 2 Tablespoons Persian Lime flavor olive oil
  OR extra-virgin olive oil
- ⅓ cup fresh squeezed orange juice
- ¼ cup fresh organic cilantro, chopped
- 1 garlic clove, minced
- 7 drops liquid stevia, to taste

Salad:
- ½ medium red beet, vegetable peeler ribbons
- ½ medium yellow beet, vegetable peeler ribbons
- ½ medium watermelon radish, vegetable peeler ribbons
- 2 organic carrots, vegetable peeler ribbons
- Cilantro for garnish

Directions:

1) In a measuring cup, combine the oil, juice, cilantro, garlic and stevia and mix well.

2) Combine beets, radish and carrots in a large salad bowl. Pour the dressing on the salad and toss well. Garnish with cilantro and serve immediately.

Surprise Spiral Salad

4 servings

Dressing:
- ¼ cup extra-virgin olive oil
- 2 Tablespoons filtered water
- 1 teaspoon cinnamon
- Pinch of nutmeg
- ⅛ teaspoon stevia, to taste
- 1 cup fresh squeezed orange juice,
  approximately 3 oranges

Salad:
- 8 cups organic spring mix greens
- 1 small-medium red onion
- 1 medium yellow beet
- 1 medium sweet potato
- ½ ripe avocado, pit removed,
  peeled and diced

Directions:

1) In a measuring cup, combine the oil, water, cinnamon, nutmeg, stevia, and orange juice.

2) Place the salad greens in a large salad bowl. Spiralize the red onion, the beet and the sweet potato into the salad bowl using a spiralizer. With kitchen shears, cut into the long lengths 3 or 4 times to make eating the spirals more manageable. Add the diced avocado.

3) Pour half or more of the dressing on the salad and toss well. Serve immediately.

Surprise! That's not carrot, its sweet potato!

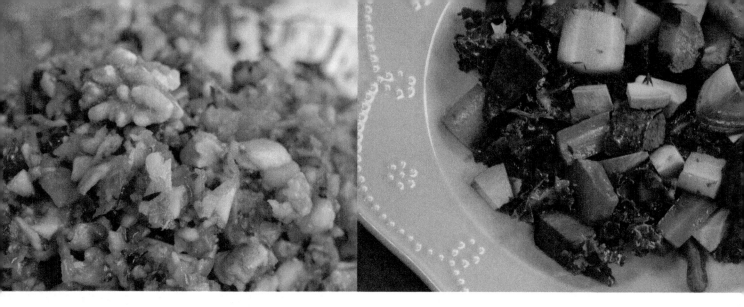

Quick Cranberry Salad

8-10 servings

Gluten Free
Grain Free
Dairy Free

- 2 cups cranberries, fresh or frozen
- 2 ½ Tablespoons raw honey
- 8-12 drops liquid stevia, to taste
- 1 organic orange, with peeling
- 1 large organic sweet apple, with peeling
- ¼ teaspoon cinnamon
- ⅓ cup walnuts OR pecans, chopped

Directions:

1) Rinse the frozen cranberries and place in a food processor. Pulse 20 times then pour into a large mixing bowl.

2) Add the honey and stevia to the cranberries and stir well to combine.

3) Wash the orange and the apple. Keep the peeling on both of them. Cut the orange in 8 pieces and remove any seeds. Cut and core the apple. Place in the food processor and pulse them 10 times then add to the cranberries and mix well to combine.

4) Add in the cinnamon and your choice of nuts. Stir to combine and serve in chilled bowls.

This salad is good with ½-¾ cup of pineapple, too.

Rooting for My Health Salad

2 servings

Gluten Free
Grain Free
Dairy Free

- 2 cups fresh kale, thinly sliced
- ¾ cup roasted vegetables
  (Getting to the Root of It, page 218)
- ¼ ripe avocado, pit removed, peeled and diced in small pieces
- 2 Tablespoons extra-virgin olive oil
- ⅓ cup fresh squeezed blood orange juice
- 2 Tablespoons filtered water
- 1 teaspoon cinnamon
- 5-10 drops liquid stevia, to taste

Directions:

1) Layer the kale, roasted vegetables and the avocado on salad plates.

2) In a measuring cup, combine the oil, juice, water, cinnamon, and stevia. Mix well.

3) Pour half of the dressing on each salad. Serve immediately.

Flourish Florets Salad

4-6 servings

Gluten Free
Grain Free
Dairy Free

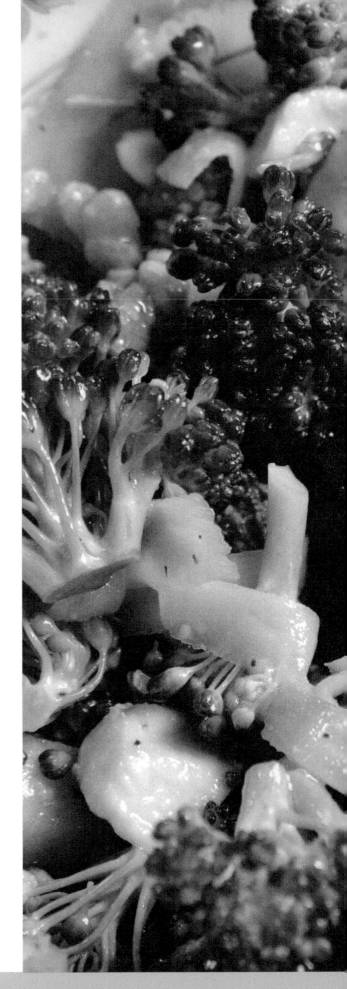

- 2 cups broccoli florets
- ½ cup broccoli stem, vegetable peeler ribbons
- ¼ cup ripe avocado, diced
- 1 small fresh garlic clove, minced
- 1 Tablespoon fresh squeezed lemon juice
- 1 ½ Tablespoon extra-virgin olive oil
- ¼ teaspoon Nature's Sunshine® sea salt
- ⅛ teaspoon ground black pepper
- ½ teaspoon coconut aminos

Directions:

1) Peel the outer skin off of the broccoli stem then proceed to use a vegetable peeler to make thin ribbons out of it. Place the broccoli, ribbons and avocado into a salad bowl.

2) In a measuring cup, combine the garlic, lemon juice, olive oil, sea salt, black pepper and coconut aminos for the dressing. Mix well. Pour the dressing on the salad and toss well.

Lemon Thyme Vinaigrette

Makes ½ cup

- 2 Tablespoons extra-virgin olive oil
- 2 Tablespoons Persian lime flavor olive oil
- 2 Tablespoons water
- ¼ cup fresh squeezed lemon juice
- ¼ teaspoon stevia (21 drops liquid stevia)
- ¼ teaspoon ground black pepper
- ¼ teaspoon organic lemon zest
- 1 Tablespoon fresh lemon thyme leaves
- ⅛ teaspoon Nature's Sunshine® sea salt
- ⅛ teaspoon guar gum

Directions:

1) Combine all ingredients into a blender and blend on high speed approximately 40 seconds until all the ingredients are mixed well. Stir well before serving as the dressing tends to separate.

Extra-virgin olive oil may be substituted for the Persian lime flavor olive oil.

Traditional Coleslaw

Makes ½ cup

- 4 cups green cabbage, shredded
- ½ cup organic carrots, shredded
- ½ cup Vegenaise®
- 3 Tablespoons organic Greek yogurt, plain whole milk
- 1 Tablespoon raw honey
- 6-8 drops liquid stevia
- 1 ½ Tablespoons fresh squeezed lemon juice
- ½ teaspoon Nature's Sunshine® sea salt
- 1 teaspoon celery seeds
- Dash ground black pepper

Directions:

1) Shred the cabbage and carrot in a food processor. Place into a large mixing bowl.

2) In a 2 cup measuring cup, combine the Vegenaise®, yogurt, honey, stevia, lemon juice, sea salt, celery seeds and pepper. Mix well and pour over cabbage and carrots. Mix well and refrigerate until ready to serve. Stir to combine and serve in chilled bowls.

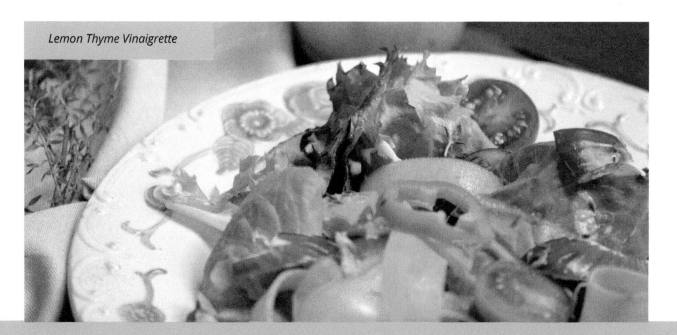

Lemon Thyme Vinaigrette

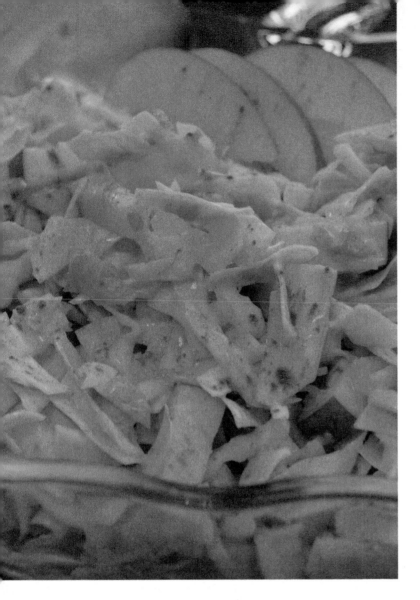

Apple Coleslaw

4 servings

- 5 cups green cabbage, coarsely sliced
- ½ cup organic carrots, shredded
- ½ cup Vegenaise®
- 3 Tablespoons organic Greek yogurt, plain whole milk
- 2 Tablespoon raw honey
- 1 Tablespoon fresh squeezed lemon juice
- ½ large organic red apple, diced
- ½ teaspoon cinnamon

Directions:

1) Place the cabbage and carrots into a large mixing bowl.

2) Add in the Vegenaise®, yogurt, honey, lemon juice and apple. Mix well to combine.

3) Sprinkle the cinnamon on top. Stir to combine and serve in chilled bowls.

Quick Fruit Salad

4-6 servings

- 2 oranges, peeled and sectioned
- 1 large banana, sliced
- 1 organic apple with peeling, chopped

- 6 organic strawberries, sliced
- ½ teaspoon cinnamon
- ¼ cup pecans OR walnuts, optional

Directions:

1) Place the orange sections in a salad bowl. Squeeze 4 of the orange sections to make juice in the bottom of the bowl. Cut the remaining orange sections in half.

2) Add the banana, apple and strawberries.

3) Add cinnamon and nuts (if desired). Stir well and serve in chilled bowls.

Appreciate the fruits for their natural flavor. IF you need some sweetener, add a little raw honey or a couple drops of liquid stevia. This is such a versatile recipe; you can try an orange, kiwi and strawberry combination. Make it with your favorite fruit!

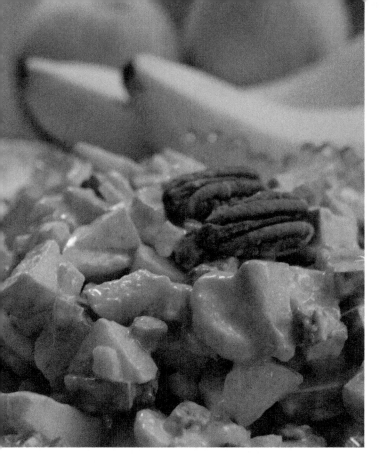

Confetti Coleslaw

6-8 servings

- 1 cup carrots, shredded
- ¼ cup onion, finely chopped
- 6 cups green cabbage, shredded or coarsely sliced
- 2 cups purple cabbage, shredded or coarsely sliced
- ½ cup Vegenaise®
- 10 drops liquid stevia
- ¼ cup organic Greek yogurt, plain whole milk
- 2 Tablespoons raw coconut nectar OR raw honey
- 2 ½ Tablespoons fresh squeezed lemon juice
- 1 ¼ Tablespoons apple cider vinegar
- ¼ cup unsweetened almond milk
- ½ teaspoon Nature's Sunshine® sea salt
- Dash ground black pepper

Directions:

1) Place cabbage, carrots and onion into a large mixing bowl.

2) Add the Vegenaise®, yogurt, your choice of raw coconut nectar or honey, stevia, lemon juice, vinegar, almond milk, sea salt, and pepper. Mix well and serve in chilled bowls.

Apple Banana Salad

4 servings

- 1 large banana, sliced
- ⅓ cup organic celery rib, sliced, optional
- 1 large organic apple, with peeling, diced
- ⅓ cup pecans OR walnuts
- 1 Tablespoons raw honey
- ½ teaspoon cinnamon
- ⅓ cup organic Greek yogurt, plain whole milk OR Vegenaise®

Directions:

1) Place the apple in a salad bowl along with the banana, celery and nuts.

2) Add your choice of Greek yogurt or Vegenaise®, honey and cinnamon. Stir well.

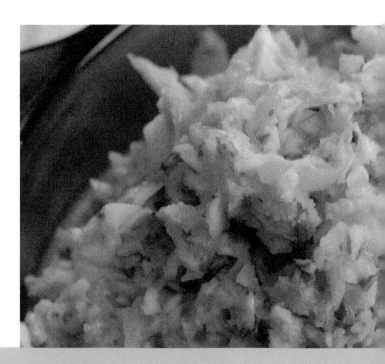

Parade of Flavors Salad – Butternut Squash

4 servings

Dressing:
- Dash ground black pepper
- ¼ teaspoon ground cumin
- ½ teaspoon curry powder
- 1 teaspoon cinnamon
- 1 teaspoon coconut aminos
- 1 teaspoon toasted sesame oil
- 2 Tablespoons extra-virgin olive oil
- ¼ cup fresh squeezed orange juice
- 2 teaspoons raw honey OR 4-8 drops liquid stevia

Salad:
- 8 cups fresh spinach, packed
- ½ cup cooked quinoa
- 2 cups butternut squash,
  bite size squares (already roasted and chilled)
- ½ cup red onion, diced
- 4 dried figs, chopped
- ½ cup whole almonds, chopped

Directions:

1) In a measuring cup combine the dressing ingredients and stir well.

2) Place spinach, quinoa, butternut squash, onion, and figs in a large salad bowl.

3) Place almonds on an unbleached parchment paper lined baking sheet and bake in preheated 350 degree oven for 8 minutes until toasted. Add to the salad bowl.

4) Pour the dressing over the salad and toss to coat.

Suggestion: Omit butternut and figs. Add 1 medium organic apple, with peeling, diced, and 1 cup organic carrot, shredded.

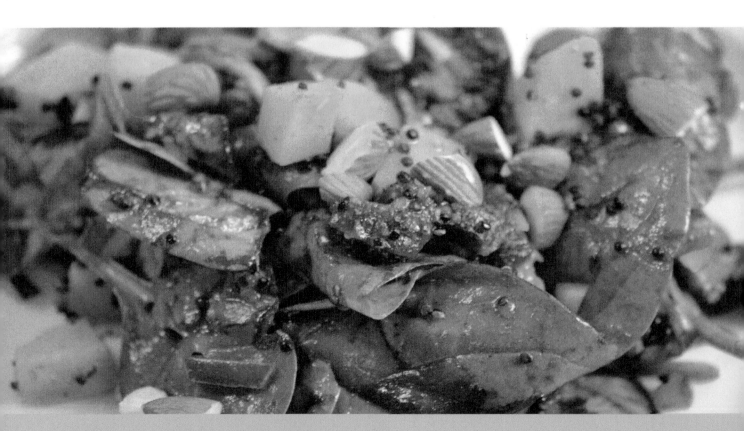

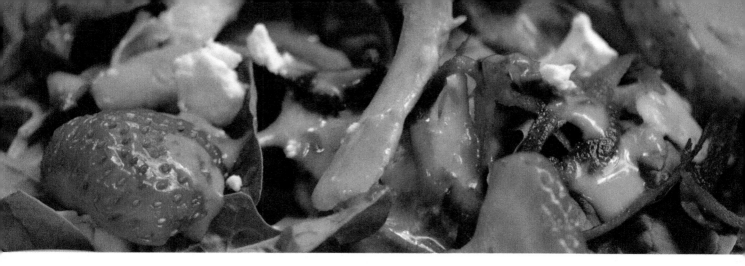

Strawberry Vinaigrette

Gluten Free
Grain Free
Dairy Free

Makes 1 cup

- 2 Tablespoons strawberry flavor vinegar OR balsamic vinegar (Napa Valley Naturals® Cherry Wood Aged Organic Balsamic Vinegar)
- ¼ cup cold filtered water
- ½ cup organic strawberries, chopped
- 1 teaspoon Dijon mustard
- ¼ cup extra-virgin olive oil
- Dash Nature's Sunshine® sea salt
- Dash ground black pepper
- 7 drops liquid stevia, to taste

Directions:

1) Blend all ingredients except oil in blender until smooth, and then add oil and pulse 5 or 6 times until combined. Stir well before serving as the dressing tends to separate.

Encourage 2 Flourish: Radish Story

One evening I was slicing radishes to go on our salads, and the Lord dropped into my heart the truth that radishes mirror the story of the gospel. The bright red outside gives way to a pure white inside, which reminds me of Psalm 51:7 that God washes our sins away and makes us white as snow, just like this radish is white as snow. I will never look at a radish the same again.

"Surely I was sinful at birth, sinful from the time my mother conceived me. Yet you desired faithfulness even in the womb; you taught me wisdom in that secret place. Cleanse me with hyssop, and I will be clean; wash me, and I will be whiter than snow... Create in me a pure heart, O God, and renew a steadfast spirit within me. Do not cast me from your presence or take your Holy Spirit from me. Restore to me the joy of your salvation and grant me a willing spirit, to sustain me."

Psalm 51:5-12 *NIV*

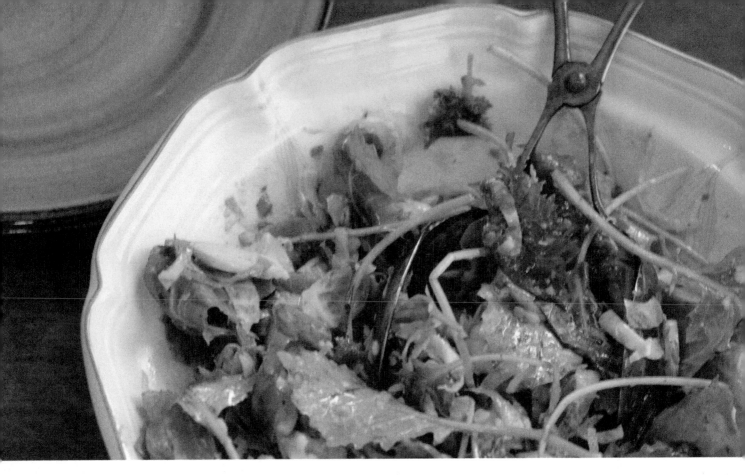

Kan't Get Enough Kale Salad

4 servings

- 2 cups Brussels sprouts, shredded
- 2 cups baby kale OR curly kale, thinly sliced
- ¼ cup walnuts OR almonds, chopped
- 1 fresh garlic clove, minced OR 4 roasted cloves, mashed
- 2 Tablespoons fresh squeezed lemon juice
- 2 Tablespoons grated parmesan cheese
- ½ teaspoon Dijon mustard, optional
- ⅓ cup extra-virgin olive oil
- ½ teaspoon Nature's Sunshine® sea salt
- ¼ teaspoon ground black pepper
- ⅛ teaspoon liquid stevia
- 1 teaspoon Bragg® liquid amino

Directions:

1) Ten Brussels sprouts weigh approximately 5 ounces and measure whole as 1 ½ cups. When processed or shredded, they yield about 2 cups. Wash and trim the Brussels sprouts. Cut them in half and then place them in a food processor and process 8 seconds.

2) Combine the Brussels sprouts, Kale and nuts in a large salad bowl.

3) In a measuring cup, combine the rest of the ingredients for the dressing. Mix well with a fork. Pour the dressing on the salad and toss well and chill before serving.

Tip: Use roasted garlic if you want a milder taste. It's not as noticeable if roasted.

For Dairy Free, Candida Friendly and lower in calories:
Omit the parmesan cheese, the Dijon mustard and the 1/3 cup extra-virgin olive oil. Replace it with:
- 2 Tablespoons ripe avocado, mashed
- 2 Tablespoons extra-virgin olive oil
- 2 Tablespoons unsweetened almond milk

Peachy Keen Salad

Gluten Free
Grain Free

4 servings

Peach Salad Dressing:

Makes ¾-1 cup dressing

• 2 Tablespoons peach flavor vinegar
  OR white balsamic vinegar
• ¼ cup cold filtered water
• 1 organic peach
• 1 teaspoon Dijon mustard
• ¼ cup extra-virgin olive oil
• 1 teaspoon cinnamon
• ¼ teaspoon ground ginger
• ⅛ teaspoon stevia

Salad:

• 8 cups fresh mixed salad greens
• 1 organic yellow beet, shredded
• 1 large organic carrot, vegetable peeler ribbons
• ¼ medium red onion, sliced
• 10 organic peach slices
• ½ cup soaked almonds
• ¼ cup feta OR goat cheese, crumbled, optional
• ½ ripe avocado, peeled and pit removed, diced, optional

Directions:

1) Blend all ingredients except oil in blender until smooth, and then add oil and pulse 5 or 6 times until combined. Stir well before serving as the dressing tends to separate.

2) In a large salad bowl place the salad greens, shredded beet, carrot ribbons and onion slices. Toss to combine. Plate the salad in individual servings. Place the peach slices on top with almonds and dressing. If desired, garnish with crumbled cheese and avocado.

Suggestion:
This salad and the peach dressing is even great with strawberry slices.

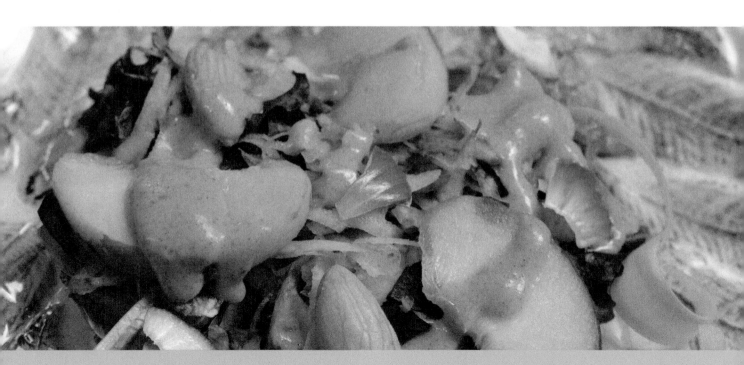

Homemade Ranch Style Dressing

Makes 1 cup

- ¼ cup unsweetened almond milk
- 1 ¼ teaspoon fresh squeezed lemon juice
- ½ cup organic Greek yogurt, plain whole milk
- ¼ cup Vegenaise®
- ¼ teaspoon guar gum
- 3 drops liquid stevia
- 5 drops Bragg® liquid aminos
- ¼ teaspoon ground black pepper
- ½ teaspoon Nature's Sunshine® sea salt
- ½ teaspoon onion granules
- ½ teaspoon garlic powder
- 1 teaspoon dried parsley OR ½ Tablespoon fresh, minced
- 1 teaspoon fresh chives, minced, optional
- ¹⁄₁₆ teaspoon dried dill

Directions:

1) Combine the almond milk and the lemon juice and set aside.

2) In a blender, combine the yogurt, Vegenaise®, stevia and liquid aminos (Be careful! The liquid comes out fast!!!).

3) Mix the guar gum into the almond milk and then pour into the blender.

4) Add the pepper, sea salt, onion granules and garlic powder then blend on medium-high for 15-20 seconds to mix in the guar gum and blend up any clumps.

5) Add in the parsley, chives (if using) and the dill. Blend on lowest speed for 5 seconds, just to stir in. Refrigerate 4-12 hours then it is ready to serve.
Stir well before serving.

Orange Sesame Dressing

Makes 1/3 cup

- ¼ cup fresh squeezed orange juice
- 2 Tablespoons toasted sesame oil
- ½ Tablespoon Bragg® liquid aminos
- ½ Tablespoon Coconut Aminos
- ½ teaspoon fresh ginger
- 1 garlic clove
- Pinch of cayenne pepper

Directions:

1) Press the fresh ginger and the garlic clove in a garlic press and place in a measuring cup.

2) Add in the orange juice, sesame oil, liquid aminos, coconut aminos and the cayenne pepper. Mix well with a fork. Pour over your choice of salad greens and toss to coat. Serve immediately.

How to make Toasted Almonds

- **Whole raw almonds**

Directions:

1) Chop desired amount of almonds. Place them on an unbleached parchment paper lined baking sheet and bake in a preheated 350 degree oven for 8 minutes.

2) Remove from oven and immediately lift the parchment paper and the almonds off of the hot baking sheet to cool.

Enjoy toasted almonds on garden salads, whipped sweet potatoes, yogurt or as a snack.

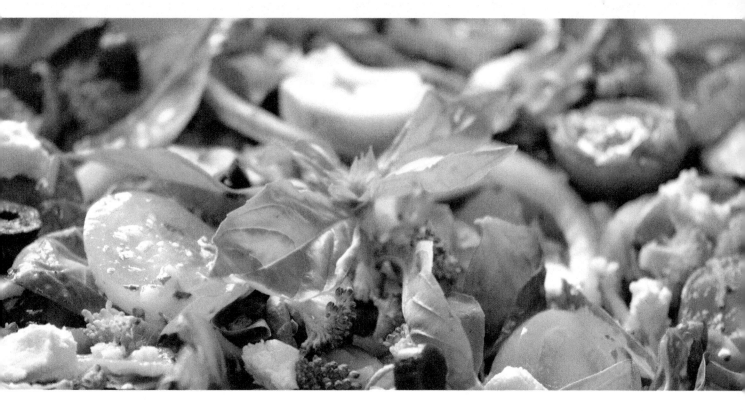

Mediterranean Salad

4-6 servings

Italian Vinaigrette Dressing:
Makes ¾ cup

- ¼ cup fresh squeezed lemon juice
- ¼ cup extra-virgin olive oil
- ¼ cup filtered water
- ½ Tablespoon Vegenaise® OR ripe avocado, mashed
- 1 garlic clove, minced
- 1 teaspoon dried Italian seasoning
- ⅛ teaspoon ground black pepper
- ¼ teaspoon Nature's Sunshine® sea salt
- ¼ teaspoon stevia (21 drops liquid stevia)

Salad:

- 8 cups salad greens
- 1 cup broccoli florets
- ½ cup organic carrots, shredded
- 10 heirloom cherry tomatoes, halved
- 6 artichoke hearts, drained and halved
- ½ red onion, sliced
- 1 small red or yellow bell pepper, sliced
- ¼ cup kalamata olives, drained and sliced
- ¼ cup feta cheese OR goat cheese, crumbled
- Fresh basil leaves, for garnish

Directions:

1) Combine all ingredients into a blender and blend on high speed approximately 30 seconds until thoroughly mixed.

2) In a large salad bowl place the salad greens and top with broccoli and carrots.

3) Pour in half of the dressing and toss well to coat. Arrange the tomatoes, artichoke hearts, onion slices, bell pepper slices and olives on the salad. Pour the rest of the dressing on top. Sprinkle with your choice of crumbled cheese and garnish with basil leaves.

Farmer's Market story-

To market to market to buy some fresh kale...home again, home again, with veggies to unveil!

Spring time brings a special joy to my heart for many reasons, one being the re-awakening of the Farmer's Market. A long winter has come to an end and the frost is mostly gone; the hibernating relationships are blossoming once again. Farmer's Markets are more than the dirt hued vegetables and dew kissed fruits, they are a place of connection between food and farmer- chef and the ingredients, a place to know people and appreciate their harvest. I am so grateful to know the people behind my food and get to know them and support them. Before you know it, you will come away with not only amazing foods, but friendships too.

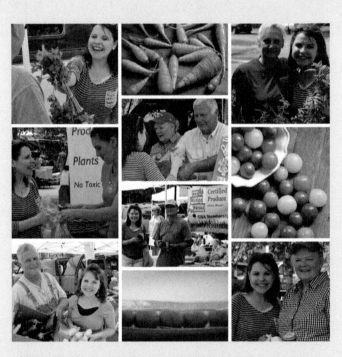

Some choice market finds:

• Kale, Swiss chard, Brussels sprout leaves and other luscious greens

• Sweet potatoes and squashes of all shapes and sizes

• Fresh cut flowers- perfect for a cheering someone's day

• Tomatoes of all sorts, sizes, and shades- heirlooms are the best!

• Seasonal treasures- fresh berries, broccoli, asparagus, snap peas, peaches and melons

• Some markets have local organically raised meats and eggs

What are heirloom plants, and why are they preferable over others?

Cultivated for years, heirlooms are seeds of plants that have been preserved for decades and even centuries for growing nourishing foods. For starters, they are eco-friendly and can be sown year after year from the seeds of the produce you harvest/grow. Palate wise, heirlooms can have a deeper more authentic flavor. Even their appearance can be rustic, earthy, or uneven which adds to their unique appeal. Explore your local farmer's market to begin reaping the benefits of these beautiful foods! And remember you can always start your own garden, even if it's on your patio.

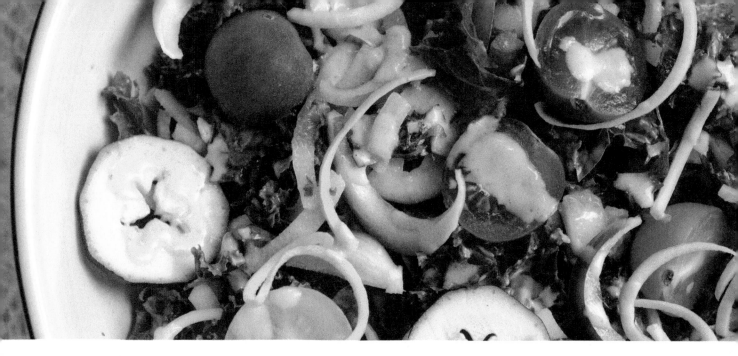

Market Me Smile Salad

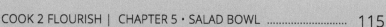

4-6 servings

Dressing:
- 1 garlic clove, minced
- 2 Tablespoons fresh organic cilantro
- ¼ teaspoon Nature's Sunshine® sea salt
- ⅛ teaspoon ground black pepper
  OR dash cayenne pepper
- 15 drops liquid stevia, to taste
- 2 Tablespoons extra-virgin olive oil
- ¼ ripe avocado, pit removed and peeled
- 2 Tablespoons fresh squeezed lime juice
- ¼ cup filtered water

Salad:
- 8 cups fresh curly kale, torn
- 1 small-medium cucumber, diced
- ½ small zucchini, sliced
- ½ small yellow squash, spiralized,
  trimmed to small pieces
- ¼ kohlrabi, spiralized, trimmed to small pieces
- ¼ cup red onion, chopped
- 8 red heirloom cherry tomatoes, halved

Directions:

1) Place all the ingredients for the dressing into a blender and blend on high speed for 30 seconds or until thoroughly mixed.

2) Combine all the kale, a portion of the cucumber, all the zucchini, all the squash, all the kohlrabi and all the onion in a large salad bowl. Pour half of the dressing over the salad and massage together for approximately 3 minutes.

3) Sprinkle the remaining cucumber and the tomatoes on top of the salad. Allow to chill before serving. Pour additional dressing on each individual salad serving (if desired).

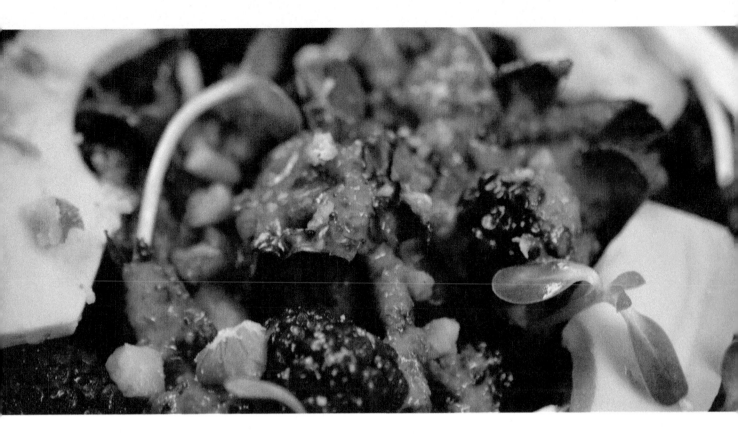

Eat It to Beet It Salad

Gluten Free
Grain Free
Dairy Free

4-6 servings

Dressing
Makes 2/3 cup

• ¼ cup extra-virgin olive oil
• ¼ cup filtered water
• 2 Tablespoon fresh squeezed lemon juice
• 1 garlic clove, minced
• ¼ cup organic red beet, shredded
• Pinch of Nature's Sunshine® sea salt
• Pinch of ground black pepper
• ⅛ teaspoon cinnamon
• ⅛ teaspoon stevia, to taste

Salad

• 8 cups fresh greens, including kale, arugula or romaine lettuce
• 1 cup fresh organic sunflower seed sprouts
• ½ organic red beet, vegetable peeler ribbons
• ¼ medium red onion, diced
• ½ cup red cabbage, thinly sliced, optional
• 1 cup organic blackberries
• ½ ripe avocado, peeled and pit removed, diced
• ⅓ cup black walnuts, chopped

Directions:

1) In a large salad bowl place the salad greens, sprouts, beet, onion and red cabbage (if using).
Pour in half of the dressing and toss well to coat.

2) Arrange the blackberries, avocado and walnuts. Pour the rest of the dressing on top.

Spotlight : Beets

A relative to quinoa, spinach, and Swiss Chard, beets are a stellar food.
Thanks to the unique phytonutrients in beets, they provide the body with:

- antioxidant properties to combat damage to cells
- anti-inflammatory benefits
- detoxification enhancement

Bolster up your minerals with beets since they offer manganese, potassium, copper, and magnesium. Folate is also a notable nutrient available from beets. To maintain these nutrients, yet keeping the flavor, the less cooking time the better. Don't throw away the tops; they are a nutritional gold mine. Simply wash them and freeze for a smoothie, juice them, or slice thinly for a salad.

Fun fact: the phytonutrient content of beets is rooted in its color; red beets supply more betalain which aid in detoxification, whereas yellow beets gift the body with superior amounts of lutein for the eyes.

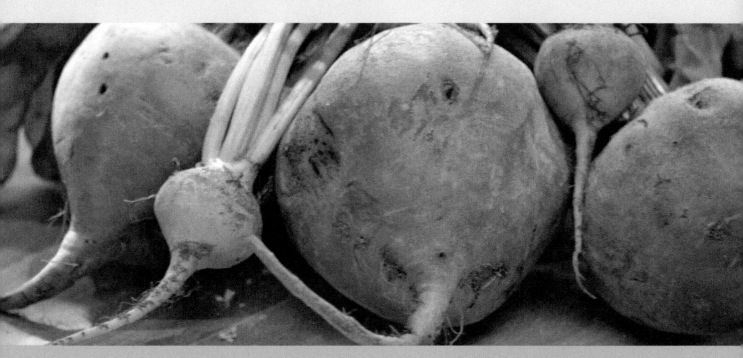

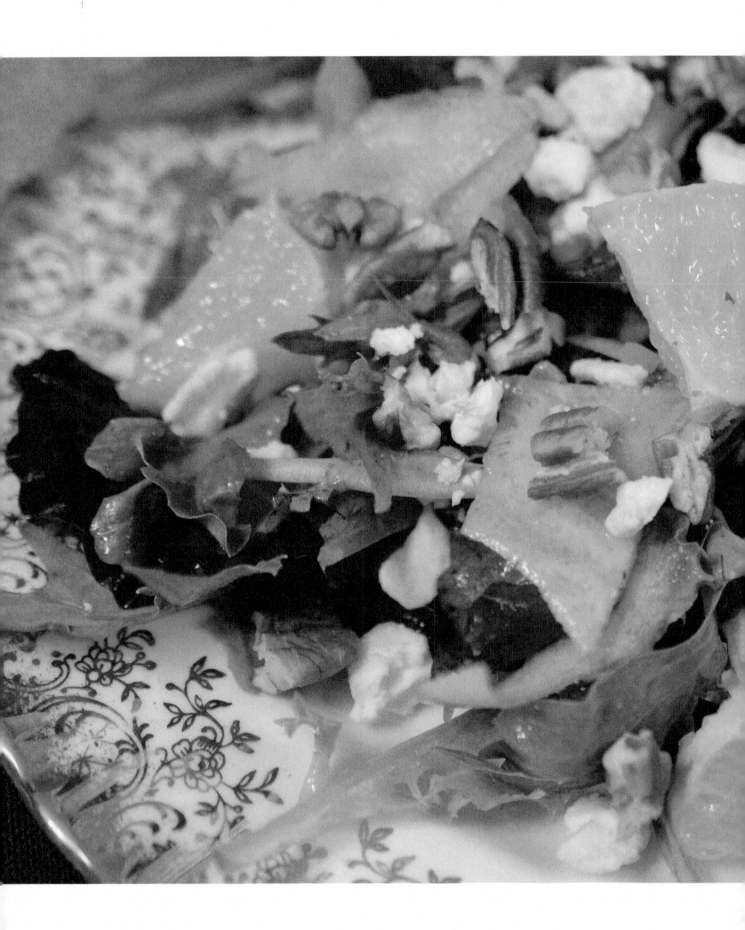

Orange Courtwarming Salad

4-6 servings

Dressing:
- ¼ cup extra-virgin olive oil
- 2 Tablespoons filtered water
- 1 teaspoon cinnamon
- Pinch of nutmeg
- ⅛ teaspoon stevia, to taste
- 1 cup fresh squeezed orange juice, approximately 3 oranges

Salad:
- 1 large fresh Romaine lettuce heart, torn
- 1 cup purple cabbage, sliced
- 1 ½ cups carrot, shredded
- 1 medium yellow beet, shredded
- ½ ripe avocado, pit removed, peeled and diced in small pieces
- Any other salad greens you enjoy
- 1 orange, peeled and sectioned, each slice cut in half
- Red onion, slices, optional
- ¼ cup goat cheese, crumbled
- ¼ cup pecans OR walnuts

Directions:

1) In a measuring cup, combine the oil, water, cinnamon, nutmeg, stevia, and orange juice.

2) Combine all salad greens and fresh vegetables and the avocado in a large salad bowl.

3) Mix the dressing and pour half or more on the salad and toss well. Plate the salad and top each one with orange pieces, red onion (if desired), goat cheese and nuts.

This sweet citrus salad commemorates the Courtwarming dance of my sophomore year where nine of my friends and I prepared and enjoyed an elegant dinner together, including this orange salad. Cooking with them was so much fun; it actually became a tradition... a delicious tradition.

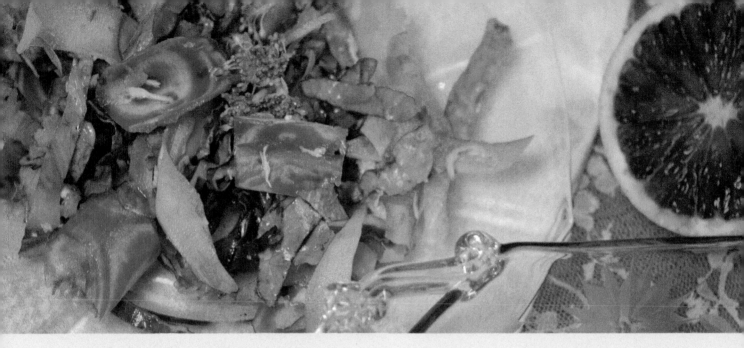

Encourage 2 Flourish: Blood Orange

Of all of the plants with abundant essential oils, oranges rank near the top; a sweet citrus mist cascades with the removal of its peel. One day while shopping, I noticed an unusual orange amongst the typical oranges; it was a blood orange. On a whim I purchased it thinking I would add some variety to my citrus consumption. Though I had forgotten I had it, the Lord had not. Before I unpeeled this colorful fruit, I had been praying and reflecting on the great sacrifice Jesus made for us on the cross. His body was broken for us, and His precious blood was spilled willingly and passionately.

Then it hit me- Jesus was a fragrant sacrifice to God by obediently surrendering His life. What wafting love, grace and mercy the Father must have smelled! It had pleased the Father to crush Jesus because in that crushing (peeling) the anguish and unparalled sacrifice became the fruitful and love-filled fragrance that could cover the sin-stench of every human being. Mind you, this fragrant orange I held in my hand was a blood orange. WOW! Yet another powerful parallel truth unveiled in the kitchen... "taste and see that the Lord is good".

Psalm 34:8

Blood Orange Salad

6 servings

Dressing:
- **2 Tablespoons extra-virgin olive oil**
- **⅓ cup fresh squeezed blood orange juice**
- **2 Tablespoons filtered water**
- **1 teaspoon cinnamon**
- **¼ teaspoon stevia (21 drops liquid stevia), to taste**

Salad:
- **1 large fresh Romaine lettuce heart, torn**
- **1 cup purple cabbage, sliced**
- **1 ½ cups organic carrot, vegetable peeler ribbons**
- **1 small-medium red OR yellow beet, vegetable peeler ribbons**
- **Any other salad greens you enjoy**
- **1 blood orange, peeled and sectioned, each section cut in half**
- **¼ red onion, sliced, optional**

Directions:

1) In a measuring cup, combine the oil, juice, water, cinnamon, and stevia. Mix well with a fork.

2) Combine all salad greens and fresh vegetables in a large salad bowl.

3) Pour half or more of the dressing on the salad and toss well.

4) Plate the salad and top each one with orange pieces and red onion slices (if desired).

Ensalada Mexicana

4-6 servings

Dressing:
- **1 garlic clove, minced**
- **2 Tablespoons fresh organic cilantro**
- **¼ teaspoon Nature's Sunshine® sea salt**
- **⅛ teaspoon ground black pepper OR dash cayenne pepper**
- **¼ teaspoon stevia (21 drops liquid stevia)**
- **½ Tablespoon Vegenaise®**
- **¼ cup extra-virgin olive oil**
- **¼ cup fresh squeezed lime juice**
- **¼ cup filtered water**

Salad:
- **1 large fresh Romaine lettuce heart, torn**
- **1 organic carrot, shredded or vegetable peeler ribbons**
- **2 cups fresh spring baby greens**
- **1 medium red OR yellow bell pepper, diced**
- **½ ripe avocado, pit removed, peeled and sliced**
- **¼ cup red onion, chopped**
- **4 radishes, diced**
- **15 red OR yellow cherry tomatoes, halved**
- **½ cup organic frozen corn, optional**
- **1 cup black beans, rinsed and drained**
- **Cilantro, for garnish**

Directions:

1) Place all the ingredients for the dressing into a blender and blend on high speed for 30 seconds or until thoroughly mixed.

2) Combine all salad greens, fresh vegetables, frozen corn (if desired) and black beans in a large salad bowl. Pour the dressing on the salad and toss well. Garnish with cilantro (if desired). Serve immediately or refrigerate until ready to serve. Toss again before serving.

Garlic Balsamic Salad

Gluten Free
Grain Free

4-6 servings

Garlic Balsamic Dressing:
Makes ⅔ cup

- ¼ cup extra-virgin olive oil
- ¼ cup balsamic vinegar (Napa Valley Naturals® Cherry Wood Aged Organic Balsamic Vinegar)
- 2 Tablespoons filtered water
- 1 garlic clove, minced
- Pinch of Nature's Sunshine® sea salt
- Pinch of ground black pepper
- 1 teaspoon Dijon mustard, optional
- ⅛ teaspoon stevia, to taste

Salad:
- 8 cups fresh greens, including spinach
- 1 organic red beet, shredded
- ½ cup red cabbage, thinly sliced, optional
- 1 medium red onion, sliced
- ½ cup walnuts, chopped
- ¼ cup feta OR goat cheese, crumbled

Directions:

1) In a large salad bowl place the salad greens, beet and red cabbage (if using).

2) Pour in half of the dressing and toss well to coat. Arrange the onion slices.

3) Pour the rest of the dressing on top. Add walnuts and your choice of crumbled cheese.

Tips:
Try this with avocado and your choice of strawberries, raspberries or blackberries!

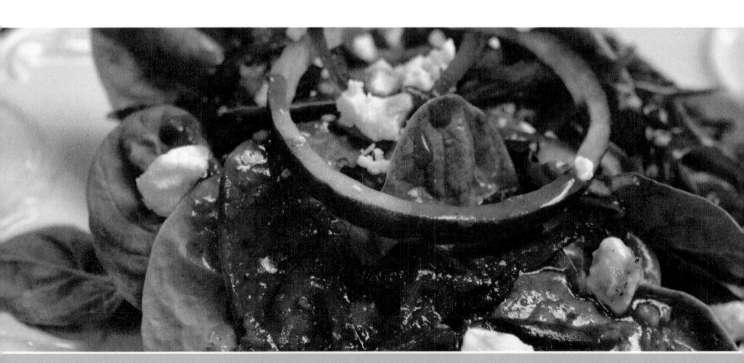

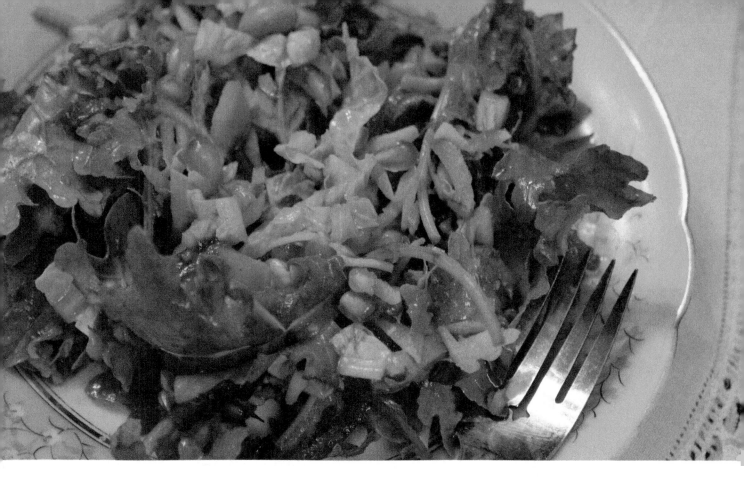

Super Food Salad

Gluten Free
Grain Free
Dairy Free

4 servings

Dressing:
Makes 1 cup

- ½ cup fresh squeezed orange juice
- ½ cup raspberries
- ¼ cup organic green tea, brewed
- 3 Tablespoons extra-virgin olive oil
- 1 Tablespoon raw honey
- 6-8 drops liquid stevia
- ½ teaspoon cinnamon

Salad:

- 6 cups fresh kale, chopped
- 1 cup Napa cabbage, thinly sliced
- ½ cup beet, shredded
- ½ cup organic carrot, shredded
- ½ cup red or orange bell pepper, diced
- ½ cup organic edamame, frozen OR ripe avocado, diced
- ½ cup pomegranate arils OR blueberries

Directions:

1) Blend all dressing ingredients in a blender and blend on high speed for approximately 30 seconds until thoroughly mixed.

2) In a large salad bowl, combine the kale, cabbage, beet, carrot, bell pepper, your choice of edamame or avocado and your choice of pomegranate arils or blueberries. Toss to combine. Pour the dressing on the salad and toss well.

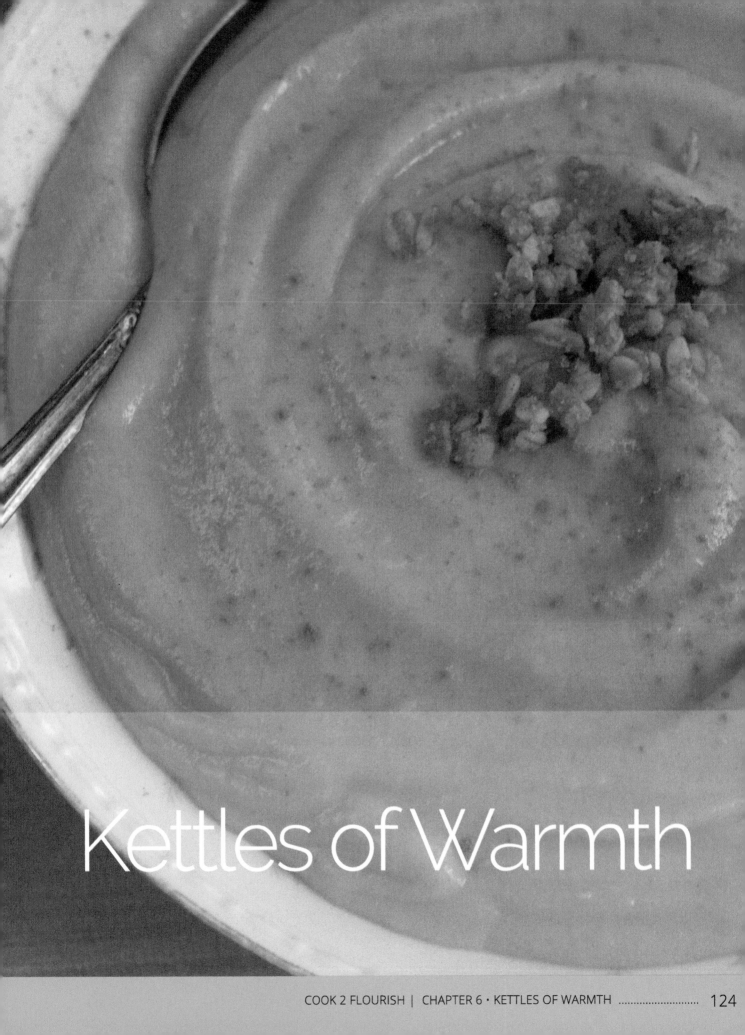

Kettles of Warmth

Butternut Curry Soup

4 servings

- ⅔ cup organic carrots
- 2 cups butternut squash, cubed (9 ounces)
- 1 cup onion, chopped
- 4 garlic cloves
- 1 Tablespoon grapeseed oil
- ½ teaspoon cinnamon
- ½ teaspoon curry powder
- ½ teaspoon coconut aminos
- ⅛ teaspoon ground ginger
- ¾ cup unsweetened coconut milk
- ¾ cup unsweetened almond milk

Directions:

1) In a 9x13x2 inch glass baking dish, cut the carrots and the butternut squash into ½ inch chunks. Add in the onion and garlic cloves. Drizzle with grapeseed oil and toss to coat. Bake in preheated 350 degree oven for 35-45 minutes, stirring once during baking.

2) Remove from oven and pour the roasted vegetables into a high speed blender along with the cinnamon, curry powder, coconut aminos, ginger and milk. Blend until smooth for 30-40 seconds. (Tip: Keep a firm hand on the lid since the contents are hot).

3) Pour soup into a saucepan and heat on medium-low until warm and ready to serve.

How to build Souper Soup

	BROTH	STOCK	CREAM
Start with base:	Organic if store bought. Broth from Crock-Pot® roast, baked chicken or roasted turkey.	Prepared from boiling beef, chicken or turkey bones and vegetables, then strained to keep the broth.	Use the cauliflower cream base on page 141.

Add vegetables:	**Raw vegetables**
	Butternut squash, organic carrots, cabbage, organic celery, organic frozen corn, frozen peas, frozen green beans, garlic, onion, organic potatoes, sweet potatoes, or zucchini.
	Roasted vegetables
	Brussels sprouts, garlic, green beans, bell pepper, mushrooms, parsnip, organic potatoes, squash, turnips.

(If adding onions and celery, sauté in grapeseed oil or broth first before adding other vegetables).

Add Protein:	Cooked Beef, cooked Chicken, cooked Turkey or organic Tofu. Beans, garbanzo beans, organic edamame or lentils.
Add Spices:	Dried spices (taste first then add sea salt last).
Add Thickener:	Tomato sauce, leftover mashed potatoes, Tomato paste (requires water to be added). Vegetable puree (sautéed onions and celery, blended to be thickened) pumpkin or butternut squash puree.
Add-In Options:	Cooked brown rice, cooked quinoa, Jovial® 100% organic Einkorn whole grain pasta, or cooked spaghetti squash 'noodles.'
Last Additions:	Fresh herbs, kale, Swiss chard, spinach, fresh tomatoes. Additional water or broth.
Toppings:	Avocado slices, goat cheese, fresh parsley, fresh organic cilantro, roasted garbanzo beans, parmesan cheese or pesto.

No Waste Chicken and Chicken Broth

- 1 organic chicken, completely thawed
- Nature's Sunshine® sea salt
- Ground black pepper
- Dried whole rosemary
- Garlic powder
- Hungarian paprika

- Dried parsley flakes
- Dash cayenne pepper, optional
- 1-1 ½ cups filtered water

- 1 sharp paring knife
- 1 9x13x2 inch (or larger) glass baking dish
- 1 medium pot with filtered water

Directions:

1) Place chicken in baking dish.

2) Begin by cutting up the chicken in pieces. Remove the legs first, and then the thighs, then the tip of the wing, then cut the wing with a chunk of breast meat included. Then divide the back from the breast. Divide the breasts and remove the bone.

3) Remove as much skin as possible off each piece as you cut up the chicken. Place the skin, fat, bone and wing tip in the pot to boil. (You may add 2 cups vegetable peelings, ½ teaspoon sea salt, and 1 teaspoon lemon juice for flavoring and nutritional benefits.)

4) Remove the giblet bag from the chicken. Place all the giblets in the pot except the neck. Place the neck in the baking dish.

5) Arrange the chicken pieces in the baking dish so they are not overlapping.

6) Season the chicken pieces generously with the spices listed above.

7) Pour 1 ½ cups of water into the baking dish (not directly on the chicken pieces, it will wash the spices away).

8) Place the chicken in preheated 350 degree oven uncovered for 1-1 ½ hours. (On Sunday we double the water so the chicken is nearly covered. It is moist, crunchy on top and ready when we get home from church 2 hours later.)

9) Season the giblets and skin in the pot with sea salt, pepper and garlic. Pour enough water into the pot until the skin is covered with water by 2 inches. Put a lid on the pan and boil for 30-45 minutes.

10) When the boiling pot is done, remove from heat and let it cool. Then pour only the broth into glass jars and refrigerate. It will keep one week. Discard the chicken skin.

11) Remove the chicken from the oven and serve immediately. After dinner, ladle out the broth into a glass jar and place in the refrigerator. It will keep one week.

Uses: Use broth instead of oil to sauté vegetables, sauté green beans, to make soup, to reheat leftovers, or to cook eggs. Use broth to boil rice, rice pilaf, quinoa, beans, or pasta. Tip: Washed organic vegetable peelings and carrot tops can be added to the boiling pot.

How to make Veggie Broth

Makes 5 cups

- 4-5 cups filtered water
- 1 organic carrot
- ⅓ onion, sliced
- 2 garlic cloves
- 2 Swiss chard stems
- 1-2 cups Brussels sprouts ends and trimmings

- 1 Tablespoon dried parsley
- 2 fresh sage stems, optional
- 4 bay leaves
- Dash cayenne pepper
- 1-2 teaspoons Nature's Sunshine® sea salt
- ½ Tablespoon brown rice miso
- 1 Tablespoon fresh squeezed lemon juice

Directions:

1) In a soup pot combine all the ingredients listed. Cover with a lid and bring to a boil then simmer on medium-low for 1 to 2 hours.

2) Remove from heat and let it cool down, then pour only the broth into glass jars and refrigerate. It will keep one week. Discard the vegetables.

Tip: When making a salad or preparing foods using washed organic vegetables, remember to keep the ends of the vegetables for broth. Place all of your trimmings, ends, roots, stems, leaves and extras in a BPA free Ziploc® style freezer bag. Then, when it is full or you are making chicken broth, add some or all of the vegetables to this broth. It is nutritious, affordable and flavorful!

Keep:

- Beet greens, tops and root trimmings
- Broccoli leaves, stems and trimmings
- Cauliflower leaves, stems and trimmings
- Swiss chard leaves and trimmings
- Celery leaves, root and trimmings

- Brussels sprouts trimmings
- Cabbage leaves and trimmings
- Kale trimmings
- Garlic cloves
- Fresh herbs

- Spinach trimmings
- Onion trimmings
- Carrot trimmings

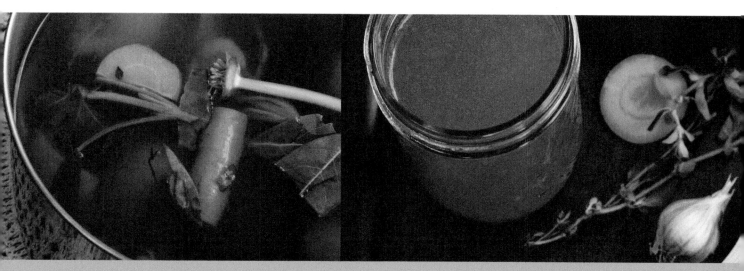

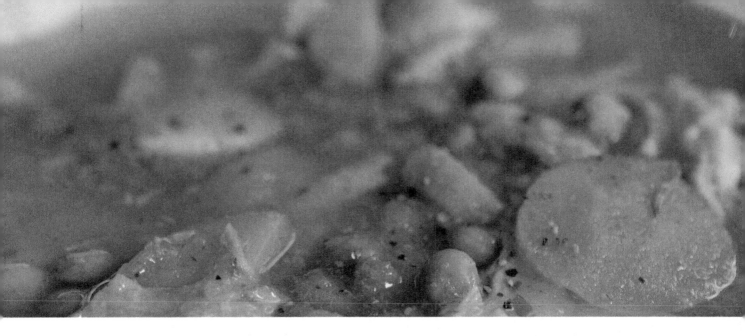

Chicken Soup

4 servings

- 1 garlic clove, minced
- 1 large onion, chopped
- 3 organic celery ribs with leaves, chopped
- 3 cups of chicken broth
- 2-3 large organic carrots, sliced
- Dash ground black pepper
- Dash cayenne pepper
- ½ teaspoon dried parsley
- ½ teaspoon garlic powder

- 1 medium organic potato, with skin, diced, optional
- ½ cup garlic spud Caul-it-Tatoes (mashed potatoes), optional (page 211)
- 1 sprig fresh thyme, optional
- ½ Tablespoon our chicken seasoning OR favorite seasoning (page 238)
- ¼ teaspoon Nature's Sunshine® sea salt
- 1 ½-2 cups cooked chicken breast, cut up into bite size pieces
- ½ cup frozen peas, optional

Directions:

1) Place garlic, onion, celery and broth into a 2 quart saucepan and sauté over medium heat for 5 minutes, or until the onion is translucent.

2) Remove 1/3 of the broth and as much of the vegetables as possible. Place in a blender or food processor and blend until smooth. Approximately 15 seconds. Pour back into the soup pot. (Tip: if using a blender, keep a firm hand on the lid since the contents are hot).

3) Add the carrots and the potatoes (if desired). Stir in the Caul-it-Tatoes (if desired).

4) Add the spices, chicken and the peas (if desired).

5) Let simmer for 15 minutes or until carrots are cooked but not mushy.

6) Ladle the soup into bowls and serve immediately.

By omitting the Caul-it-Tatoes this soup is dairy free as well.

Vegetable Soup

Gluten Free
Grain Free
Dairy Free

4-5 servings

- ½ cup broth, beef OR chicken
- 3 garlic cloves, minced
- 1 large onion, diced
- 2 organic celery ribs with leaves, chopped
- 4 cups broth, beef OR chicken
- 2-3 large organic carrots, sliced
- 1 leek, sliced, optional
- 1 ½ cups green cabbage, chopped
- Dash ground black pepper

- ¼ teaspoon Nature's Sunshine® sea salt
- 1 (14.5 ounce) can Muir Glen® organic fire roasted tomatoes OR whole tomatoes
- Avocado slices, for serving
- 4 cups total of vegetables:
    - organic potatoes, roasted turnips, roasted Brussels sprouts, roasted parsnips, kale, frozen peas, frozen green beans OR mushrooms

Directions:

1) Pour the broth into a large soup pot and sauté garlic, onion and celery over medium heat for 5 minutes, or until the onion is translucent.

2) Add the broth, carrots, leek (if desired), cabbage, your choice of vegetables and seasonings. Let simmer for 15 minutes or until carrots are cooked but not mushy.

3) Add the tomatoes last so they are not overcooked.

4) Ladle the soup into bowls and garnish with avocado slices.

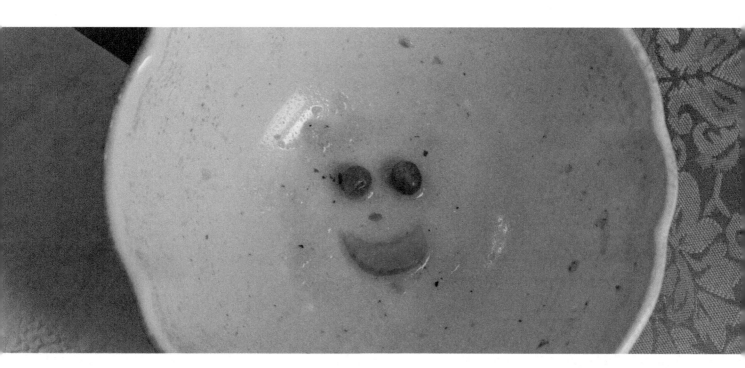

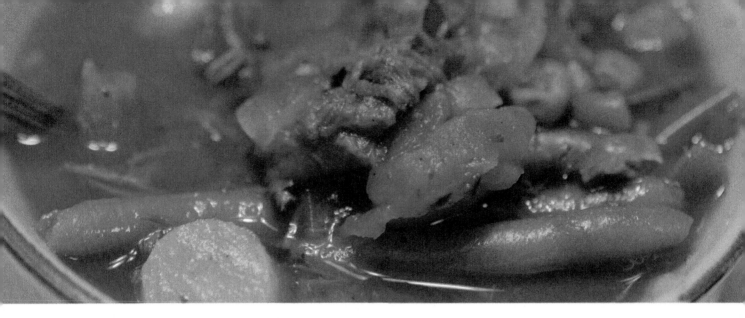

Beef Stew

6-8 servings

- 2 Tablespoons grapeseed oil
- 1 (2 pound) organic lean grass fed beef OR venison roast
- ½ cup filtered water
- 1 large onion, diced
- Ground black pepper, to taste
- 1-2 teaspoons Nature's Sunshine® sea salt
- 3 cups filtered water
- 2 cups organic potatoes, with peeling, cubed
- 2 cups organic carrots, sliced
- 1 ½ cups filtered water

- 1 ½ teaspoons garlic powder
- 1 teaspoon dried whole rosemary, crushed
- 1 teaspoon dried oregano
- 2 teaspoons Italian seasoning
- 2 bay leaves, whole
- 1 (6-ounce) tomato paste
- 1 (14.5-ounce) can Muir Glen® Organic fire roasted tomatoes
- 1 ½ cups frozen peas
- 1 cup frozen green beans, broken into 1 inch pieces
- 1 ½ cups vegetables: mushrooms, zucchini, bell pepper, squash, beans, etc.

Directions:

1) Drizzle oil into a large soup pot and brown the roast for 4 minutes on each side, adding ½ cup water as needed.

2) Add onion, pepper, sea salt and 3 cups of water. Cover and simmer on low for 1 to 1 ½ hours until meat is tender.

3) Remove the roast from the pot and turn off the burner. Place the roast on a meat cutting board and trim off the fat and cut into 1-inch cubes. Return the roast to the soup pot.

4) Add the potatoes and carrots and 1 ½ cups of water. Simmer on medium for 8 minutes.

5) Add the garlic powder, rosemary, oregano, Italian seasoning, bay leaves, tomato paste, tomatoes, peas, green beans and your choice of vegetables.

6) Let simmer for 15-25 minutes until vegetables are cooked but not mushy. Add additional water if needed.

7) Remove and discard the bay leaves before serving. Ladle the soup into bowls and serve immediately.

> **Tip:** If using a leftover roast or a Crock-Pot® roast, skip steps 1 and 2 and use beef broth instead of the water.

Chili

· · · · · · · ·

4-6 servings

- Dash Nature's Sunshine® sea salt
- 1 large onion, chopped
- 2 garlic cloves, minced
- ¼ cup filtered water
- ½ teaspoon ground cumin
- 1 teaspoon garlic powder
- 1 Tablespoon chili powder
- 1 (10 ounce) can Rotel® diced tomatoes and green chilies
- ½ - 1 cup fresh red or yellow bell pepper, chopped
- 1 (14.5 ounce) can Muir Glen® Organic petite diced tomatoes fire roasted
- 1 (15 ounce) can organic kidney beans, drained
- 1 (15 ounce) can organic black beans, drained
- 2 (8 ounce) cans tomato sauce, no sugar added

Directions:

1) In a 2 quart sauce pan, brown the meat over medium heat until it is thoroughly cooked. If the meat needs to be drained, do so.

2) Add in the sea salt, onion, garlic and bell pepper. Sauté for about 5 minutes.

3) Add the rest of the ingredients, and put a lid on the pot. Let it come to a boil then decrease to a simmer.

4) Let simmer for 15 minutes or until carrots are cooked but not mushy.

5) Ladle the chili into bowls and serve immediately.

Suggestions: Serve with "Mulegrain" cornbread, faux cornbread, carrot sticks or apple slices. The fire roasted tomatoes give this chili depth and the tomatoes and green chilies make it spicy. It is important to purchase BPA Free canned goods, especially canned tomatoes.

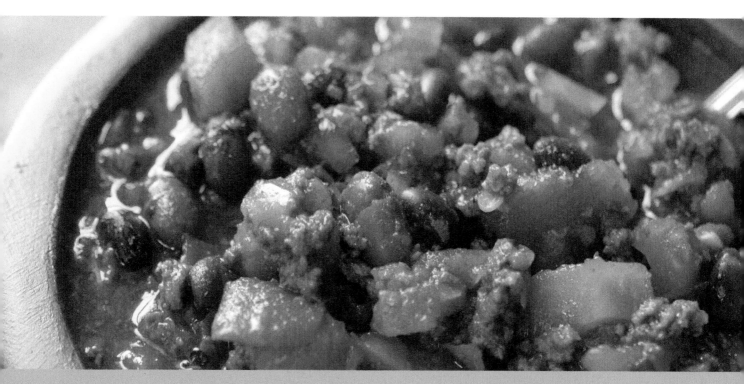

Creamy Herbed Tomato Soup

4 servings

- ⅓ cup red OR yellow bell pepper
- 1 ¼ cup fresh tomatoes
- 8 garlic cloves
- 1 cup onion, chopped
- 1 Tablespoon grapeseed oil
- ¼ teaspoon Nature's Sunshine® sea salt
- ¼ teaspoon ground black pepper

- 6 fresh basil leaves
- 7 fresh oregano leaves
- ½ cup unsweetened almond milk
- ½ cup avocado
- ⅛ teaspoon ground black pepper
- ¼ teaspoon garlic powder
- ½ teaspoon Nature's Sunshine® sea salt

Directions:

1) Combine the bell pepper, fresh tomatoes (if using), garlic and onion in a 9x9x2 inch glass baking dish and toss with the oil, sea salt and pepper.

2) Bake in preheated 350 degree oven for 25-30 minutes.

3) Remove the roasted vegetables from oven and place in a high speed blender along with the basil, oregano, milk, avocado, pepper, garlic and sea salt. Blend until smooth for 30-40 seconds. Keep a firm hand on the lid since the contents are hot. Clean the sides of the blender once or twice if needed, then blend again.

4) Pour soup into a saucepan and let simmer on medium-low until hot.

5) Ladle the soup into bowls and serve immediately.

Suggestion: If you do not have fresh tomatoes, you could substitute Muir Glen® organic fire roasted tomatoes by placing in the blender with the other ingredients.

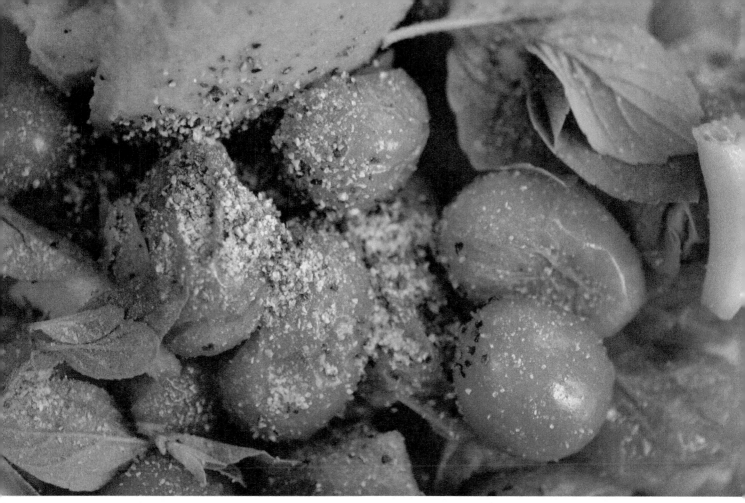

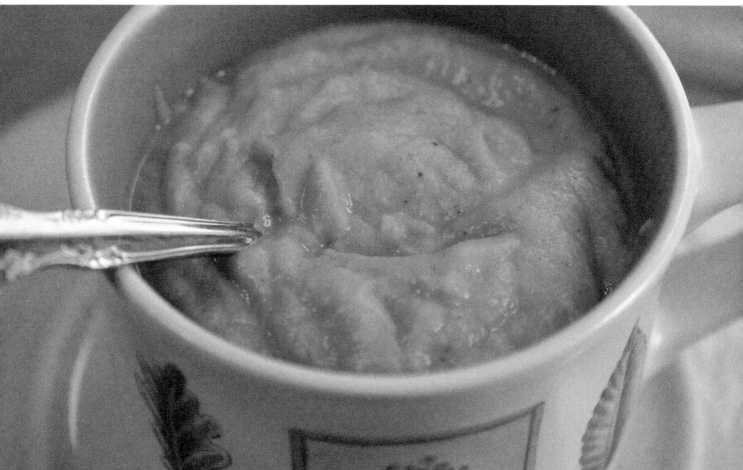

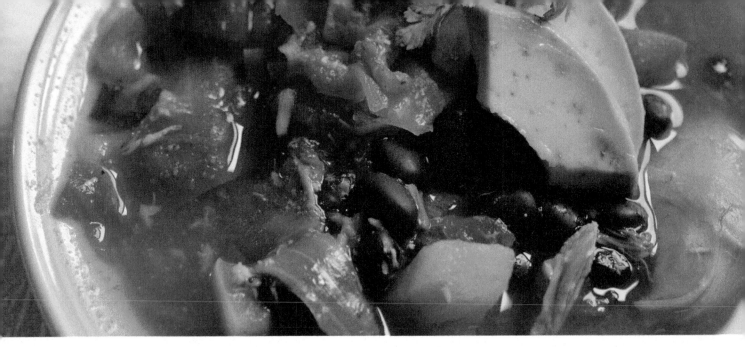

Fiesta Fajita Soup

4 servings

- 1 medium onion, chopped
- ½ medium red or yellow bell pepper, chopped
- ½ teaspoon extra-virgin coconut oil
- 2 teaspoons smoked paprika
- 2 teaspoons ground cumin
- ½ Tablespoon garlic powder
- Dash cayenne pepper
- 3 cups chicken broth
- ½ (15 ounce) can black beans, drained and rinsed
- ½ teaspoon Nature's Sunshine® sea salt
- 1 (14.5 ounce) can Muir Glen® fire roasted tomatoes
- 1 ½ cups chicken fajita leftovers OR cooked chicken
- ½ teaspoon ground turmeric
- 2 Tablespoons fresh organic cilantro, minced
- ⅓ cup avocado, diced

Directions:

1) Sauté the onion and bell pepper in coconut oil in a 2 quart saucepan over medium heat for 7-10 minutes.

2) Add to the saucepan the tomatoes, broth, your choice of chicken, black beans, paprika, cumin, garlic powder, sea salt, cayenne pepper, turmeric and cilantro. Cover and bring to a boil then reduce heat to simmer.

3) Garnish with diced avocado and serve OR if you want a creamier soup, remove 1 cup of the soup broth from the saucepan (no chicken or vegetables). Place in a blender or food processor with the diced avocado and blend until smooth. Approximately 15 seconds. Pour back into the soup pot and heat through. (Tip: if using a blender, keep a firm hand on the lid since the contents are hot). Ladle into soup bowls and serve hot.

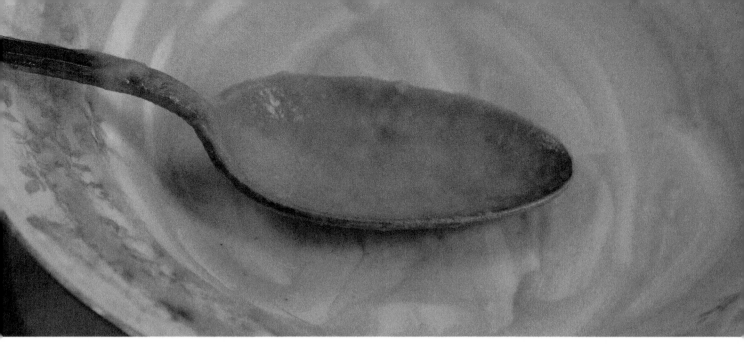

Sunshine Soup

4 servings

- **2 cups butternut squash (9 ounces)**
- **1 medium onion, chopped**
- **1 cup organic carrots, sliced**
- **3 garlic cloves**
- **1 Tablespoon extra-virgin coconut oil**

- **½ teaspoon Nature's Sunshine® sea salt**
- **¼ teaspoon ground black pepper**
- **1 teaspoon fresh sage, chopped**
- **3 cups chicken broth, divided**

Directions:

1) Peel and cut the butternut squash into 1 inch chunks. Place the squash in a 9x9x2 inch glass baking dish with the onion, carrots and garlic.

2) Toss with the oil, sea salt, pepper and sage.

3) Bake in preheated 350 degree oven for 25-35 minutes or until soft and tender.

4) Place the vegetables in a high speed blender with 1 ½ cups of broth and blend 40 seconds until smooth. Keep a firm hand on the lid since the contents are hot. Pour into a 2 quart saucepan.

5) Pour the remaining 1 ½ cups of broth into the blender and blend on high for 15 seconds to clean the pitcher. Then pour into the saucepan and stir well.

6) Simmer on medium-low until hot. Ladle the soup into bowls and serve immediately.

Tip: To make a butternut soup, omit the onion and carrot and use 4 cups (18 ounces) of butternut squash and use only 1 garlic clove. Follow the rest of the recipe as described.

Compassion Soup

4-6 servings

Veggie broth:
- **6 cups filtered water**
- **⅓ cup onion**
- **1 organic carrot**
- **2 garlic cloves**
- **3-4 cups vegetable trimmings**
- **4 bay leaves**
- **2 fresh sage OR thyme stems, optional**
- **1 Tablespoon dried parsley**
- **Dash cayenne pepper**
- **1 teaspoon Nature's Sunshine® sea salt**
- **½ Tablespoon brown rice miso**
- **1 Tablespoon fresh squeezed lemon juice**

Directions:

1) Bring all the ingredients to a boil in a 2 quart saucepan over medium heat. Then lower the heat and simmer for 1-2 hours.

Tip: You could simmer the vegetable trimmings in a Crock-Pot® all night long on low.

2) Then strain the broth and set aside. Discard the vegetable trimmings.

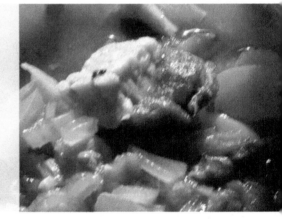

Friendship is priceless, and even the simple gift of soup can encourage a friend on the mend. Simple acts of kindness are the best; never underestimate the potential you have to bless someone. God has given us each unique gifts and this soup is one way that I got to use mine.

Roasted Tempeh

- **1 (8 ounce) package gluten free tempeh**
- **1 cup garbanzo beans, drained and rinsed**
- **2 garlic cloves, minced**
- **½ Tablespoon avocado oil OR grapeseed oil**
- **½ teaspoon Nature's Sunshine® sea salt**
- **¼ teaspoon fennel seeds**
- **¼ teaspoon ground black pepper**

Directions:

1) Cut the tempeh into ¼ inch cubes.

2) Combine the tempeh, garbanzo beans, garlic and your choice of oil, sea salt, fennel and pepper in a small mixing bowl then toss to coat.

3) On an unbleached parchment paper lined stainless steel baking sheet, bake the tempeh and garbanzo beans in preheated 375 degree oven for 25 minutes until they have a golden brown crust. Roasting the tempeh causes it to take on a milder flavor and will season the soup well.

Soup base

4-6 servings

- **6 cups veggie broth, divided**
- **1 cup onion, diced**
- **4 Swiss chard stems and leaves, diced**
- **2 cups organic carrots, diced**
- **1 cup organic celery, diced**
- **½ - 1 Tablespoon Bragg® liquid aminos**
- **½ Tablespoon brown rice miso**
- **2-3 Tablespoons tomato paste**
- **⅓ cup sundried tomatoes in extra-virgin olive oil, drained and chopped**
- **1 teaspoon extra-virgin coconut oil OR grapeseed oil**

Directions:

1) In the 2 quart saucepan, simmer the onion, Swiss chard, carrots, and celery in your choice of oil with 1 cup of the veggie broth until the onions are translucent and the veggies are tender.

2) Scoop out 1 cup of the simmering veggies and puree them with 1 more cup of veggie broth in a high speed blender. Keep a firm hand on the lid as the contents are hot. Add back into the 2 quart saucepan.

3) Pour the remaining balance of the veggie broth into the 2 quart saucepan along with the liquid aminos, miso, tomato paste, and sundried tomatoes.

4) Add in the roasted tempeh and garbanzo beans. Stir to combine. Let all the veggie goodness simmer for 20-30 minutes until hot. Ladle the soup into bowls and savor or you may like a more smooth and creamy soup. If so, pour all the soup contents into a high speed blender and blend until smooth. Keep a firm hand on the lid as the contents are hot.

Tip: If you already have veggie broth or chicken broth on hand this will cause the soup to come together much quicker. This is much easier than it looks! Use your favorite veggies and greens if you don't care for the ones listed above; it's all about variety, color and taste!

Suggestion: Substitute cooked chicken breast or turkey for the tempeh which will eliminate the roasting step. The garbanzo beans do not have to be roasted; they can just be added to the soup in step 3. Substitute your favorite beans for the garbanzo beans.

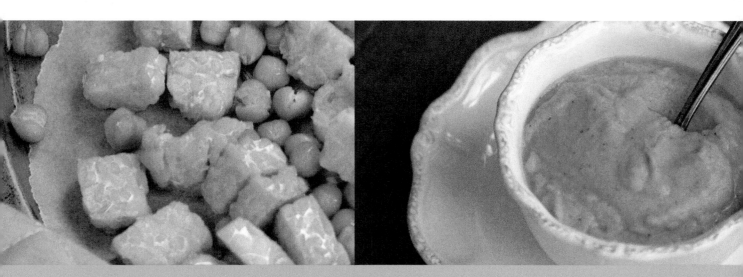

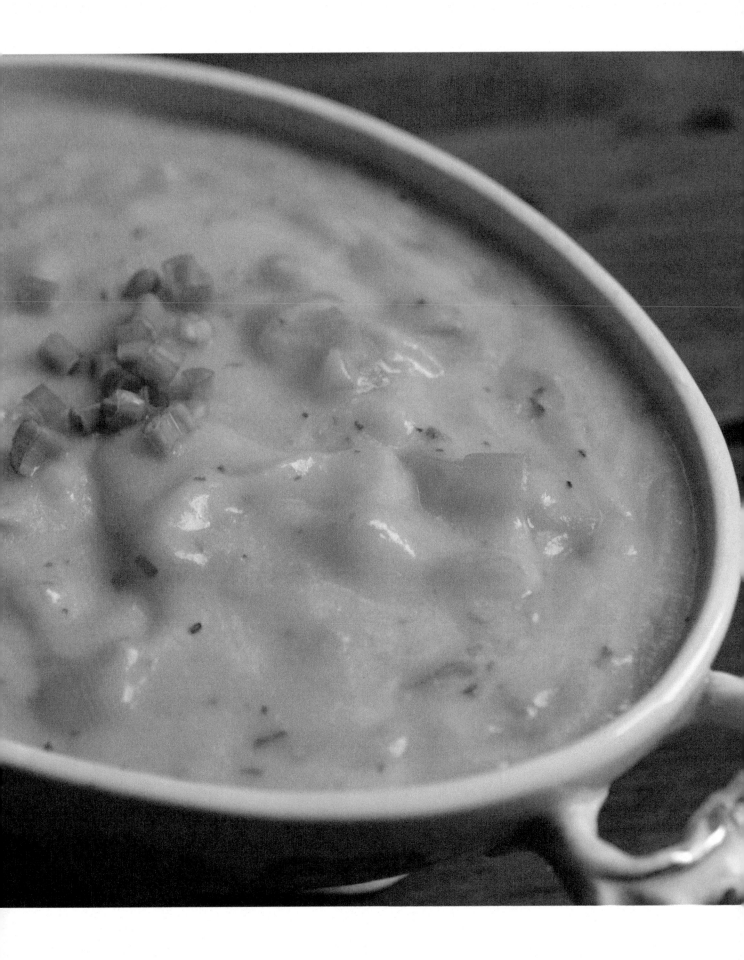

Creamy Comfort Soup

4-6 servings

- 8 cups cauliflower florets
- ½ cup unsweetened almond milk

Veggies:
- 2 garlic cloves, minced
- 1 ½ cups onion, diced
- 1 cup organic celery ribs with leaves, diced
- ½ cup organic carrots, diced
- ½ cup organic potato, with skin, diced, optional
- ¼ cup of chicken broth OR filtered water
- ½ cup (3 ounces) uncured organic turkey bacon, diced

Roux:
- 2 Tablespoons organic butter, no substitutes
- 1 Tablespoon garbanzo bean flour
- 1 Tablespoon arrowroot powder
- 1 ½ cups unsweetened almond milk
- ½ teaspoon Nature's Sunshine® sea salt
- ½ teaspoon ground black pepper
- 1 teaspoon dried parsley
- Chives, for garnish

Directions:

1) Bring water to a boil in a 2 quart saucepan with steamer basket in it. Steam the cauliflower over boiling water for 10-12 minutes. Drain the water.

2) Place garlic, onion, celery, carrots, potato (if desired, it's not needed) and broth into a 2 quart saucepan and sauté over medium heat for 5 minutes, or until the onion is translucent. Add in the turkey bacon and sauté for 2 minutes.

3) Remove the sautéed veggies from the saucepan and place in a bowl to keep warm. Add the butter to the pan. Once melted, add in the flour and the arrowroot and stir with a whisk to make a roux. Pour in the almond milk and continue stirring. Add the veggies back into the saucepan. Cover and simmer on low.

4) Puree the cauliflower and almond milk in a high speed blender on High. Keep a firm hand on the lid since the contents are hot. Clean the sides of the blender once or twice if needed, then blend again. This makes 4 cups. Pour into the saucepan with the veggies.

5) Let simmer for 15 minutes on low.

6) Ladle the soup into bowls and serve immediately. Garnish with chives (if desired).

Suggestion: This recipe could easily make clam chowder. If you have a leftover baked potato or a ½ cup roasted potatoes, use in this recipe. Quite honestly, the first time we made this soup, we forgot to put the potato in it!
And it was delicious! That's why potato is optional in the above recipe. Chicken pot pie: add chicken, peas, green beans and the buttery spelt pie crust! (page 287)

Suggestions on what to eat:

- Echinacea tea and/or tea with lemon and raw honey and ginger

- Vitamin C rich foods: kiwi, strawberries, red bell peppers, raspberries,

  cauliflower, broccoli

- Herbs: oregano, parsley, thyme

- Spices (can help break up mucus): cayenne pepper, ginger, garlic, cinnamon

- Tip: if you can't tolerate the cayenne easily,

  try adding it to guacamole page 243 or salsa page 249

- Greens: Smoothies such as Strawberry Kiwi Smoothie page 13

- Homemade chicken broth and soup with veggies page 130

- Lots of onions and garlic- fajitas page 150

  with cayenne added to your guacamole page 243

- Lighter proteins to give the body an easier time breaking down

  the food so it can spend more energy attacking the congestion.

- WATER! Aim for ½ your body weight in ounces, up to 100 ounces.

1. What to Avoid

(these instigate mucus production and quell the immune system):

- Wheat, white flour products, glutinous grains and products
- Sugar and sugary foods (except fruit)
- Dairy- milk and cheese, especially. Organic plain yogurt in moderation.
- Fried foods/ canola oil/ hydrogenated oils in foods

....

2. While you are recuperating:

- Epsom salt foot soak with ½ cup baking soda, ½ cup plain Epsom salt, and ½ Tablespoon ground ginger
- James 5:14-15a NIV "Is anyone among you sick?
  Let them call the elders of the church to pray over them and anoint them with oil in the name of the Lord. And the prayer offered in faith will make the sick person well; the Lord will raise them up…"

....

3. Nature's Sunshine products to have in your herbal cabinet
(www.n2flourish.mynsp.com)

- Silver Shield® liquid
- Solstic® Immune drink
- Essential Shield essential oil blend
- VS-C®
- If you are "backed-up" or constipated: LBS-II® to get things moving again; it is important to have the elimination channels open.

For educational use only. These suggestions are not to take the place of a doctor or medical attention. The reader assumes full responsibility for his/her health; this information is not intended to diagnose, treat, prevent or cure disease.

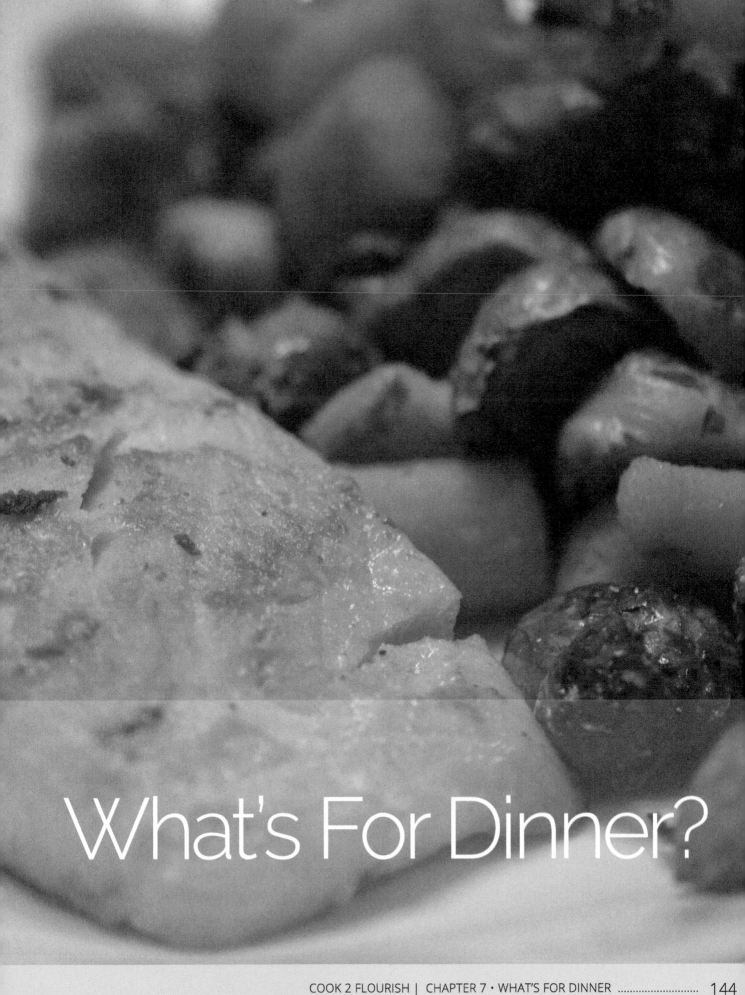

What's For Dinner?

Perfectly Delicious Salmon

4 servings

- **4 (4 ounce) pieces of fresh OR completely thawed salmon**
- **Nature's Sunshine® sea salt, to taste**
- **Ground black pepper, to taste**
- **1 teaspoon garlic powder, divided**
- **1 teaspoon of grapeseed oil**
- **2 Tablespoons of filtered water, divided**

Directions:

1) Season each piece with salt and pepper to taste and ¼ teaspoon of garlic powder.

2) Drizzle the oil over the salmon pieces then turn seasoned side down in a stainless steel skillet. Turn the burner on to medium heat and pour 1 Tablespoon of water into the pan.

3) Cover the salmon with a lid or a piece of unbleached parchment paper.

4) Cook for 5 minutes then turn the salmon over.

5) Add 1 more Tablespoon of water.

6) Cook for approximately 3-5 more minutes. Make sure it is done. Remove from the heat. Keep covered and serve immediately.

My husband and I were at a business convention and we went to the restaurant in the hotel, Ruth's Chris® and ordered salmon. We remarked to the waiter how good it was and he said "it's simply seasoned with salt and pepper".

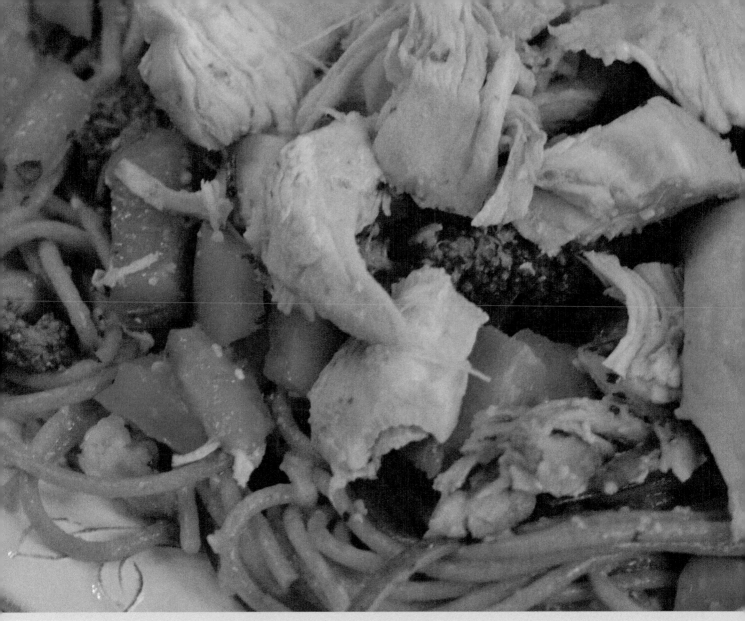

Chicken Vegetable Pasta

Chicken Salad

Makes 2½ cups

- 1½ cups cooked chicken breast, diced
- 1 cup organic celery, diced
- ⅓ cup Vegenaise®
- 1 Tablespoon sesame seeds
- 1 teaspoon onion flakes
- ½ teaspoon Nature's Sunshine® sea salt
- ½ teaspoon garlic powder

- Dash ground black pepper
- Dash cayenne pepper

Directions:

1) Combine all ingredients in a mixing bowl and stir well.

Tip: This is tasty in a lettuce wrap, on a salad, or as a dip for veggies and crackers.

Chicken Vegetable Pasta

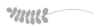

4 Servings

- 4 boneless skinless chicken breast halves
- 1 teaspoon paprika
- 1 teaspoon garlic powder
- 1 teaspoon dried rosemary
- ¼ teaspoon Nature's Sunshine® sea salt
- Dash ground black pepper
- Dash cayenne pepper
- 1 cup chicken broth, divided

- ½ box (6 ounces) Jovial® 100% Organic Einkorn whole wheat pasta
- 1 medium zucchini
- 1 ½ cups broccoli florets
- 3 medium carrots, thinly sliced
- 2 large garlic cloves, minced
- ½ onion, chopped
- 1½ teaspoons garlic rosemary flavored extra-virgin olive oil
- ½ cup black olives, sliced
- 2 Tablespoons grated parmesan cheese

Directions:

1) Place chicken breasts in a stainless steel skillet over medium heat and season with paprika, garlic powder, rosemary, sea salt, pepper, and cayenne. Add ½ cup chicken broth and cover with a lid. Cook chicken for 15 minutes or until juices run clear.

2) Reduce heat to warm. Using a sharp knife, cut up the chicken into 1 inch pieces.

3) Prepare pasta according to package directions. Reserve hot water for blanching the zucchini noodles. Using a vegetable spiralizer, spiralize the zucchini. When finished spiralizing, the zucchini will be one very long noodle. Make one or two cuts to make the noodles shorter. Approximately 6 to 8 inches in length.

4) Add ¼ cup broth to the skillet and turn heat up to medium. Add the broccoli and carrots to the chicken in the skillet. Cover and cook 5 to 8 minutes until al dente.

5) Pour chicken, broccoli and carrots into a bowl and cover to keep warm.

6) To the skillet add ¼ cup remaining chicken broth. Over medium heat add minced garlic and onion and sauté with pan drippings for 2 minutes. Add the prepared pasta.

7) Blanche the zucchini noodles into the hot water from the pasta for 30 seconds. Then add to the garlic, onion and pasta. Sauté together for 2 to 3 minutes to get warm.

8) Pour the chicken, broccoli and carrots back into the skillet. Add the garlic rosemary flavored extra-virgin olive oil, olives and the parmesan cheese. Toss to coat and serve immediately.

Suggestions: For gluten-free, use Jovial® Gluten Free 100% organic brown rice pasta, spiralized zucchini or spaghetti squash. For dairy-free, omit the parmesan.

Tip: If you don't have garlic rosemary flavored extra-virgin olive oil, substitute extra-virgin olive oil. If you have leftover chicken you can make this dish in a flash.

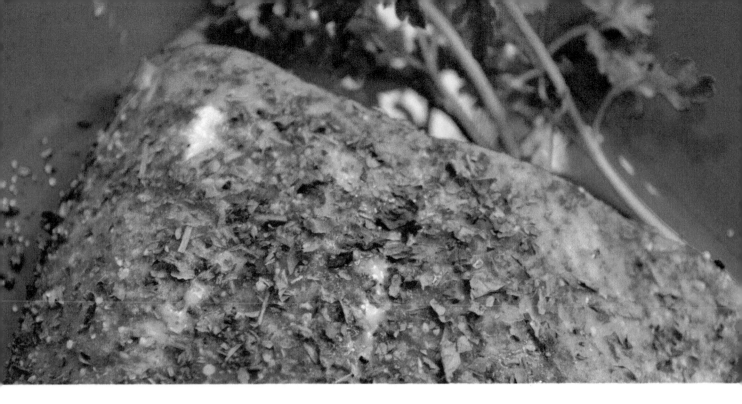

Blackened Wild Salmon

Gluten Free
Grain Free
Dairy Free

6 servings

- 1-2 pound filet of salmon, cut into 2 inch strips lengthwise
- 1 Tablespoon blackened fish seasoning, to taste
- 1 Tablespoon garlic powder
- 1 Tablespoon grapeseed oil
- 2-3 Tablespoons filtered water

Directions:

1) In a stainless steel skillet, season each piece with blackened fish seasoning and garlic powder. Drizzle the oil over the salmon pieces. Turn the pieces over so seasoned side is down.

2) Turn the burner on to medium heat and cover the salmon with a lid or a piece of unbleached parchment paper. Cook for 5 minutes.

3) If the fish has the skin on it, peel off the skin then turn the salmon over.

4) Pour water into the pan. The water will sizzle and coat the fish with the seasoning in the bottom of the pan. Cover.

5) Cook for approximately 3-5 more minutes. Make sure it is done. Remove from the heat. Keep covered and serve immediately.

To bake in the oven, season each piece with blackened fish seasoning and garlic powder. Drizzle the oil over the salmon pieces. Turn the pieces over so seasoned side is down in a glass baking dish. Bake in preheated 350 degree oven for 12-18 minutes depending on the thickness of the fish. Remove from the oven; if the fish has the skin on it, peel it off, and place seasoning side up on the plate. Serve immediately.

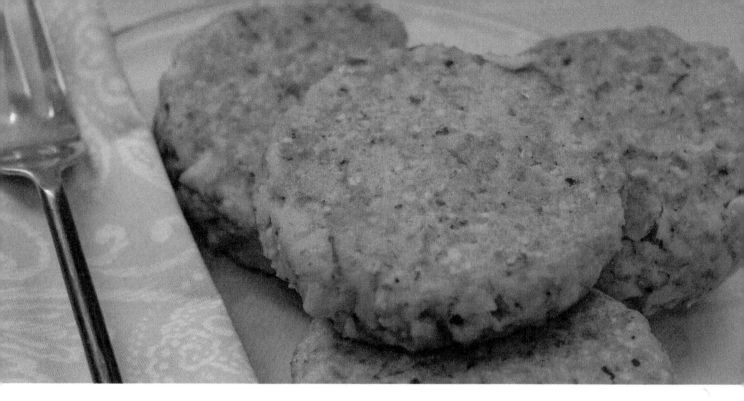

Salmon Patties

4 servings

- 1 (14.75 ounce) can wild salmon
- 2 Tablespoons liquid from the canned salmon
  (omit if using cooked quinoa)
- ¼ cup organic gluten free old fashioned rolled oats
  OR cooked whole white quinoa

- 1 organic egg
- Dash Nature's Sunshine® sea salt, to taste
- Dash ground black pepper, to taste
- ½ teaspoon dried parsley
- 1 Tablespoon dried onion flakes
- 2 teaspoons grapeseed oil

Directions:

1) Open the salmon and measure out the liquid and pour into a mixing bowl. Drain out the rest of the liquid into the sink. Empty the salmon into the bowl and remove the skin as best possible. Wash your hands.

2) To the mixing bowl, add your choice of rolled oats or cooked quinoa, egg, sea salt, pepper, parsley, and onion. Mix well with a fork to combine.

3) Preheat a stainless steel skillet on medium low with 1 teaspoon of the grapeseed oil.

4) Form the salmon into four patties about ½ inch thick and 3 inches wide. Place the patties in the skillet and turn heat up to medium. Cook for 7 minutes.

5) Drizzle the remaining grapeseed oil over the top of the four patties then turn them over in the pan. Cook for 5-7 more minutes or until golden brown. Serve immediately.

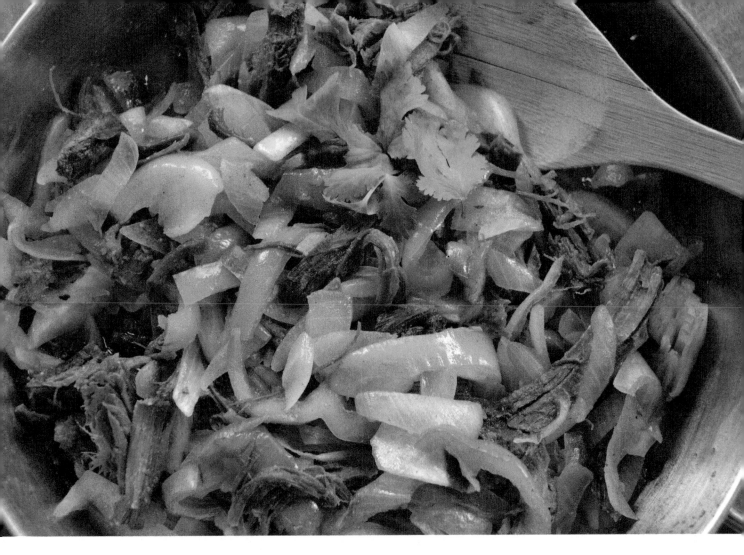

Leftover Venison Fajitas

4 servings

- **2 large sweet onions, sliced**
- **1 organic bell pepper, sliced**
- **3 garlic cloves, minced**
- **⅓ cup chicken broth**
- **1 Tablespoon extra-virgin coconut oil**
- **2 Tablespoons taco spice, to taste**
- **2 ½-3 cups leftover venison roast**
- **Fresh organic cilantro, for garnish**

Directions:

1) In a stainless steel skillet over medium heat combine the onions, bell pepper, garlic and chicken broth. Simmer stirring often until onions are translucent.

2) Add the coconut oil, taco spice, and venison roast. Stir to combine.

3) Cover with a lid and reduce the heat to medium low. Once the venison is warm it is ready to serve. Garnish with cilantro (if desired).

Suggestion: Serve with shredded carrots and lettuce, salsa, guacamole, black beans or brown rice.
Tip: Leftover chicken or turkey can be used for this same recipe.

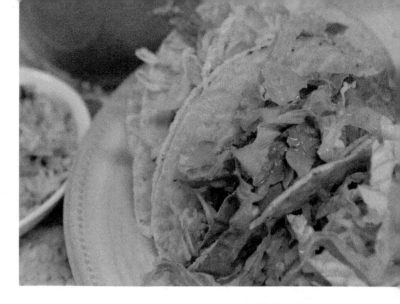

Spicy Chicken

• 3 organic chicken breasts
• Dash cayenne pepper
• ¼ teaspoon sea salt
• ½ teaspoon paprika
• ½ teaspoon ground turmeric
• ½ teaspoon garlic powder
• ½ teaspoon cumin
• ½ cup water

Directions:

1) Place the chicken breasts in a medium stainless steel skillet.

2) Combine and mix all spices together. Sprinkle the spices on the chicken.

3) Cook in the skillet on medium heat for10 minutes then turn each piece over and add the water. Cook for an additional 10-20 minutes until juices run clear. Turn the chicken every 10 minutes until caramelized and tender. Reduce heat to simmer to keep warm until ready to serve.

Tip: Use 6-8 chicken tenders and cook for 20 minutes, or until juices run clear. This will be quicker than using chicken breasts. Serve with Ensalada Mexicana salad (page 121), Southwest Chicken Enchiladas (page185) or Chicken Fajitas (page 150).

I cook 4 whole large chicken breasts at one time (you could also use frozen chicken breast or chicken tenderloins). Once cooked, I divide the chicken into two meals for 6 servings and one smaller snack meal for 3 servings. Then I put the chicken in BPA free Ziploc® style baggies and freeze them in the freezer, labeled "Spicy Chicken large" and "Spicy Chicken small". Then it is easy to reach in the freezer and quickly add vegetables to make a nutritious meal in a few minutes.

Tacos

4-6 servings

• 1 ½ pounds organic lean grass fed ground beef, buffalo OR venison
• ½ cup onion, chopped
• 1 garlic clove, minced
• 1-2 Tablespoons taco seasoning, to taste
• ¼ cup filtered water
• 3 ½ - 4 cups Crock-Pot® cooked black beans
  OR 2 (15 ounce) cans organic black beans, drained
• ½ teaspoon ground cumin

Directions:

1) In a large stainless steel skillet, brown the meat over medium heat until it is thoroughly cooked. If the meat needs to be drained, do so.

2) Add in the onion, garlic, taco seasoning and water. Sauté for about 5 minutes then put a lid on the pan. Decrease burner to simmer.

3) Move the meat over to one side of the skillet to make room for the beans. Drain any excess liquid. Pour in the black beans and season with cumin. Put the lid on the skillet and simmer until the beans are hot.
Serve immediately.

Suggestion: Serve with sliced Romaine lettuce, shredded carrots, diced bell pepper, salsa, and Spanish rice (page 227) or Mexican pasta (page 209). Make taco shells or serve as taco salad. Leftovers are an easy breakfast or snack in a wrap.

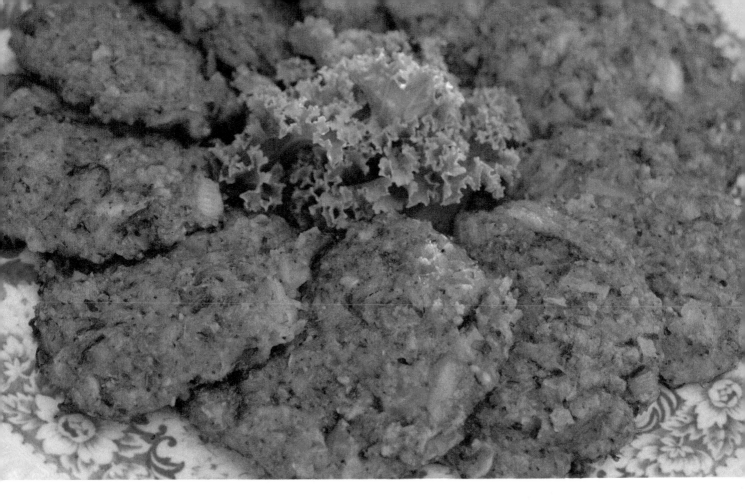

Crab Cakes

4 servings

- 1 teaspoon grapeseed oil
- 1 garlic clove, minced
- ¼ cup onion, very finely chopped
- ¼ cup organic celery rib with leaves,
  very finely chopped
- ¼ cup organic orange bell pepper, very finely chopped
- ½ teaspoon Nature's Sunshine® sea salt
- ¼ teaspoon ground black pepper
- ½ teaspoon Dijon mustard
- 1 teaspoon old bay seasoning
- 1 teaspoon dried parsley
  OR 1 Tablespoon fresh parsley, finely chopped
- ¼ cup Vegenaise®
- 1 ½ cups loosely packed crab meat
- ⅓ cup Crunchmaster® cracker crumbs (15 crackers)
- 1 large organic egg
- 3 Tablespoons organic oat bran OR almond flour

Directions:

1) Sauté the garlic, onion, celery, bell pepper, sea salt and pepper together with the grapeseed oil in a stainless steel skillet for approximately 7 minutes or until onions are translucent.

2) Pour the contents of the skillet into a large mixing bowl and add the rest of the ingredients in the order given. Mix well to combine.

3) Shape into round patties about ½ inch thick and 3 inches in diameter.

4) Bake crab cakes in preheated 350 degree oven for 20-27 minutes on a stainless steel baking sheet lined with unbleached parchment paper.

For a gluten free option, use almond flour in place of the organic oat bran.

Almond Crusted Cod

2 servings

- 1 teaspoon grapeseed oil
- 2 (4 ounce) pieces of fresh
  or completely thawed cod
- Nature's Sunshine® sea salt, to taste

- Ground black pepper, to taste
- ½ teaspoon garlic powder, divided
- ½ teaspoon fresh lemon thyme leaves, divided
- ¼ cup whole almonds, chopped, divided

Directions:

1) Place cod pieces in a glass baking dish, lightly greased with grapeseed oil.

2) Season each piece with salt and pepper to taste.

3) Season each piece with ¼ teaspoon of garlic powder and ¼ teaspoon lemon thyme.

4) Sprinkle 2 Tablespoons of almonds on each piece.

5) Bake in preheated oven at 350 degrees for approximately 12 minutes. If the cut of fish is thick, it may need 15 to 17 minutes. The fish should flake and be cooked all the way through. Remove from oven. Serve immediately.

> **Almond Crusted Salmon:** Use recipe above and drizzle 1 Tablespoon of peach flavor balsamic vinegar over the fish then season with salt, pepper, garlic, thyme and almonds.

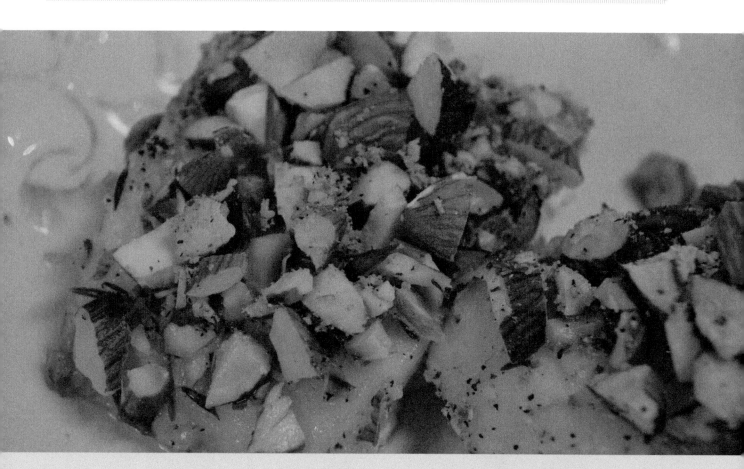

Homemade Pizza

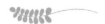

Makes two 12 inch pizza crusts

- 2 teaspoons active dry yeast
- 1 teaspoon raw honey
- ¼ cup warm water (110-115 degrees)
- 3 cups whole sprouted spelt flour, sifted
- ½ teaspoon Nature's Sunshine® sea salt
- ½ cup + 2 Tablespoons warm water (110-115 degrees)
- 1 Tablespoon grapeseed oil OR extra-virgin coconut oil, for rising

Directions for dough:

1) Combine yeast, honey, and ¼ cup warm water in a small bowl; stir to combine. Let stand for 5 minutes, mixture should double in size.

2) In a food processor with dough blade, add the flour and salt. Pour in the yeast mixture. Use the remaining warm water to rinse all yeast mixture from the small bowl; pour into the food processor. Process on "dough" until dough forms a ball and cleans the sides of the processor bowl.

3) Dough should be a little sticky and elastic. Remove from mixer and knead briefly in a bowl drizzled with grapeseed oil or coconut oil. Form dough into a ball, cover and let rise in a warm place for 30 minutes. (Begin fixing the toppings).

4) Punch dough down. Divide into 2 pieces. Roll each piece out about ¼ inch thick on round baking sheets coated with non-stick grapeseed oil spray. Let rise in a warm place for 15-30 minutes. (Continue to let rise while making the sauce and finishing the toppings). Roll out dough onto a stainless steel pizza pan lightly coated with non-stick grapeseed oil spray or on a stoneware pizza pan.

Directions for toppings:

5) 1 pound ground sirloin seasoned with ½ teaspoon fennel seeds, ½ teaspoon onion flakes & ½ teaspoon Italian seasoning. Once cooked, you could add 4 or 5 cleaned, chopped fresh mushrooms, if desired.

6) Red or green bell peppers, diced

7) Black olives, sliced

8) Mushrooms, sliced

9) Grated white cheeses – Monterey Jack OR Mozzarella

Directions for sauce:

10) 2 (8 ounce) cans of tomato sauce

11) ½ teaspoon onion flakes

12) Pinch dried basil

13) ½ teaspoon Italian seasoning mix

Directions for baking:

14) Preheat oven to 425 degrees. Bake the pizza crust with sauce only for about 10 minutes on 400 degrees. Then top with desired toppings and bake at 400 degrees for 20-25 minutes until crust is golden and cheese is melted.

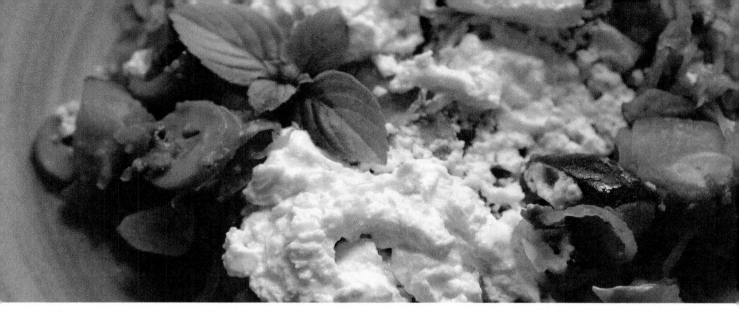

Flavorful Spaghetti Squash Lasagna

2 servings

- ½ cup organic lean grass fed ground beef, buffalo OR venison, fully cooked and drained
- 2 cups spaghetti squash noodles, cooked
- ½ medium onion, chopped
- ¼ red bell pepper, diced
- 2 Tablespoons roasted garlic cloves, chopped
- 3 artichoke hearts in water, drained and chopped
- 4 sundried tomatoes in extra-virgin olive oil, drained and chopped

- ½ cup black olives, sliced
- 1 teaspoon Italian seasoning
- 1 teaspoon fennel seeds
- ½ Tablespoon fresh basil leaves, sliced
- 2 Tablespoons tomato paste
- Dash Nature's Sunshine® sea salt
- Dash ground black pepper
- ¼ cup goat cheese, crumbled

Directions:

1) In a large stainless steel skillet, fully cook and drain the meat.

2) Steam the spaghetti squash in a steamer basket in pot with boiling water. Remove squash from heat and let cool slightly. Scoop out the noodles with a fork into a 9x13x2 inch glass baking dish sprayed with grapeseed oil non-stick spray and set aside.

3) Sauté the onion and bell pepper with the meat for 5 minutes. Remove from heat and drain the liquid. Add to the spaghetti squash.

4) Add in the garlic, artichoke hearts, sundried tomatoes, olives, Italian seasoning, fennel seeds, basil leaves and tomato paste. Stir to combine.

5) Season with sea salt and pepper to taste.

6) Sprinkle goat cheese on top.

7) Bake in a preheated 350 degree oven for 15-20 minutes until heated through.

Tip: To steam the spaghetti squash, cut in half and then cut each half into 4 pieces. Cover and steam in a steamer basket over boiling water for 15 minutes or until noodles are easily scooped out. Use spaghetti squash noodles in place of pasta.

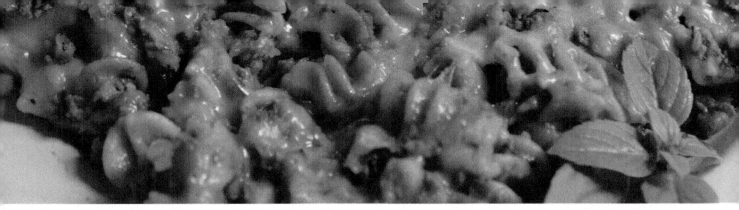

Italian Garden Casserole

6 servings

- ½ -¾ pound organic lean grass fed ground beef, buffalo OR venison, fully cooked and drained
- ½ package (6 ounces) Jovial® 100% organic Einkorn whole wheat penne pasta
- 1 medium-large onion, chopped
- 1 garlic clove
- 1 red bell pepper, sliced
- 8 medium-large button mushrooms, cut in half, optional

- ½ medium zucchini, sliced
- 1 cup black olives, sliced
- 8 pieces of uncured turkey pepperoni, diced
- 1- 1 ½ Tablespoons Italian seasoning
- 1 Tablespoon fennel seeds
- 1 (14.5 ounce) can Muir Glen® diced tomatoes with basil & garlic
- 8-15 ounces tomato sauce, no sugar added
- 1 cup shredded cheese: mozzarella, Monterey jack OR fresh mozzarella cheese

Directions:

1) In a large stainless steel skillet, fully cook and drain the meat.

2) Cook pasta according to package directions. Drain. Set aside.

3) In a food processor, pulse to finely chop the onion and garlic clove. Add to the skillet.

4) Pulse the bell pepper slices to finely chop them. Add to the skillet.

5) Pulse the mushroom halves, (if using) to finely chop them. Add to the skillet.

6) Pulse the zucchini to finely chop. Add to skillet.

7) Sauté the vegetables with the meat for 5 minutes. Remove from heat and drain the liquid.

8) In a large bowl, add the olives, pepperoni, Italian seasoning, fennel seeds, cooked pasta and the meat-vegetable mixture.

9) In the food processor, pulse the diced tomatoes until fine. Pour the tomatoes and the desired amount of tomato sauce into the large bowl and stir to combine.

10) Pour into a large 9x13x2 inch glass baking dish sprayed with grapeseed oil non-stick spray and sprinkle with cheese.

11) Bake in a preheated 350 degree oven for 30 minutes until cheese is melted and dish is bubbly.

> **Tip:** Turn this into Chicken Mostaccioli by replacing the ground meat with 3 cups cooked chicken breast, diced. Traditional lasagna has ricotta cheese in it. If you want that type of dish, add an 8 ounce carton organic full fat cottage cheese, rinsed and drained to step 8.
>
> Why Muir Glen® tomatoes? This brand of tomatoes is sweeter than store canned tomatoes which are usually sour and more acidic. Muir Glen® tomatoes are also in BPA free cans, which is especially important when it comes to tomatoes!

Spicy Crusted Fish Filets

4 servings

- **4 (6 ounce) wild fish filets**
- **¾ cup almond flour OR organic cornmeal**
- **3 teaspoons paprika**
- **½ teaspoon dried thyme**
- **½ teaspoon Nature's Sunshine® sea salt**
- **¼ teaspoon ground black pepper**
- **1 teaspoon garlic powder**

- **1½ teaspoons dried parsley**
- **Dash cayenne pepper, optional**
- **1 Tablespoons grated parmesan cheese, optional**
- **1 ½ Tablespoons organic Greek yogurt, plain whole milk OR 1 organic egg, beaten**
- **2 Tablespoons grapeseed oil**

Directions:

1) Take a piece of fish and pat it dry with paper towels. If it was frozen pat out excess water.

2) In a dish with a 1 inch rim, place your choice of the almond flour or the cornmeal. Add in the spices and parmesan cheese (if desired).

3) In another dish with a 1 inch rim, place your choice of the yogurt or the egg.

4) Coat both sides of the fish with the yogurt and then with the spice mixture.

5) Cook in a stainless steel skillet with grapeseed oil on medium heat until golden brown. Approximately 4 to 5 minutes on each side, depending on the thickness of the fish or bake in preheated oven at 350 degrees for 12-17 minutes depending on the thickness of the fish.

> **Tip:** Coat the fish with a thin layer of yogurt with a basting brush. A good white fish is wild cod, wild halibut or fresh caught fish from a lake or stream. Catfish, however, is not best because it feeds on the toxic debris on the bottom floor of the lake. Tilapia is most always farm raised and can be full of toxins, often coming from China.

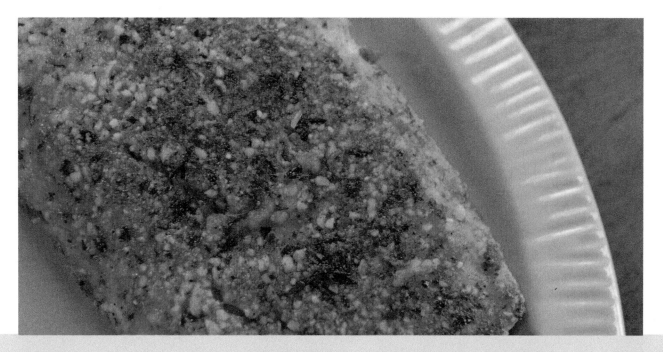

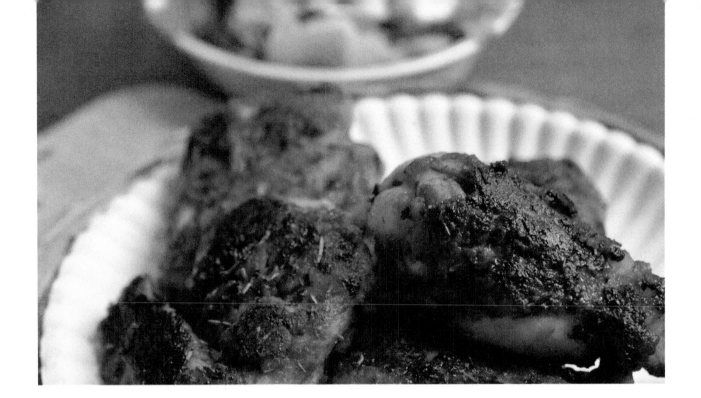

Parmesan Crusted Chicken

4-6 servings

- ¼ cup grated parmesan cheese
- 3 teaspoons Hungarian paprika
- ½ teaspoon dried thyme
- ½ teaspoon whole rosemary, crushed
- 1 teaspoon garlic powder

- ½ teaspoon Nature's Sunshine® sea salt
- 1½ teaspoons dried parsley
- 2 Tablespoons organic Greek yogurt, plain whole milk
- 4 boneless skinless chicken breasts OR 6-8 chicken thighs/legs
- 1-2 Tablespoons grapeseed oil

Directions:

1) In a dish with a 1 inch rim, place the parmesan cheese, paprika, thyme, rosemary, sea salt, garlic powder and parsley.

2) In another dish with a 1 inch rim, place the yogurt.

3) Coat both sides of the chicken with a thin layer of the yogurt using a basting brush and then press the chicken into the spice mixture.

4) Cook in a stainless steel skillet with grapeseed oil on medium heat until cooked through. Approximately 15 minutes for chicken breasts or 20-25 minutes for thighs/legs. Cover the pan with a lid for the first 7-10 minutes then finish the cooking time without a lid. Bake in preheated oven in a glass or stoneware baking dish coated with grapeseed oil at 350 degrees for 25-40 minutes depending on the thickness of the chicken.

. . . .

Breaded chicken breast (similar to round processed chicken patties) omit grapeseed oil. Spray 15x10x1 inch stoneware bar baking pan with non-stick grapeseed oil spray. Add ¼ cup coconut flour and ½ teaspoon more sea salt to the spice mixture above. Bake in preheated 350 degree oven for 25-40 minutes depending on the thickness of the chicken. Dry breaded outside and juicy on the inside. Leftovers can be sliced and placed on a salad or made into a sandwich.

Italian Chicken Fingers

4 servings

- ½ cup Crunchmaster® cracker crumbs
- ¼ teaspoon Nature's Sunshine® sea salt
- ½ teaspoon garlic powder
- 1 teaspoon Italian seasoning
- Dash cayenne pepper
- 2 whole organic chicken breasts
- 2 Tablespoons organic Greek yogurt, plain whole milk
- 1 teaspoon filtered water

Directions:

1) Preheat the oven to 350 degrees and line a stainless steel baking sheet with parchment paper.

2) Using a food processor, process approximately 22 crackers until they are fine crumbs.

3) In a small glass dish with two-inch sides, place the cracker crumbs, sea salt, garlic powder, Italian seasoning and cayenne pepper.

4) In another small glass dish with a two-inch side, place the two whole chicken breasts. Cut each chicken breast into six long strips. Wash hands and work area thoroughly with soap and hot water.

5) Add the yogurt and the water to the chicken pieces and stir with a fork to combine and coat the chicken.

6) Line up the chicken dish next to the cracker crumb dish next to the unbleached parchment paper lined baking sheet.

7) Take a chicken strip and coat one side in the cracker crumbs. Place crumb side up on the parchment paper. Repeat until all pieces are coated on one side. Bake in 350 degree oven for 17-20 minutes. Serve immediately.

Suggestion: If you want both sides coated, double the crackers and seasonings and add 5 minutes to the baking time. Turn the pieces over half way through the baking time.

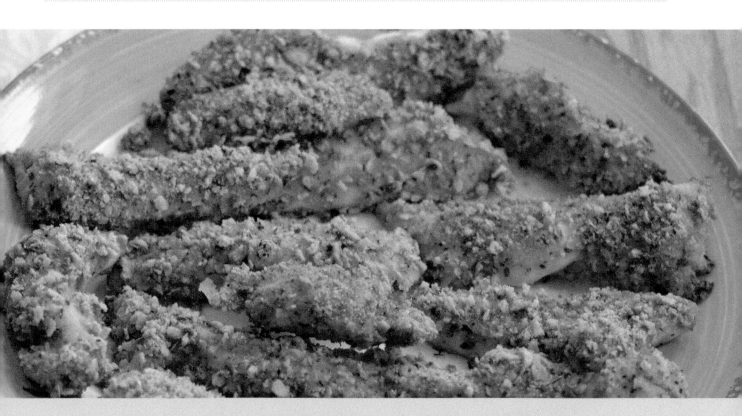

Simmer Down Dinner (Chicken or Roast)

5-8 servings

- 1 fresh organic chicken, cut up and skinned OR 1 (3-4 pound roast)
- ⅓ cup filtered water
- 1 Tablespoon chicken seasoning (page 241)
- 2 cups onion, chopped
- 1 ½ cups mushrooms, cleaned and sliced
- 1 cup fresh kale
- ¼ cup fresh basil, chopped

- ½ Tablespoon fresh oregano, chopped
- 2 garlic cloves, minced
- 1 (14.5 ounce) can Muir Glen® Fire Roasted Tomatoes
- 2 Tablespoons tomato paste
- ½ Tablespoon chicken seasoning (page 241)
- ¼ teaspoon Nature's Sunshine® sea salt
- ¼ teaspoon ground black pepper

Directions:

1) Place the chicken in a large stainless steel skillet with the water and chicken seasoning. Cover with a lid. Cook on medium heat for 25 minutes, turning once during cooking.

2) Meanwhile, combine the tomatoes, tomato paste, chicken seasoning, sea salt and pepper. Mix well and set aside.

3) Add to the chicken, the onion, mushrooms, kale, basil, oregano and garlic. Pour the tomato mixture over the veggies and cover with a lid. Cook 25 more minutes on medium.

4) Reduce the heat to medium-low and simmer for 10 minutes. Serve hot.

Crock-Pot® method:
Cover all the ingredients with the lid, set on high setting for 6 hours.

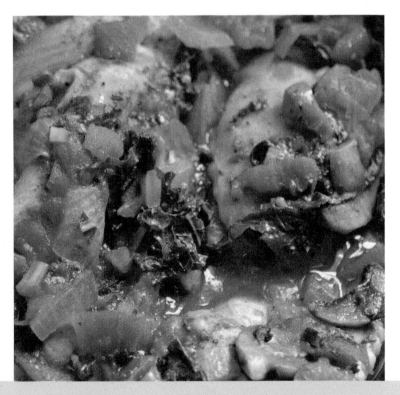

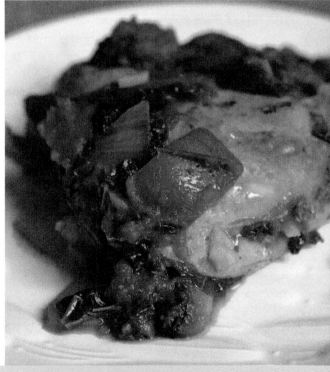

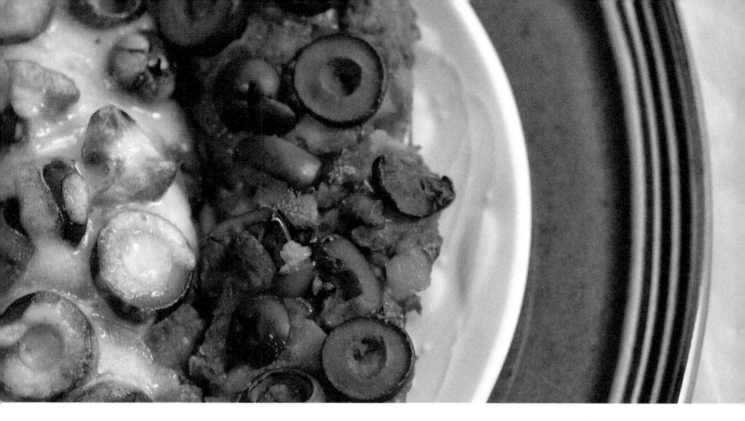

Pizza Boats

. . . .

2 servings

- 1 medium zucchini (approximately 8 inches x 2 inches)
- ½ teaspoon grapeseed oil
- ¼ teaspoon garlic powder
- Pinch Nature's Sunshine® sea salt
- ¼ pound organic lean grass fed ground beef, buffalo OR venison
- ⅓ cup red bell pepper, diced
- ⅓ cup red onion, diced
- 1 teaspoon extra-virgin coconut oil

- ½ teaspoon fennel seeds
- ½ teaspoon Italian seasoning
- Pinch Nature's Sunshine® sea salt
- ⅛ teaspoon garlic powder
- ⅛ teaspoon dried sweet basil
- ⅛ teaspoon ground cumin
- ¼ cup tomato paste
- 3 slices turkey pepperoni, optional
- ¼ cup black olives, sliced
- ¼ cup mozzarella cheese, optional

Directions:

1) Slice the zucchini in half and scoop out the pulp and seeds. Set them aside in a small bowl. Coat the zucchini halves really well with the grapeseed oil. Place in a glass baking dish and season the center with the garlic powder and sea salt. Place in preheated 350 degree oven for 15 minutes.

2) In a medium stainless steel skillet, cook the ground venison until done and crumbly. Drain off any fat. Place venison in a bowl and set aside.

3) To the warm skillet, add the zucchini pulp, bell pepper, onion and coconut oil. Sauté for 3-5 minutes then add the seasonings, tomato paste and cooked venison. Cook for 3 more minutes stirring to mix well.

4) Remove zucchini halves from oven and fill them with a portion of the tomato mixture. Top with the pepperoni, if desired, olives and cheese, if desired, or with your favorite pizza toppings. Bake for 10 minutes until cheese is melted and the pizza boat is hot. Serve immediately.

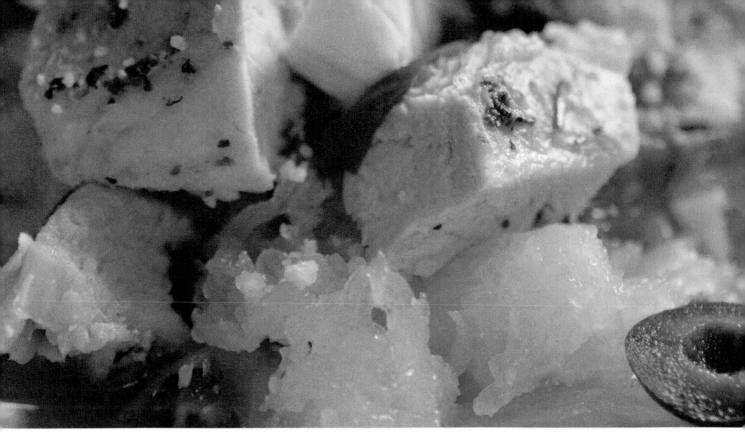

Chicken Pomodoro

Gluten Free
Grain Free

2 servings

- 2 organic chicken breasts
- 4-6 Tablespoons chicken broth
- ½ teaspoon garlic powder
- 1 teaspoon Italian seasoning
- ½ Tablespoon whole rosemary
- Dash Nature's Sunshine® sea salt
- Dash ground black pepper

- 2 cups prepared marinara sauce (see page 183)
- 4 cups spaghetti squash noodles, cooked
- 4 roasted garlic cloves, chopped
- 4 fresh basil leaves, torn
- 10 black olives, sliced
- 4 sundried tomatoes in extra-virgin olive oil, chopped
- 2 (½ inch) slices fresh mozzarella cheese, diced
- 1 Tablespoon grated OR shredded parmesan cheese, optional

Directions:

1) In a medium stainless steel skillet, place the chicken breasts, chicken broth, garlic powder, Italian seasoning, rosemary, sea salt and pepper. Cook over medium heat until thoroughly cooked through. Remove one at a time and slice into chunks. Return the chicken to the pan and add the marinara sauce. Simmer to heat through.

2) Divide the cooked spaghetti squash noodles on to two plates.

3) Add the roasted garlic, the torn basil leaves, olives, sundried tomatoes, fresh mozzarella cheese.
Then pour the hot marinara sauce and chicken over the top.

4) Sprinkle with parmesan cheese (if desired). Serve immediately.

Tip: The spaghetti squash noodles have a tendency to get cold quickly.
You might want to warm your plates in the oven before plating. It would help keep the dish warmer longer while eating it.

COOK 2 FLOURISH | CHAPTER 7 • WHAT'S FOR DINNER 162

Meatballs

Makes 3 dozen

- 1 ½ pounds organic lean grass fed ground beef, buffalo OR venison
- 1 cup total: whole grain bread, organic oat bran, organic gluten free old fashioned rolled oats
- ½ cup shredded cheese: mozzarella OR Monterey jack
- ⅓ cup grated parmesan cheese

- 1 garlic clove, minced
- 3 large organic eggs, beaten
- 1 ½ Tablespoons dried parsley OR ¼ cup fresh parsley
- 1 ½ teaspoons fennel seeds
- 1 ½ teaspoons dried onion flakes
- 1 ½ teaspoons Italian seasoning
- **Dash ground black pepper**

Directions:

1) Place the ground meat in a large bowl.

Select your choice of or a combination of bread crumbs, oat bran and dry rolled oats to equal 1 cup. Pour into the bowl.

2) Add in the shredded cheese of your choice, parmesan cheese, garlic, eggs, parsley, fennel, onion, Italian seasoning and pepper. Mix all the ingredients together with a fork until well combined. Shape into small golf ball size meatballs then place on a stainless steel or stoneware baking sheet with a ½ inch rim (in case of grease spillage or rolling) lined with unbleached parchment paper.

3) Bake in preheated 350 degree oven for 30-40 minutes. Serve immediately.

Tip: *There are enough meatballs for two or three meals. These are even great for a snack with veggies. Let the meatballs cool and stack them in a BPA free Ziploc® style freezer bag and store them in the freezer. Then take out however many you need for your meal or snack.*

Meatball Burgers:

Omit shredded and parmesan cheese. Add ⅓ cup bell pepper and ¼ cup sesame seeds.

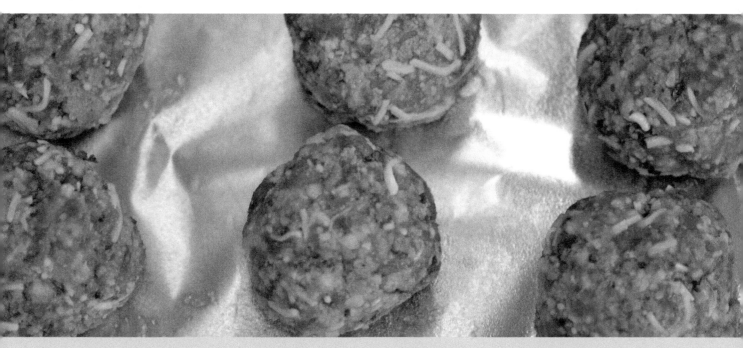

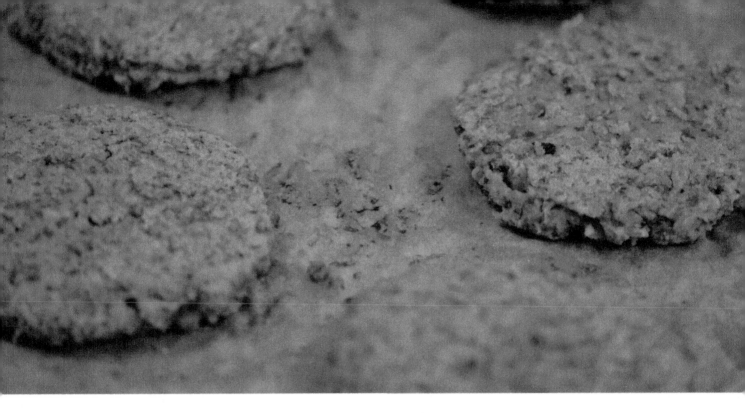

Chic-P Nibbles

Gluten Free
Grain Free
Dairy Free

4 servings

- ½ cup pine nuts OR English walnuts
- 2 cups fresh curly parsley
- 3 garlic cloves
- 1 Tablespoon onion, chopped
- 1 sundried tomato in extra-virgin olive oil

- 2 Tablespoons fresh squeezed lime juice
- 1½ teaspoons ground cumin
- ½ teaspoon Nature's Sunshine® sea salt
- Dash ground black pepper
- 1 (15 ounce) can garbanzo beans, drained and rinsed

Directions:

1) Combine nuts, parsley, garlic, onion, tomato, lime juice, and seasonings in food processor and process 15 seconds until the mixture is fine and smooth.

2) Add the garbanzo beans and pulse approximately 8 to 10 pulses until mixture is combined. It will be slightly chunky.

3) Form into 2 ½ inch patties and place on an unbleached parchment paper lined stainless steel baking sheet. Mixture should make eight patties.

4) Place in a preheated 350 degree oven and bake until golden brown, approximately 30 minutes, turning them once halfway through the baking time.

Suggestion: These are my version of traditional falafel. Serve them with a salad and refrigerate any leftovers. Consume within two days or freeze them individually. Re-heat leftovers or frozen Chic-P Nibbles in the oven.

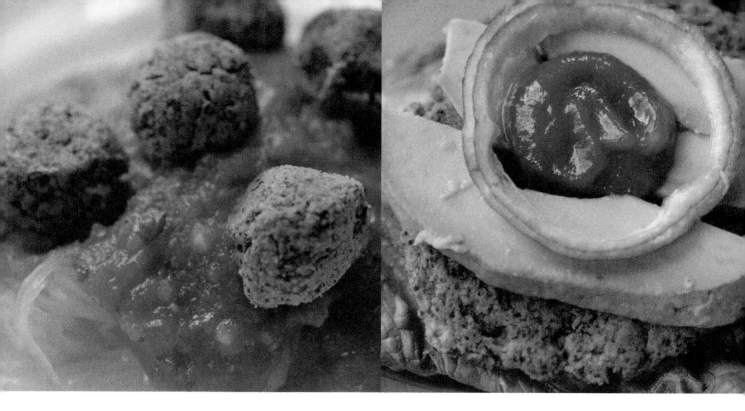

Black Bean Burgers

Makes 4 burgers, 2 servings

- 1 cup black beans (Crock-Pot® prepared page 224)
- ¼ cup almond flour
- 1 Tablespoon onion, chopped
- 1 teaspoon garlic powder
- 1 teaspoon dried parsley

- ½ -1 teaspoon Bragg® liquid aminos, to taste
- ½ Tablespoon ground cumin
- Pinch cayenne pepper
- 2 teaspoons grapeseed oil, divided

Directions:

1) Place the cooled black beans in a food processor along with the almond flour, onion, garlic powder, parsley, liquid aminos, cumin and cayenne pepper.

2) Process until mixture is fine and smooth. Scrape the sides of the bowl once or twice between processing. Form into patties which should stick together and hold their shape.

3) Drizzle 1 teaspoon of the grapeseed oil in an approved Green® non-stick skillet. Add the patties and press them down in the skillet to flatten them then cook on medium heat for approximately 8 minutes. Drizzle the remaining grapeseed oil on top of each patty then turn them over in the skillet and cook for about 8 more minutes. The black bean burgers should be golden brown.

Suggestion: This recipe can also be rolled into marble size meatballs, which makes approximately 25 black bean meatballs. Cook in the skillet as instructed above to brown them then bake in preheated 350 degree oven for 20-30 minutes. Serve with marinara sauce and spaghetti squash.

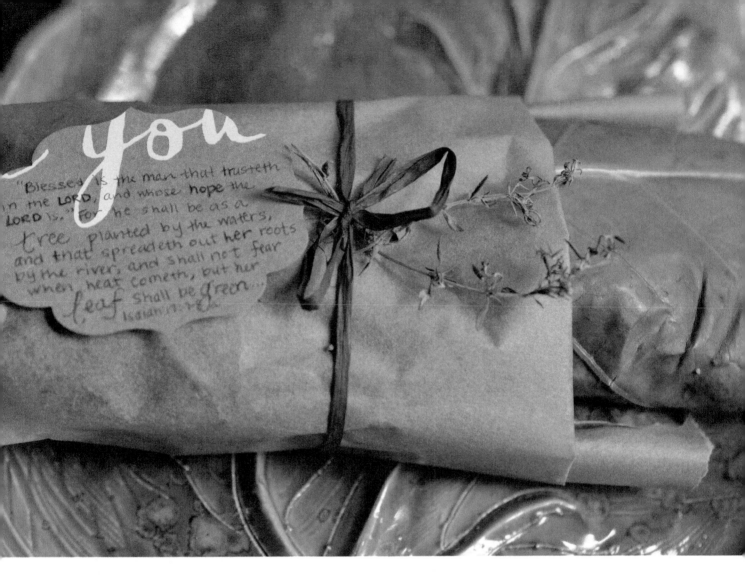

Favorito Burrito

Gluten Free
Grain Free
Dairy Free

1-2 servings

- **2 large collard leaves
  (Swiss Chard or cabbage), washed**
- **½ cup Caul-it-Rice (page 225)**

- **½ - ¾ cup fully cooked chicken**
- **½ - 1 cup cooked OR raw veggies, chopped**
- **¼ ripe avocado, pit removed and peeled, mashed**

Directions:

1) If you have not already cooked your cauliflower rice, simply place the green leaves over the steaming pot for 30 seconds to 1 minute to soften the leaves- do this one at a time. If you have cooked the Caul-it-Rice, simply place water in medium sauce pan and bring to a boil. When it is steaming, place the leaf over the rim of the pan and cover for 30 seconds to 1 minute.

2) Pat the greens with a paper towel to dry the steam and place on a piece of parchment paper. Mash the avocado gently onto the leaves then add the Caul-it-Rice and your choice of veggies.

3) Roll up the leaves like you would roll up a burrito and place in an air tight container or bag to keep fresh or enjoy immediately.

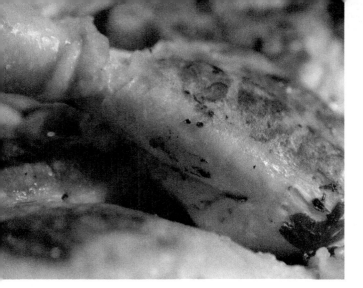

Tea Time Marinade for Chicken or Salmon

Makes ¾ cup

- 1 teaspoon dried thyme
- 1 teaspoon dried basil
- 1 teaspoon garlic powder
- ¼ teaspoon oregano
- 2 garlic cloves, minced
- 1 ½ Tablespoons avocado oil
- ¼ teaspoon whole rosemary, crushed
- 1 Tablespoon dried parsley
- 1 Tablespoon fresh squeezed lemon juice
- 1 teaspoon Nature's Sunshine® sea salt
- ½ teaspoon ground black pepper
- ⅔ cup organic green tea, brewed

Directions:

1) Combine all ingredients and pour over meat and marinade for 1 hour or overnight in the refrigerator. A glass dish or a BPA free Ziploc® style bag works best. Discard marinade.

2) Chicken - Bake, fry in stainless steel skillet with water or grill chicken until completely done and juices run clear.

3) Salmon - Bake, cook in a stainless steel skillet or grill salmon. Don't overcook it. Fish doesn't take very long to cook, 4-5 minutes each side depending on the thickness.

Tender BBQ Roast

6-8 servings

- 1 (4 pound) organic grass fed beef roast OR venison
- 3 garlic cloves, minced
- 2 cups filtered water
- 1 large onion, chopped
- 1 cup tomato sauce
- ¼ cup raw honey
- 2 Tablespoons molasses
- 3 Tablespoons Bragg® liquid aminos
- ¼ cup fresh squeezed lemon juice
- ½ teaspoon Nature's Sunshine® sea salt
- 2 teaspoons arrowroot powder
- 2 teaspoons smoked paprika
- 1 teaspoon chili powder
- 1 teaspoon garlic powder
- 1 teaspoon ground cumin
- ¼ teaspoon cayenne pepper

Directions:

1) In a large Crock-Pot®, place all ingredients except the roast. Stir well to combine.

2) Place the roast in the pot and turn it over to coat with BBQ sauce.

3) Cover and cook on high for 6-8 hours. If possible, turn the roast one or two times during the cooking to coat it with the sauce. If not, do it before serving. Refrigerate any leftovers.

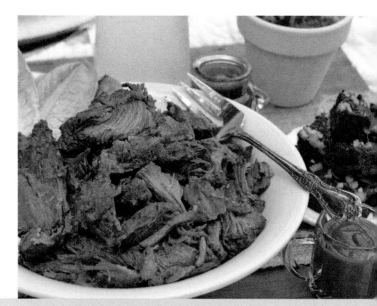

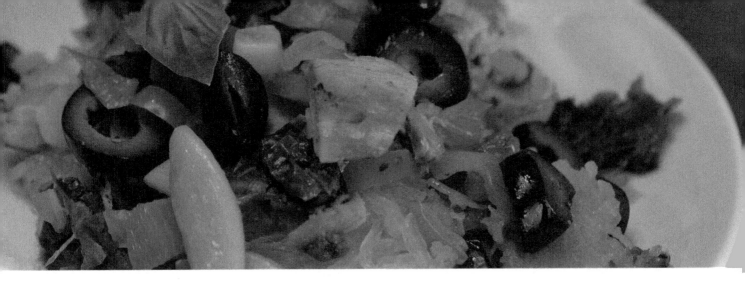

Panzetti

2 servings

- 4 cups steamed spaghetti squash noodles
- 4 roasted garlic cloves, chopped
- ¼ cup roasted onion, chopped
- ¼ cup roasted red pepper, chopped
- 2 cups leftover baked or grilled chicken breast, sliced
- ½ cup black olives, sliced
- 4 sundried tomatoes in extra-virgin olive oil, chopped
- 2 Tablespoons oil from sundried tomatoes
- 2 (½ inch) slices fresh mozzarella cheese, diced
- Fresh basil leaves, for serving

Directions:

1) In a medium stainless steel skillet, place the spaghetti squash noodles over medium heat. Add in the roasted garlic, roasted onion and roasted peppers. Cover with a lid while getting the rest of the ingredients.

2) Add in the chicken, olives, sundried tomatoes and the oil from the sundried tomatoes. Cover with lid and cook for 25 minutes or simmer on low for up to 1 hour. Do not stir.

3) Divide the contents of the pan onto two plates. Top with fresh mozzarella cheese and fresh basil leaves. Serve immediately.

Tip: This is a great dish to make with leftover steamed spaghetti squash, leftover roasted vegetables and leftover chicken breasts. Easy and delicious!

Tortilla Pizza

1 or 2 per person

- **Tomato paste**
- **Rudis® gluten free tortillas, Ezekial 4:9® sprouted whole grain tortillas or brown rice tortillas**
- **Your choice of pizza toppings: onion, bell pepper, black olives, fully cooked and seasoned pizza meat, uncured turkey pepperoni, mozzarella cheese, etc.**

Directions:

1) Spread a layer of tomato paste on each tortilla and place on an unbleached parchment paper lined stainless steel baking sheet. Place in preheated 350 degree oven for 7 minutes then remove from oven and top with your choice of desired toppings. Return to oven for 10-12 minutes until toppings are heated through and cheese is melted.

Butternut Bites (Pizza or Taco)

2-4 servings

- **2 cups butternut squash**
- **½ Tablespoon grapeseed oil**
- **½ teaspoon Nature's Sunshine® sea salt**
- **½ teaspoon ground black pepper**
- **½ teaspoon garlic powder**
- **Tomato paste**

Directions:

1) Peel and cut the butternut squash into ¼ inch slices.
In a mixing bowl combine the squash, oil, sea salt, pepper and garlic powder. Toss to coat.

2) Place in a 9x13x2 inch glass baking dish coated with non-stick grapeseed oil spray.

3) Bake in preheated 350 oven for 25 minutes until the squash is tender, but not over cooked.

4) Remove from oven and spread a thin layer of tomato paste on each slice then top with your choice of cooked and seasoned pizza or taco meat and any toppings you would like. Then bake for 15-20 minutes until the toppings are warmed all the way through, but be careful to not let them burn.

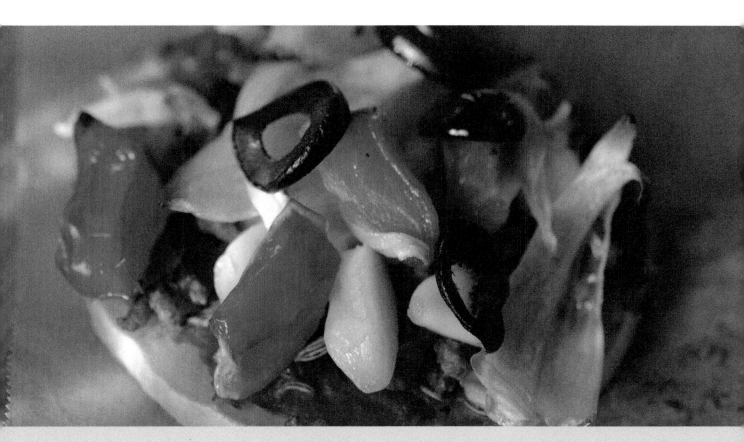

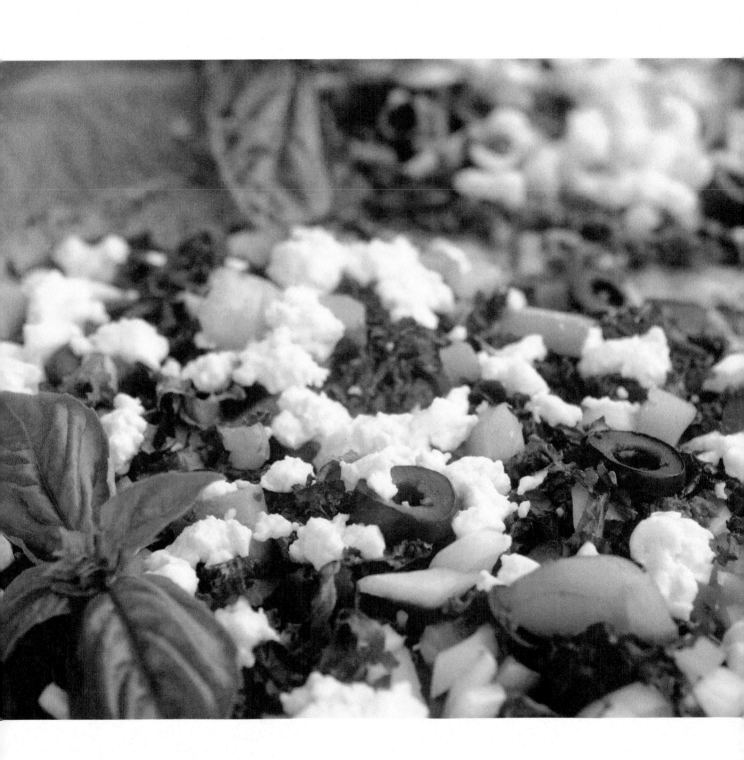

Caul-it-Pizza

Gluten Free
Grain Free

Makes two 12 inch crusts

Dough recipe:
- **4 cups cauliflower, bite size florets (14 ounces)**
- **3 large organic eggs**
- **2 Tablespoons coconut flour**
- **1 teaspoon garlic powder**
- **1 teaspoon Italian herb seasoning**
- **½ teaspoon Nature's Sunshine® sea salt**
- **⅛ teaspoon ground black pepper**
- **¼ cup sundried tomatoes in extra-virgin olive oil, drained**
- **cheese cloth, to drain cauliflower**

Directions for dough:

1) Process the cauliflower florets in a food processor until fine granules that look like snow. Pour the cauliflower granules into the cheese cloth. Gather the four corners of the cheese cloth and gently twist and continue twisting the cauliflower granules to release excess water. Twist and squeeze as much water out as possible! You may drain as much as a ½ cup of water out of the cauliflower. This is very, very important, otherwise the dough will not be able to be picked up and eaten.

2) Place the cauliflower granules back into the blender along with the eggs, coconut flour, garlic powder, Italian herb seasoning, sea salt and pepper. Drain the sundried tomatoes. Add in only the tomatoes. Process 40 seconds or until well combined.

3) Pour the batter onto a parchment paper lined stoneware pizza pan or stainless steel baking sheet.

4) Bake in preheated 400 degree oven for 15-20 minutes until golden brown. Some thin areas may brown first or burn a little. Remove from oven and test to see if the dough is able to hold together when lifted up off edge of the parchment paper.

5) Immediately slide the dough off of the parchment paper and onto a cooling rack. Do not let it sweat! Otherwise it will get soggy. Looks hard, but it's not!

Directions for toppings:

1) 2 cups cooked grass fed ground beef seasoned with: ½ teaspoon fennel seeds, ½ teaspoon onion flakes, ½ teaspoon Italian seasoning, dash cumin and sea salt to taste.

2) 2 cups sliced roasted vegetables - red bell peppers, onions and mushrooms

3) ½ cup sliced black olives OR kalamata olives

4) ¼ cup oil packed sundried tomatoes, drained and chopped

5) ½ - 1 cup crumbled feta OR goat cheese

6) Fresh basil leaves, for serving

Directions for sauce:

1)   Mix together:
- 1 (6 ounce) can of tomato paste
- ½ teaspoon onion flakes
- ½ teaspoon Italian Seasoning
- ½ teaspoon dried basil.

Directions for baking:

Bake pizza in preheated 400 degree oven for 10-15 minutes (enough time to warm through and heat the toppings).

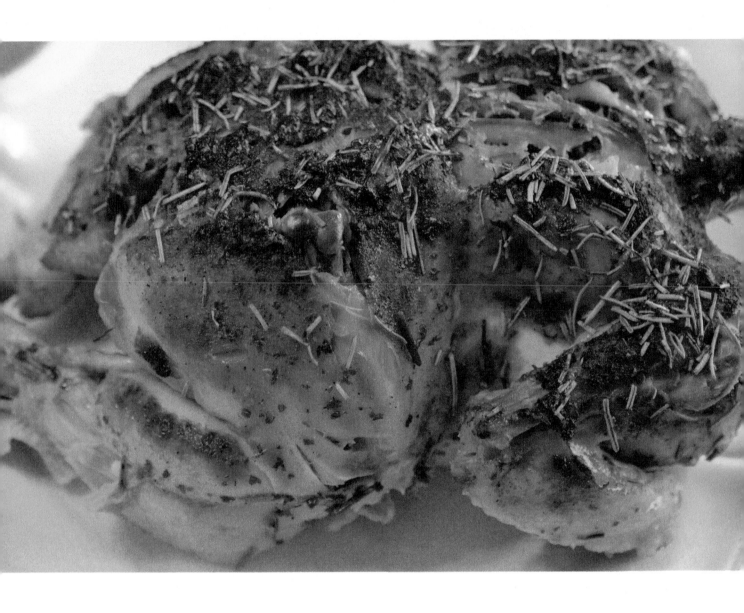

Chicken on the Fly
. . . .

Old school skills meet modern fast pace life... When asked to give a "how to" demonstration speech in 10th grade, out of the free range of ideas, my mom chose to present "how to cut up a chicken." Although her class about flew the coop watching her clip it's wings, this old school skill has equipped her to make chicken dinner on the fly many times... and she did get an A+!

Life is so busy and before you dash out the door, take 8 minutes and prepare this chicken.

When you return in a few hours, the house smells amazing and the chicken is so delicious!!!

I have done this numerous times.

Your kids get out of school and need to be at practice then you come home starved and tired.....

you enter the house, it smells incredible and voilà you have delicious chicken for dinner!

Quickest Delicious Chicken

Gluten Free
Grain Free
Dairy Free

6 servings

- 1 (4 pound) organic chicken
- 2 cups filtered water
- 2 Tablespoons Chicken Seasoning (page 241)

Directions:

1) Place chicken in a 9x13x2 inch glass baking dish. With a sharp knife, remove as much skin as possible.

2) Gently pour the water over the whole chicken.

3) Generously season the chicken with the chicken seasoning.

4) Put in the oven and turn the heat to 350 and bake uncovered for 2 hours.

Tasty Satisfying Chicken

6-8 servings

- **1 organic fresh chicken**
- **1 ½ cups filtered water, divided
  (for water fried chicken)**
- **½-1 teaspoon Nature's Sunshine® sea salt**

- **½-1 teaspoon Hungarian paprika**
- **½ teaspoon ground black pepper**
- **¼ teaspoon cayenne pepper**
- **½-1 Tablespoon garlic powder**
- **1 Tablespoon dried parsley**
- **½-1 Tablespoon dried whole rosemary (for baked chicken)**

Directions:

1) Use a sharp knife to begin cutting the chicken in pieces. Remove the legs first, and then the thighs, then the tip of the wing, then cut the wing and include a chunk of breast meat attached. Then divide the back from the breast. Divide the breasts and remove the bone.

2) Remove skin off each piece as you cut up the chicken except for the drumsticks. Leave some skin on them at the bone area.

3) If you desire to make broth, see instructions below (#9)

4) Remove the giblet bag from the chicken. Your choice, place the pieces in the broth pot or in the skillet/baking dish.

5) Arrange the chicken pieces in the skillet/baking dish so they are not overlapping.

6) Generously season the chicken pieces with the spices listed above to taste OR if it is easier, use 2-3 Tablespoons of the Chicken seasoning on page 241.

Directions for Water Fried Chicken:

7) Place seasoned chicken pieces in skillet and pour 1 cup of the water into the pan then cover with a lid. Cook covered on medium-high until water has cooked down and the chicken begins to pop. Reduce heat to medium and add ¼ cup water. Cover quickly because the pan drippings will sizzle and steam! Once it settles down, turn chicken pieces over and remove the lid.

Let the water cook down again. If you're satisfied with the look of the chicken, serve immediately or add the remaining ¼ cup water and let cook down one more time. This water fried chicken recipe only works with dark and white meat. It will not work with all white meat unless you add 1 or 2 Tablespoons of grapeseed oil to the water.

Directions for Baked Chicken:

8) Place seasoned chicken pieces in a 10x15x2 inch glass baking dish and pour 2 cups of water into the dish. Place in preheated 350 degree oven for 1:15 to 1:30.

Barbecue Chicken:

Use a spoon or a basting brush to coat the baked chicken with barbecue sauce (page 247) and bake an additional 15 minutes. *(This recipe with the Barbecue sauce is not dairy free.)*

Directions for broth:

9) Place the skin, fat, bones, giblets and wing tips in the pot to boil for broth. You may also add 2 cups washed vegetable trimmings, if desired. For nutritional benefits and flavoring, season the chicken trimmings in the pot with ½ teaspoon sea salt, ½ teaspoon ground black pepper, 2 garlic cloves and 1 teaspoon fresh squeezed lemon juice.

Pour enough water into the pot until the trimmings are covered with water by 2 inches. Put a lid on the pan and boil for 30 minutes. When the boiling pot is done, remove from heat and let it cool. Discard the chicken trimmings. Once it is cooled, then pour the broth into glass jars and refrigerate. The fat will rise to the top as the broth cools and seal the broth. It will keep one week. The lemon is added to pull minerals out of the bones.

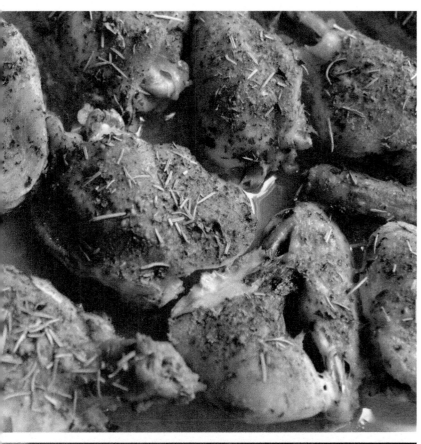

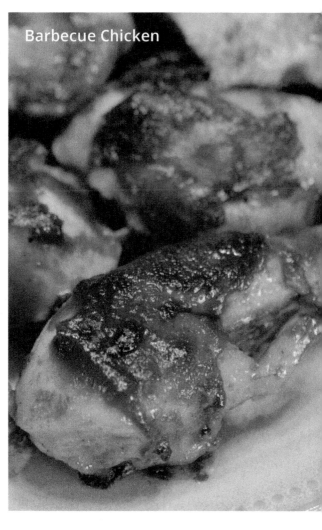

Barbecue Chicken

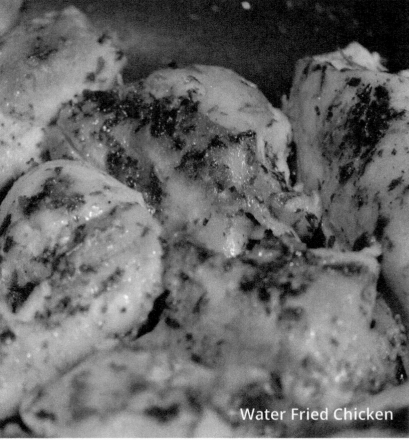

Water Fried Chicken

How to prepare a Turkey
. . . .

Purchase a frozen whole organic turkey approximately 20 pounds. Put it in the refrigerator in a large dishpan or on a large tray to thaw. As it thaws, sometimes the package leaks and it is a mess to clean up. It will take 3 or 4 days for the turkey to thaw. Once you think it is thawed, you are ready to prepare it.

Directions:

Get your spices out first and place in small bowls:

Bowl # 1 to season the broth:
- 1 Tablespoon Nature's Sunshine® sea salt
- ½ teaspoon ground black pepper
- ½ Tablespoon garlic powder

Bowl #2 to season the turkey:
- 1 teaspoon Nature's Sunshine® sea salt
- ½ teaspoon ground black pepper
- ½ Tablespoon garlic powder
- 2 Tablespoons poultry seasoning

Have a clean counter and no dishes in the sink. Bring large dish pan with turkey to the sink. Have your trash can right next to your hip. You'll need a sharp knife and two paper towels. Have your turkey roasting pan nearby. Remove the top oven rack from the oven so that the roasting pan will fit in the oven. You'll need a 10 inch wide piece of unbleached parchment paper and a much larger piece of heavy duty foil to cover the turkey and seal the edges of the pan.

Cut open the netting and throw it away. Take a bit of liquid soap and wash the tight fitting plastic bag that the turkey is in. Rinse and drain the water out of your dishpan. Now cut away ¼ of the plastic bag around the top of the turkey and make a long slit down the front of it. First remove the wire that is holding the leg bones together by pulling one leg bone out and then the other.

Then squeeze together the wire inside the turkey to get it out. Take both leg bones in hand and push out ward to stretch them apart so you can work. Take your knife and begin to remove as much skin and fat from the breast, back, tail, and thighs as possible and throw away.

Reach inside the turkey opening and pull out the bag that is in there. Open and (use paper towel to turn the water on) rinse the pieces of meat: the neck, gizzard, heart and liver. Place them in the roasting pan along with bowl #1 seasoning. Now turn water on and rinse the cavity of the turkey, pour water out. Place the turkey in the roasting pan breast side down. Remove all trash, skin, fat, etc. out of the dishpan and sink. Careful not to drip any turkey juice on the floor. Use the paper towel to turn on the water and to get some soap to thoroughly wash your hands. Season turkey with bowl #2 and add 3 inches of water to the roasting pan. Bake in preheated 350 degree oven for 5 hours.

Now what do I do with all of this turkey??? Glad you asked. . .

Attend to the leftover turkey as soon as possible. Take the leftover large piece of breast meat and divide it into two pieces. Wrap each piece in unbleached parchment paper and then put in a BPA Free freezer bag and put in the freezer. Next, pour off some of the broth, one ladle at a time through a wire mesh strainer into a large glass bowl or jars. (You will pour the rest off after the meat and bones are taken out of the roaster. Sometimes you will have enough broth for two bowls). Now, separate the dark meat from the bones. Put the bones, skin and "stuff" into the lid of the roaster and place all the small pieces of meat in a bowl. Divide the leftover meat, keep some for your next meal or for a sandwich and then put the rest into "main dish baggies" (approx. 3 cups each) and freeze in the freezer for quick meals later.

If you want to, put the bones back into the roasting pan and pour 3 cups of hot water over them. Swish them around to rinse them for 30 or 40 seconds. Remove the bones and place in the trash. Pour the broth through the wire mesh strainer into the broth bowl or jars. There will be enough broth to keep one in the refrigerator and freeze the rest. To freeze broth, you would let it completely cool then pour into BPA free Ziploc® style baggies or BPA free containers and place in the freezer.

Uses for the broth:
- Use to sauté vegetables, green beans and onions
- Use instead of water to cook rice, pasta, quinoa
- Use to make soup
- Use to reheat leftovers, instead of using oil or water

"Main dish baggies" examples of use:
- Turkey Quesadilla
- Turkey Fajitas
- Turkey Enchiladas
- Pot pie (note page 141)
- Enchilada Brown Rice Casserole
- Substitute for chicken in any recipe
- Turkey and Brown Rice
- Turkey Salad
- Soup

Tender Crock-Pot® Chicken

Gluten Free
Dairy Free

4-6 servings

- **1 (1 ½ pound) package chicken thighs OR whole chicken, skin removed**
- **2 cups filtered water**
- **½ teaspoon Nature's Sunshine® sea salt**
- **½ teaspoon ground black pepper**
- **½ teaspoon smoked paprika**
- **½ teaspoon dried thyme**
- **1 teaspoon dried parsley**
- **1 teaspoon dried whole rosemary**
- **2 garlic cloves, minced OR 2 teaspoons garlic powder**

Dinner Option:
- **6 large organic carrots cut in chunks**
- **1 large onion, quartered**
- **1 cup soaked organic long grain brown rice, rinsed and drained**
- **1 teaspoon our chicken seasoning OR vegetable herb seasoning (Page 237, 241)**
- **½ teaspoon dried thyme**
- **1 ½ cups broccoli florets OR frozen green beans**

Directions:
1) In a large Crock-Pot®, pour the water over the skinless chicken. Season the chicken with the salt, pepper, paprika, thyme, parsley, rosemary and garlic. Cover and cook on high. Chicken thighs need 3 to 4 hours. Whole chicken can cook 4 hours up to 8 ½ hours

Dinner Option Directions:
2) Approximately 45 minutes before serving, remove 2 cups of broth to prepare the rice on the stove. Place carrots, onion and your choice of broccoli or green beans in the pot with the chicken.
3) Pour broth into 2 quart saucepan on medium-high heat. Add in the rice, thyme and seasoning of your choice. Cook covered for 20-25 minutes or until all liquid is absorbed and the rice is tender. Keep warm.
4) Plate the four servings with the rice on the bottom with the vegetables and chicken on top. Refrigerate any leftovers.

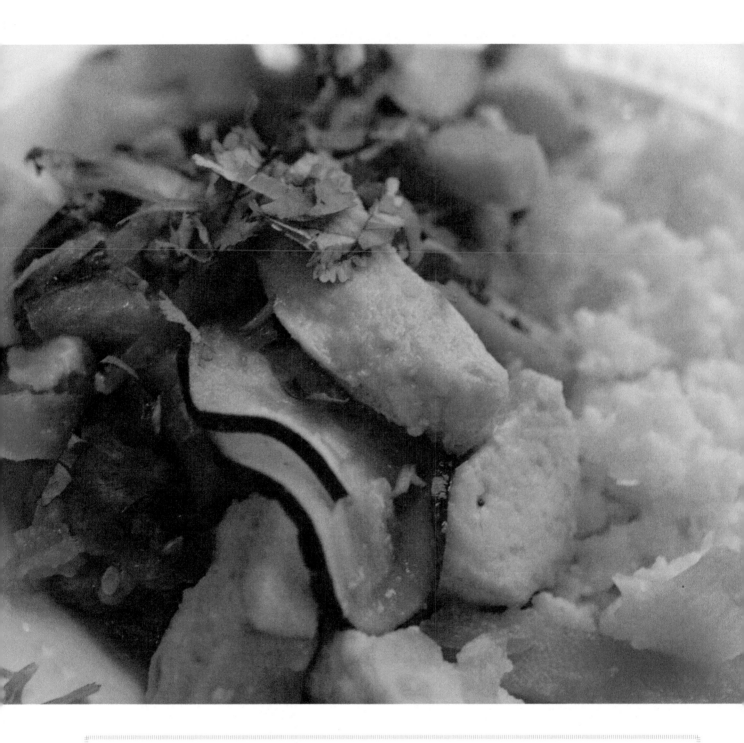

The basic way to make a stir-fry is to have your rice, your lightly seasoned vegetables and your chicken then add in as much or as little Bragg® liquid aminos (soy sauce replacement) as you like. If you want a bolder stir-fry try the ginger sauce for the vegetables or add in the optional toppings. Serve with a salad and seaweed chips. Bell pepper, baby bok choy or cilantro would also be good additions in this dish. For a grain free and gluten free option, substitute Caul-it-Rice (page 225) for the brown rice.

Simple Stir Fry

Gluten Free
Dairy Free

4 servings

- 1 ½ cups organic long grain brown rice
- 3 cups chicken broth OR filtered water
- 2 organic chicken breasts OR 6-8 chicken tenders
- ¼ cup filtered water
- Nature's Sunshine® sea salt, to taste
- Ground black pepper, to taste
- 1 teaspoon garlic powder
- ½ Tablespoon Bragg® liquid aminos
- 3 organic carrots, sliced or diced
- 2 cups broccoli florets
- 1 small onion, chopped
- ¼ teaspoon ginger, minced
- ½ teaspoon garlic, minced
- ¼ cup chicken broth OR filtered water
- 1 teaspoon extra-virgin coconut oil
- 1 cup frozen peas OR snow peas
- 2 organic eggs, beaten
- 1 teaspoon extra-virgin coconut oil
- Dash cayenne pepper
- Dash Nature's Sunshine® sea salt

Optional Toppings:
- Bragg® liquid aminos
- Sesame oil
- Raw sesame seeds
- Raw cashews
- Raw kelp seasoning

Ginger Sauce for vegetables, optional
- 2 teaspoons fresh squeezed orange juice
- ½ teaspoon brown rice miso
- ½ teaspoon coconut aminos
- ½ Tablespoon Bragg® liquid aminos
- 1 teaspoon sesame oil
- ½ teaspoon ginger, minced
- ½ teaspoon garlic, minced
- Add up to ½ Tablespoon coconut flour
  to thicken the broth in the vegetables at left.

Directions:

1) Soak the rice in water overnight (see page 25). Rinse and drain. In a 2 quart saucepan on medium high heat, add the rice and 3 cups of your choice chicken broth or water. Bring to a boil. Then cover and reduce heat to medium and let simmer until all the broth is absorbed and the rice is tender.

2) In a stainless steel skillet, cook the chicken and water on medium heat until juices run clear and it's done all the way through. Season as desired with sea salt and pepper, garlic powder and liquid aminos.

3) After the chicken is cooked, cut into bite size pieces and add the carrots, broccoli, onion, ginger, garlic, coconut oil and ¼ cup your choice of broth or water. Cover with lid and lightly steam the veggies for 7 minutes. Add peas then turn heat to low to keep warm.

4) In a small approved Green® non-stick skillet, add the coconut oil and eggs. Season with cayenne pepper and sea salt. Cook over medium-low heat 3 minutes then flip over with large spatula and cook approximately 3 more minutes until cooked through. The eggs should be one large circle. Place on a plate and cut into tiny pea size squares using a pizza cutter.

5) Add the eggs to the cooked rice. Stir lightly to combine.

6) Divide the rice, veggies and chicken among the four servings. Plate the rice on bottom, then add the veggies and chicken then top with your choice of toppings. If using liquid aminos or sesame oil, drizzle on top to taste.

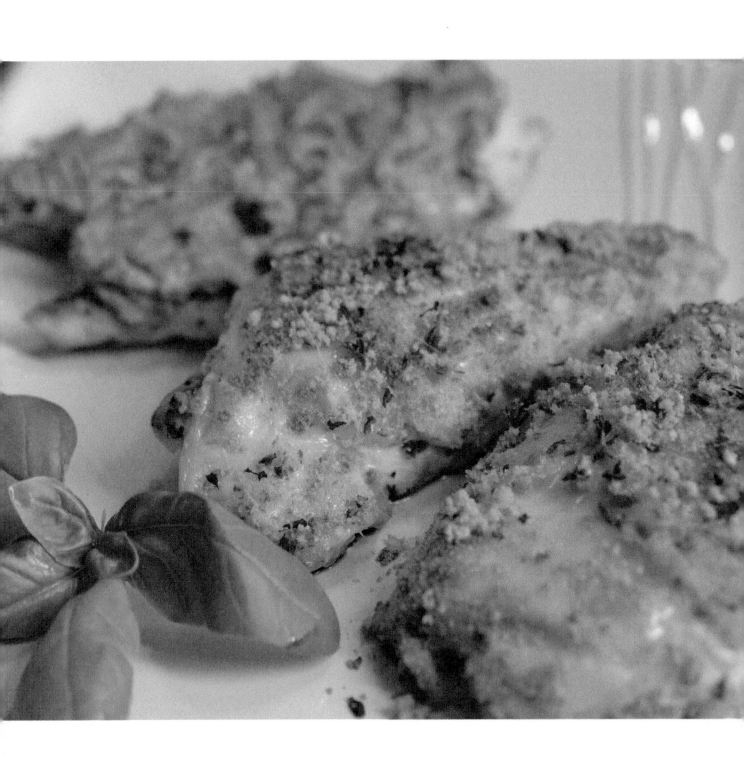

Creamy Parmesan Crusted Chicken Breast

Eat in Moderation

4 servings

- **4 boneless skinless chicken breasts**
- **2-4 ounces sliced cheese:**
  Monterey Jack, Mozzarella, Provolone

Marinade:
- **2 Tablespoons fresh squeezed lemon juice**
- **2 Tablespoons grapeseed oil**
- **½ teaspoon sea salt**
- **½ teaspoon ground black pepper**
- **½ teaspoon dried whole rosemary, crushed**
- **½ teaspoon Bragg® liquid aminos**
- **1 teaspoon onion granules**
- **2 teaspoons dried parsley**
- **2 teaspoons garlic powder**

Creamy spread:
- **2 ½ Tablespoons Vegenaise®**
- **2 Tablespoons grated parmesan cheese**
- **½ teaspoon garlic powder**
- **1 teaspoon dried parsley**
- **¼ teaspoon Nature's Sunshine® sea salt**

Crumb topping:
- **5 Tablespoons dry Ezekiel® bread crumbs**
- **1 teaspoon dried parsley**
- **2 teaspoons grated parmesan cheese**

Directions:

1) In a glass dish or a BPA free Ziploc® style gallon bag, mix up the marinade and add the chicken breasts. Place in the refrigerator for 30 minutes to 1 hour.

2) In a small mixing bowl, mix together the creamy spread.

3) In another small mixing bowl, place the dry bread crumbs, dried parsley and grated parmesan cheese.

4) Grill the chicken breast with as much of the marinade as you like. Cook approximately 5-7 minutes on each side, depending on the thickness of the chicken or until juices run clear.

5) Remove from grill and place on a baking sheet with a ½ inch rim, lined with unbleached parchment paper. (Juices may run, so make sure to have a large enough piece of parchment paper).

6) Top each chicken breast in this order: spread 2 teaspoons of creamy spread, ½ - 1 ounce of sliced cheese of your choice and sprinkle 1 ½ Tablespoons of the bread crumb mixture on top.

7) Place under broiler for only 3 minutes to lightly brown the bread crumbs and melt the cheese. Serve immediately.

• •

One of our old favorite local restaurants served a parmesan crusted chicken which was my son's favorite dish to order. It was loaded in calories and very addictive, so I came up with a healthier version.

Dairy Free option:

Top grilled chicken with Avocado Spread:
- 1 cup ripe avocado, chopped
- ¼ cup sundried tomatoes in extra-virgin olive oil, drained and chopped
- 1 teaspoon garlic, minced
- 2 teaspoons fresh thyme, minced
- 1 ½ Tablespoons fresh basil, chopped
- ¼ teaspoon Nature's Sunshine® sea salt, to taste
- ¼ teaspoon ground black pepper

Mash well and spread on hot grilled chicken breasts. Serve immediately.

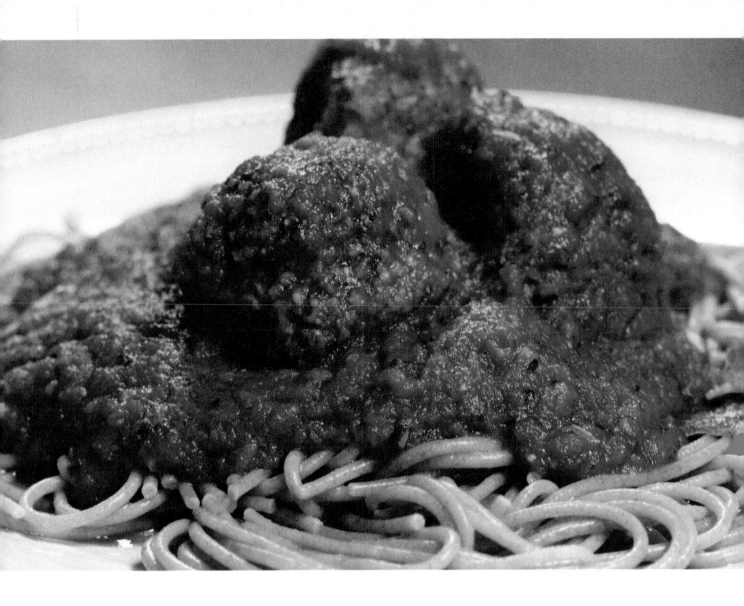

The Meat Ball Mishap...

One night my mom and I had rushed home from work to warm up spaghetti and meatballs for dinner. While she was making the sauce, I went to find the meatballs in the freezer. Seeing the frozen balls, I plopped them into the sauce. The food was now hot and on the table, and my dad asked "what meat is this?" My mom replied in jest not sure if it was bison or beef "Oh it's mystery meat." Another bite led to a perplexed look and disappointed palate; I took a bite and woefully realized the "mystery meat" was a batch of round pumpkin muffins. Lesson learned: always label frozen food.

Veggie Spaghetti Sauce

6-8 servings

- 1 medium-large onion, quartered
- 2 large garlic cloves OR ½ Tablespoon garlic powder
- ½ medium zucchini
- ½ medium red bell pepper
- 2 (8 ounce) cans tomato sauce
- 1 (28 ounce) can Muir Glen® tomatoes
- 2 (6 ounce) cans tomato paste
- 1 teaspoon dried basil, optional
- ¾ cup filtered water

- 1 Tablespoon oregano
- 1 Tablespoon Italian seasoning
- 1 Tablespoon dried parsley
- 1 Tablespoon extra-virgin olive oil
- ½ Tablespoon fennel seeds
- 2 Tablespoons grated parmesan cheese, optional
- ¼ teaspoon stevia (or more to taste)
- 3 dried bay leaves, whole
- ½-1 pound cooked and drained ground venison OR prepared meatballs

Directions:

1) Use a large bowl food processor with the sharp blade to chop the vegetables for the sauce. Wipe out the processor bowl with a spatula after each use and re-use. Process the onion and garlic cloves (if using) until chopped then put into a large pot.

2) Next process the zucchini and red pepper until they are finely chopped, then add to the large pot. Cook and stir on medium heat until the onions are translucent.

3) Pour the tomato sauce into the pot. Cover with a lid.

4) Process the Muir Glen® tomatoes, tomato paste and water in the food processor for 35 seconds then add to the pot. Cook and stir for 3 minutes.

5) At this point the sauce may seem chunky. If you like it more smooth, pour all the vegetables and tomatoes back into the food processor and process until smooth. Pour back into the large pot.

6) Add in the basil, oregano, Italian seasoning, parsley, olive oil, fennel seeds, parmesan cheese (if desired) and stevia. Stir well to combine. Add in the bay leaves and cover with a lid.

7) If you are using meatballs, add them now and simmer with a lid for 25-45 minutes or until it is ready to be served.

Tip: Enjoy over whole grain spaghetti, spiralized zucchini or spaghetti squash. For a gluten free and grain free option, use the ground meat and spaghetti squash or spiralized zucchini for the "pasta."

Gluten Free
Grain Free
Dairy Free

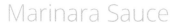

Marinara Sauce

Makes 6 cups

- 2 (28 ounce) cans Muir Glen® Organic Tomatoes
- 1 Tablespoon garlic, minced
- ½ cup onion, chopped
- 2 teaspoons dried oregano

- 1 Tablespoon dried parsley
- 1 ½ Tablespoons fresh basil, chopped
- ¼ teaspoon Nature's Sunshine® sea salt
- Dash ground black pepper
- 2 Tablespoons extra-virgin olive oil

Directions:

1) In a large food processor, process one can of tomatoes by 15 pulses. Pour into a 2 quart sauce pan on medium.

2) Add the second can of tomatoes to the food processor along with the minced garlic, chopped onion, oregano, parsley, chopped basil, sea salt and pepper. Process by 30 pulses. Pour into the sauce pan.

3) Add the olive oil and stir to combine. Cover with a lid. Reduce the heat to medium-low and simmer for 2 hours, stirring every 20 minutes.

Tip: Do not turn the heat very high because of the olive oil. Refrigerate any leftovers. This is great with meat balls or Chicken Pomodoro (page 162-163)

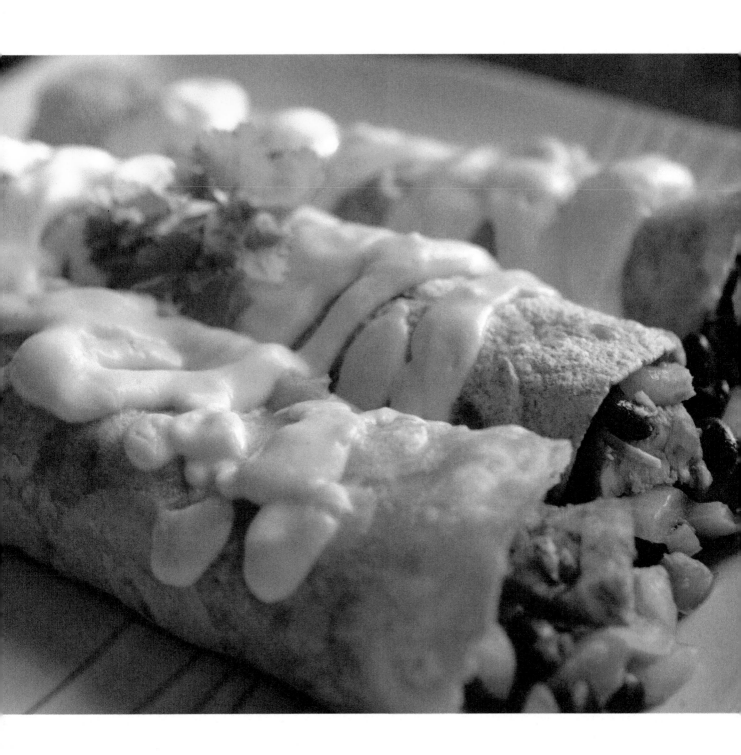

Southwest Chicken Enchiladas

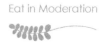

4-6 servings

- 2-2 ½ cups fully cooked chicken
- 1 yellow or red bell pepper, diced
- 1 sweet onion, diced
- 1 garlic clove, minced
- 1 teaspoon extra-virgin coconut oil
- 1 (15 ounce) can black beans, drained and rinsed well
- 2 Tablespoons fresh organic cilantro, chopped
- ½ Tablespoon ground cumin

- ¼ teaspoon Nature's Sunshine sea salt
- ½ teaspoon smoked paprika
- ¼ - ½ cup salsa, liquid drained
- ½ cup organic frozen corn, optional
- 1 cup shredded cheese: Monterey jack, pepper jack, Colby jack, fresh goat cheese
- 6 organic whole grain tortillas, 10 inch diameter

Directions:

1) Place bell pepper, onion, garlic and oil in a skillet and sauté together until onions are clear. Add in the diced leftover chicken or prepared Spicy Chicken (page 151). When using fully cooked leftover chicken, add ½ Tablespoon taco seasoning to the skillet. Heat chicken until warm.

2) In a large mixing bowl combine the black beans, cilantro, cumin, sea salt, paprika, salsa, corn (if using), 1 cup of your choice of cheese and the sautéed vegetables and chicken. Stir well to combine.

3) Take the first tortilla and fill it with 1/6 of the diced chicken mixture. Roll it up tightly and place it in a 9x13x2 inch glass baking dish coated with non-stick grapeseed oil spray. Repeat this process until all the tortillas are filled and in the dish.

4) Bake in a preheated 350 degree oven for 15-20 minutes.

5) If desired, drizzle Cheese Sauce (page 254) on top. Serve hot.

Serve with shredded carrots and lettuce, salsa, guacamole and cheese sauce.

Tortillas substitution: Rudi's® gluten free plain tortillas, organic brown rice tortillas OR Applegate® oven roasted turkey breast for a low carb option. Substitute leftover turkey for the chicken.

To Make Enchilada Casserole
Serves 8

Omit the tortillas or sliced turkey breast and step 4).

Add 3 cups cooked brown rice or quinoa to step 3) and pour into a 9x13x2 inch glass baking dish coated with non-stick grapeseed oil spray. Bake in preheated 350 degree oven for 20-30 minutes. Serve hot.

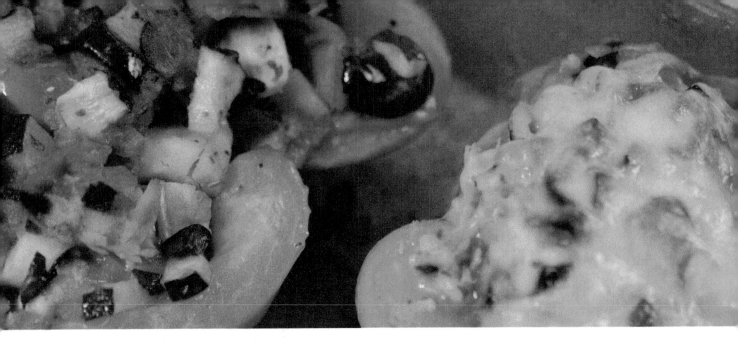

Stuffed Peppers

2 servings

- 2 red bell peppers, halved and seeded
- ¼ cup chicken broth
- ½ teaspoon grapeseed oil

- ½ teaspoon garlic powder
- ¼ teaspoon Nature's Sunshine® sea salt

Mexican Filling
- ½ cup onion, diced
- 2 Tablespoons chicken broth
- Nature's Sunshine® sea salt, to taste
- ¼ teaspoon garlic powder
- ¼ teaspoon ground cumin
- ½ teaspoon taco seasoning (page 237)

- ⅓ cup black beans, drained and rinsed
- ⅓ cup salsa
- ½ cup cooked organic long grain brown rice
- 2 Tablespoons organic cilantro, chopped
- 1 cup fully cooked chicken OR grass fed ground beef
- ¼ cup mozzarella cheese, shredded, optional

Directions:

1) In a 9x9x2 inch glass baking dish, place the four pepper halves cut side down. Add the ¼ cup broth and bake in preheated oven at 400 degrees for 15 minutes. Remove peppers from oven and drain the liquid from the baking dish. Massage them all over with the grapeseed oil then season them with ½ teaspoon garlic powder and ¼ teaspoon sea salt. Place them back in the baking dish for filling.

Directions for Mexican Filling:

1) Sauté onions in broth for 2 or 3 minutes over medium heat. Add seasonings, black beans, salsa, brown rice, cilantro and your choice of cooked meat. Mix and sauté for 2 more minutes. Remove from heat.

2) Choose whether you want the cheese (if using) mixed into the filling or sprinkled on top of the filling. For dairy free option, omit the cheese. If you want the cheese mixed into the filling, add it now and fill each pepper with ¼ of the mixture. If you want the cheese sprinkled on top, add it after you fill the peppers. Bake in 350 degree oven for 20 minutes. Serve immediately.

Italian Filling

2 servings

- 1 cup fully cooked chicken OR grass fed ground beef
- ⅓ cup onion, diced
- ⅔ cup zucchini, diced
- 2 Tablespoons chicken broth
- Nature's Sunshine® sea salt, to taste
- ¼ teaspoon garlic powder
- 1 Tablespoon fresh basil leaves, sliced
- ½ cup sundried tomatoes in extra-virgin olive oil, drained, chopped
- ⅓ cup black olives, sliced
- ½ teaspoon Italian seasoning (page 240)
- ¼ cup tomato sauce
- ¼ cup mozzarella cheese, shredded, optional

Directions:

1) Sauté the onions and zucchini in broth for 2 or 3 minutes over medium heat. Add seasonings, tomatoes, olives, Italian seasoning, tomato sauce and your choice of cooked meat. Mix and sauté for 2 more minutes. Remove from heat.

2) Choose whether you want the cheese (if using) mixed into the filling or sprinkled on top of the filling. For dairy free option, omit the cheese. If you want the cheese mixed into the filling, add it now and fill each pepper with ¼ of the mixture. If you want the cheese sprinkled on top, add it after you fill the peppers. Bake in 350 degree oven for 20 minutes. Serve immediately.

Chicken Filling

2 servings

- 1 cup fully cooked chicken
- ⅓ cup onion, diced
- ½ cup organic celery, diced
- 2 Tablespoons chicken broth
- Nature's Sunshine® sea salt, to taste
- Ground black pepper, to taste
- ¼ teaspoon garlic powder
- ⅓ cup organic carrot, shredded
- ½ cup cooked organic long grain brown rice

Directions:

1) Sauté the onions and celery in broth for 2 or 3 minutes over medium heat. Add seasonings, chicken, carrots and brown rice. Mix and sauté for 2 more minutes. Remove from heat and fill each pepper with ¼ of the brown rice mixture.

2) Bake in 350 degree oven for 20 minutes. Serve immediately.

Suggestion: Frozen peas would be a great addition to this recipe.

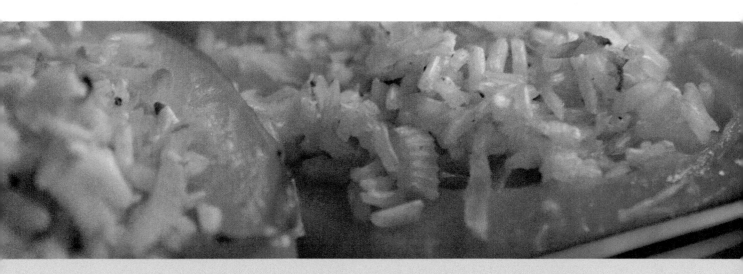

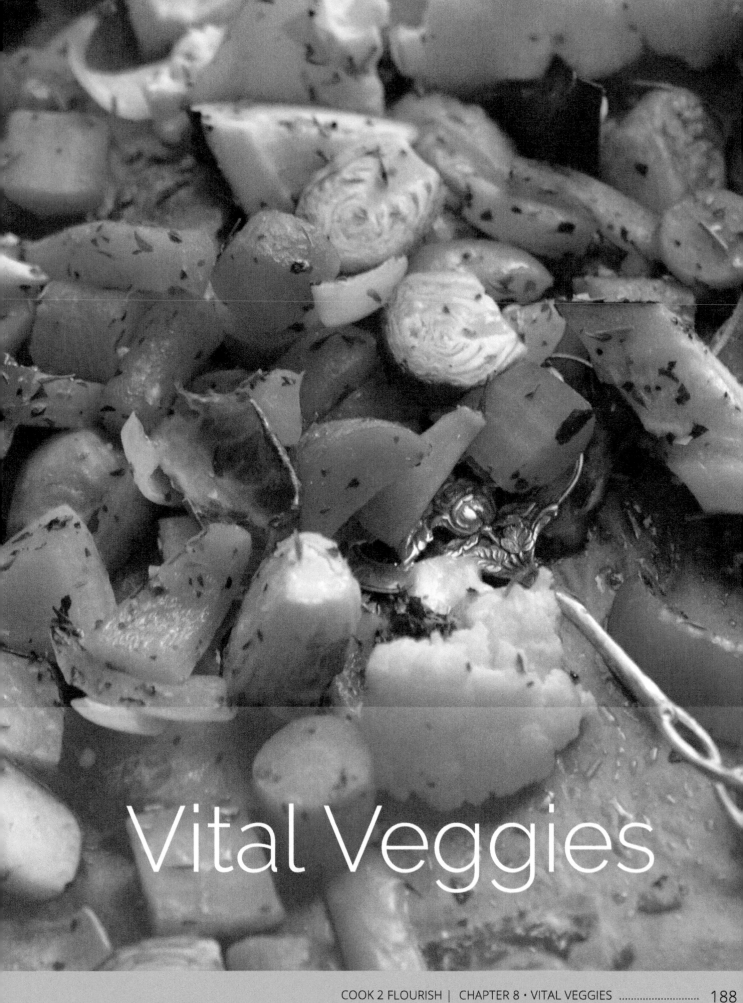

Vital Veggies

Roasted Vegetables

Gluten Free
Grain Free
Dairy Free

6 servings

- 1 large organic potato, cut into chunks
- 3 cups organic baby carrots
- 1 medium onion, cut into chunks
- 1 red bell pepper, cut into chunks
- 1 zucchini, cut into chunks
- 1 cup Brussels sprouts, washed, trimmed and cut in half
- 5-6 mushrooms, cleaned and cut in half, optional
- ⅓ cup grapeseed oil

- ½ Tablespoon dried oregano
- ½ Tablespoon dried thyme
- ½ Tablespoon dried parsley
- ½ Tablespoon dried whole rosemary
- ½ teaspoon Nature's Sunshine® sea salt
- ½ teaspoon ground black pepper
- 3 garlic cloves, pressed in a garlic press

Directions:

1) In a medium-large pot, steam the potato chunks and baby carrots until almost cooked.

2) While the potatoes and carrots are steaming, select a large 9x13x2inch glass baking dish.

3) Cut up vegetables into the glass baking dish. Add the potatoes and carrots.

4) Mix the oil, herbs and garlic together in a measuring cup and pour over the vegetables, toss to coat.
Bake in preheated 350 degree oven for 25-30 minutes, stirring once during baking. Serve immediately.

Tip: Be creative! Season them how you like. If the oregano and thyme are too much, then omit them. Roast your favorite vegetables: asparagus, broccoli, cauliflower, tomatoes, sweet potatoes, garlic cloves, squash, peppers, or green beans. Freeze leftovers and use them in a soup, whole or pureed. You could also top the soup with a spoonful of pesto.

Suggestion: Add 1 cup cooked quinoa to hot roasted vegetables, toss and serve in a bowl.

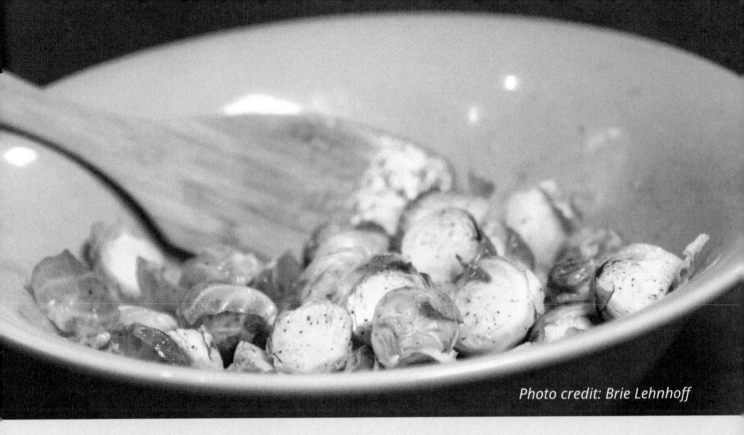

Spotlight : Brussels Sprouts

I admit, I have not always enjoyed Brussels sprouts. Even while eating healthy and becoming a health coach, they had not yet made it to my plate. In fact, these baby cabbages were not on my nutrition radar until my friend and co-worker Joyce brought them for lunch one day. Curious what to attribute the delicious aroma to, I perked up asking, "Joyce, what are you eating today?" I was not expecting to hear Brussels sprouts and certainly was not anticipating trying them. She asked me if I wanted one of her little cabbage treasures, and with hesitation I partook. Astonished, my mouth was full of a delectable depth of deliciousness sure to revisit again. That, my friend, was the origin of becoming a connoisseur of Brussels sprouts.

So what do these baby cabbages have going for them?

- *Fantastic source of fiber, folate, and vitamin C*
- *Support healthy detoxification*
- *Stellar source of toxin tackling antioxidants*

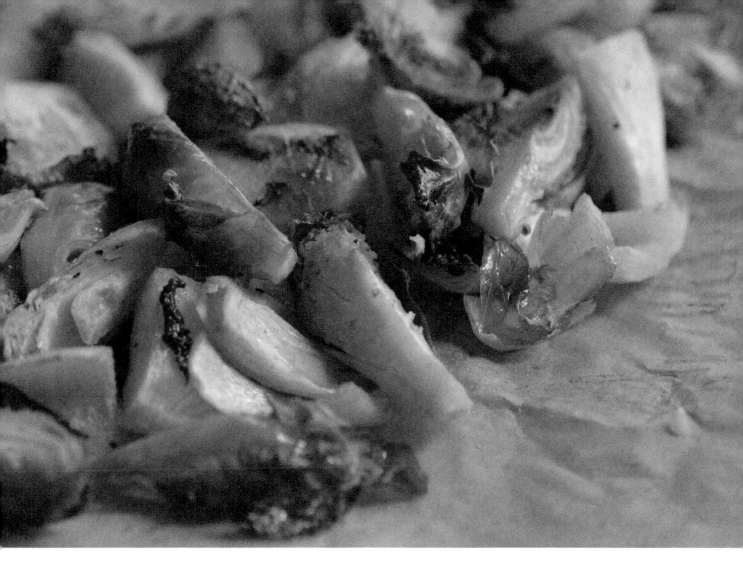

Roasted Brussels Sprouts

. . . .

Gluten Free
Grain Free
Dairy Free

4 servings

- **3 cups Brussels sprouts, trimmed and halved (4 cups before trimming)**
- **1 Tablespoon avocado oil OR grapeseed oil**
- **1 garlic clove, pressed**
- **½ teaspoon Nature's Sunshine® sea salt**
- **¼ teaspoon ground black pepper**
- **Dash cayenne pepper, optional**

Directions:

1) Place the trimmed Brussels sprouts in a large bowl. Pour in the oil. Toss to coat.

2) Add in the seasonings. Toss well to coat. Spread them out in a glass baking dish or onto an unbleached parchment paper lined stainless steel baking sheet and bake in preheated 350 degree oven for 30-35 minutes until golden brown. Serve immediately.

Braving the Brussels sprouts... and loving them!

Brussels sprouts? Yes! Give this forsaken vegetable a second chance!

With loads of nutrients beneath each leaf, they have a lot to offer, and not just nutrients, but FLAVOR!

Tossed with care and seasoned with love, they are sure to be enjoyed!

Sautéed Asparagus

4-6 servings

- 12 ounces fresh Asparagus, cut in 3 inch pieces
- 2 Tablespoons chicken OR vegetable broth
- 1 garlic clove, minced
- ¼ teaspoon ground black pepper
- ¼ teaspoon Nature's Sunshine® sea salt, to taste
- ½ Tablespoon extra-virgin olive oil
- ½ Tablespoon organic butter

Directions:

1) In a medium-large stainless steel skillet with a lid, steam-sauté the asparagus in the broth for approximately 5-7 minutes until tender.

2) Mix the rest of the ingredients together in a small bowl and pour over the asparagus. Mix to coat. Remove from heat and keep covered. Serve immediately.

Marinated Greens

4 servings

- 8 cups your choice of greens:
  Kale, Swiss chard, beet greens, spinach
- 1 Tablespoon fresh squeezed lemon juice
- 1 Tablespoon coconut aminos
- ½ Tablespoon Bragg® liquid aminos
- 2 Tablespoons extra-virgin olive oil
- ⅛ teaspoon ground black pepper
- 1 garlic clove, pressed in a garlic press

Directions:

1) Slice the greens of your choice and place in a glass serving bowl.

2) Mix the lemon juice, aminos, olive oil, pepper and garlic together in a measuring cup and pour over the greens. Toss to coat then massage the greens with your hands until wilted and reduced in size. Cover the bowl and marinate 4-6 hours or overnight. Serve chilled.

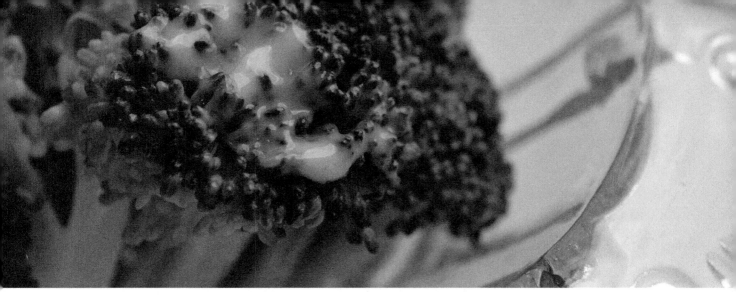

Easy Seasoned Broccoli

4 servings

- 4 cups broccoli florets
- 2 Tablespoons extra-virgin olive oil
- 1 teaspoon garlic powder
- ¼-½ teaspoon Nature's Sunshine® sea salt
- ¼ teaspoon ground black pepper
- 1 teaspoon fresh squeezed lemon juice, optional

Broccoli with cheese sauce (page 254).

Directions:

1) Pour ½ inch water in a 2 quart saucepan with a steamer basket inside. Bring water to a boil then add the broccoli. Steam over boiling water for 6-10 minutes until al dente' tender.

2) Drain. Remove the steamer basket and leave broccoli in the saucepan.

3) Drizzle the olive oil over the broccoli. Add the garlic powder, sea salt, pepper and lemon juice (if desired). Toss to coat and serve immediately.

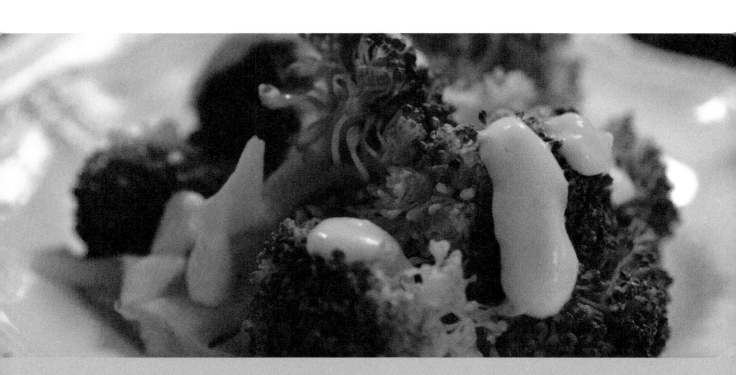

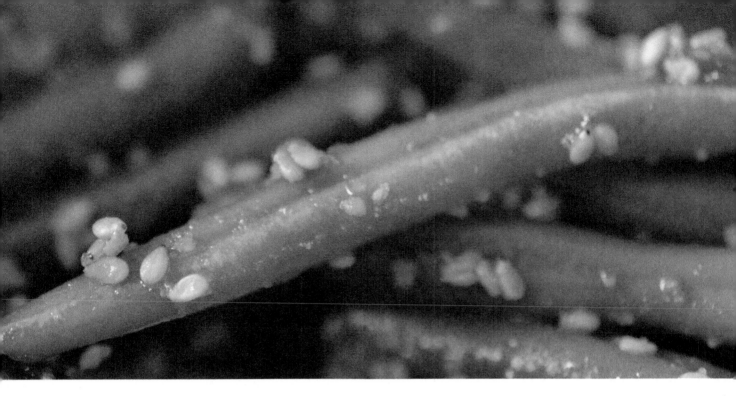

Sesame Green Beans

2 servings

- 2 ½ cups green beans, frozen
- ¼ cup chicken broth
- 1 teaspoon sesame oil
- 1 teaspoon garlic powder
- ½ teaspoon coconut aminos
- ½ teaspoon fresh ginger, grated
- 2 teaspoons sesame seeds

Directions:

1) Rinse green beans if they have frost on them and place in a medium-large stainless steel skillet. Add the broth and cover with a lid. Cook on medium heat for 10-15 minutes or until tender.

2) Season with sesame oil, garlic, coconut aminos, ginger and sesame seeds. Toss to coat. Serve immediately.

Roasted Green Beans

4 servings

- 6 cups green beans, frozen
- ½ Tablespoon grapeseed oil
- ½ teaspoon garlic powder
- ½ teaspoon Nature's Sunshine® sea salt
- ¼ teaspoon ground black pepper
- Dash cayenne pepper

Directions:

1) Rinse green beans if they have frost on them and place in a large 9x13x2inch glass baking dish along with the oil, garlic, sea salt, pepper and cayenne pepper.
2) Mix well to coat.
3) Bake in preheated 350 degree oven for 30-35 minutes, stirring once during baking. Serve immediately.

Glorious Green Beans

Gluten Free
Grain Free

4 servings

- **2 (16 ounce) packages frozen green beans**
- **¼ cup chicken broth**
- **½ teaspoon Nature's Sunshine® sea salt**
- **¼ teaspoon ground black pepper**
- **1 Tablespoon extra-virgin olive oil**
- **1 Tablespoon organic butter,**
  for serving (optional)

Directions:

1) Rinse green beans if they have frost on them and place in a medium-large stainless steel skillet. Add the broth and cover with a lid. Cook on medium heat for 10-15 minutes or until tender.

2) Season with sea salt, pepper and olive oil. Stir together. Place in serving bowl and top with butter, if desired. Serve immediately.

Gardening with PePa as a young sprout...

Besides the attempts at building tire swings and tree houses, vivid memories of gardening with my grandpa color my childhood. I remember picking grapes off the vine and how PePa stooped down to teach me what it looked like to plant green beans in a straight line. The sound of snapping peas and the plump blackberries are such fond memories ...the start to my green thumb.

I marvel at the journey from seed to sprout and how it arrives on our plates. Looking back, the seed was planted in me to enjoy gardening, appreciate its toil, and give thanks to the Lord for the harvest. As the Scriptures say, "For ground that drinks the rain which often falls on it and brings forth vegetation useful to those for whose sake it is also tilled, receives a blessing from God..." Hebrews 6:7 NASB

Making memories such as these can be as simple as strolling through the farmer's market or potting your own herb garden on your patio.

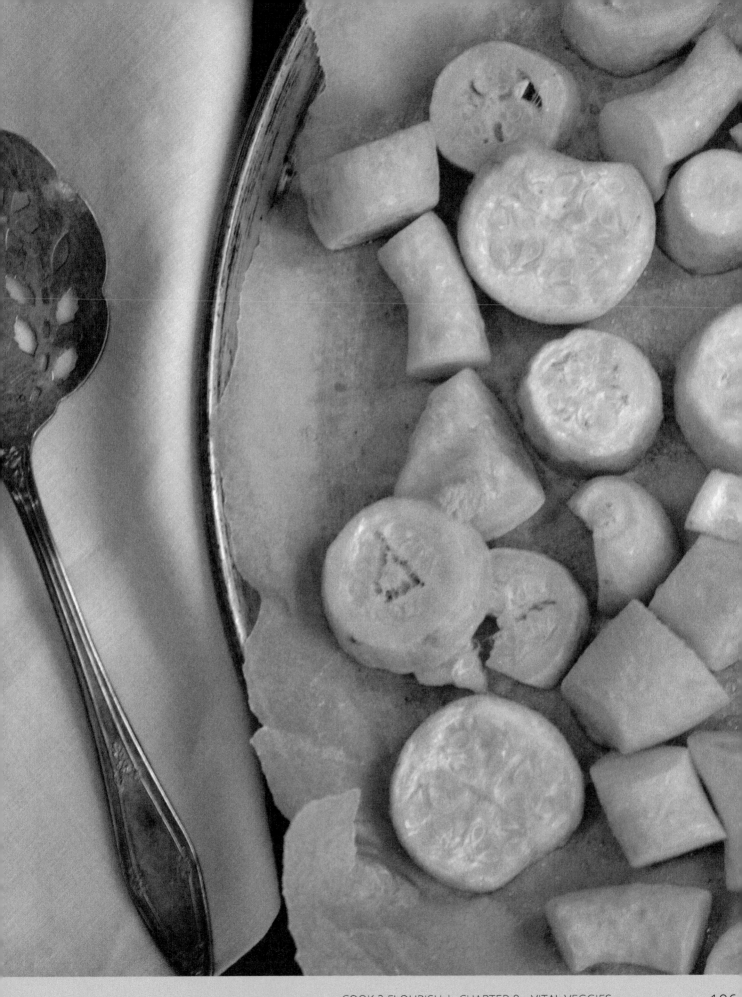

Roasted Yellow Squash

4 servings

- **6 cups tender yellow squash**
- **1 Tablespoon extra-virgin coconut oil**
- **½-1 teaspoon garlic powder**
- **¼ teaspoon Nature's Sunshine® sea salt**

Directions:

1) Wash the squash and trim the ends. Cut into ½ inch to 1 inch chunks.

2) Place in a bowl with coconut oil. With clean hands, begin to massage the squash with the coconut oil. Sprinkle in the garlic powder and sea salt. Massage again to coat.

3) Spread out the squash in a glass baking dish or on an unbleached parchment paper lined stainless steel baking sheet.

4) Bake in preheated 325 degree oven for 30 minutes. Serve immediately. These are surprisingly good!

Italian Roasted Veggies

6-8 servings

- **4 cups zucchini, unpeeled and chopped**
- **4 cups yellow squash, unpeeled and chopped**
- **4 cups eggplant, unpeeled and chopped**
- **3 cups onion, chopped**
- **1 teaspoon Italian seasoning (page 240)**
- **½ teaspoon ground black pepper**
- **½ teaspoon Nature's Sunshine® sea salt**
- **2 Tablespoons grapeseed oil**
- **2 garlic cloves, minced**

Directions:

1) Wash and chop all the veggies into 1 ½ - 2 inch diameter rounds or wedges. Place vegetables into a 9x13x2 inch glass baking dish.

2) Combine the Italian seasoning, pepper, sea salt, oil and garlic in a measuring cup. Drizzle over the vegetables and toss to coat.

3) Bake in preheated 350 degree oven for 40-45 minutes or until the veggies are tender. Serve immediately.

When your garden is at its peak, this is a great way to enjoy your bounty. This recipe would be great with Brussels sprouts, cauliflower, bell peppers or carrots.

Roasted Pepper Jack Cauliflower

4-6 servings

- **7 cups cauliflower florets (1 medium head)**
- **2 Tablespoons avocado oil OR grapeseed oil**
- **2 Tablespoons grated parmesan cheese**
- **½ Tablespoon dried parsley**
- **½ Tablespoon garlic granules**
- **½ teaspoon Nature's Sunshine® sea salt**
- **¼ teaspoon ground black pepper**
- **Dash cayenne pepper**
- **½ cup organic pepper jack cheese, grated**

Directions:

1) Place the cauliflower florets in a large bowl. Pour in the oil. Toss to coat.

2) Combine the parmesan cheese, parsley, garlic, sea salt, black pepper and cayenne pepper in a small bowl and stir well. Sprinkle over the cauliflower while tossing and stirring until well coated with the seasonings.

3) Spread out the florets onto an unbleached parchment paper lined stainless steel baking sheet and bake in preheated 350 degree oven for 25 minutes.

4) Remove from oven and sprinkle the cheese on each floret. Put back in the oven for 5 more minutes. Serve immediately.

> This recipe has flavor and zip! For those who haven't liked cauliflower in the past, try it again and perhaps this time.... you'll like it! For dairy free, omit the cheese.

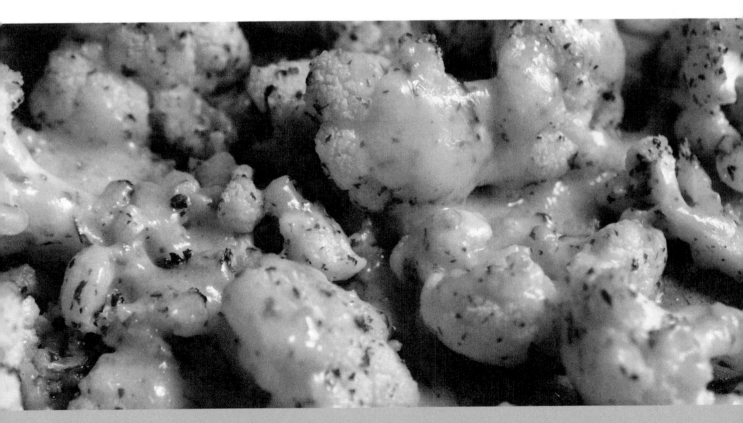

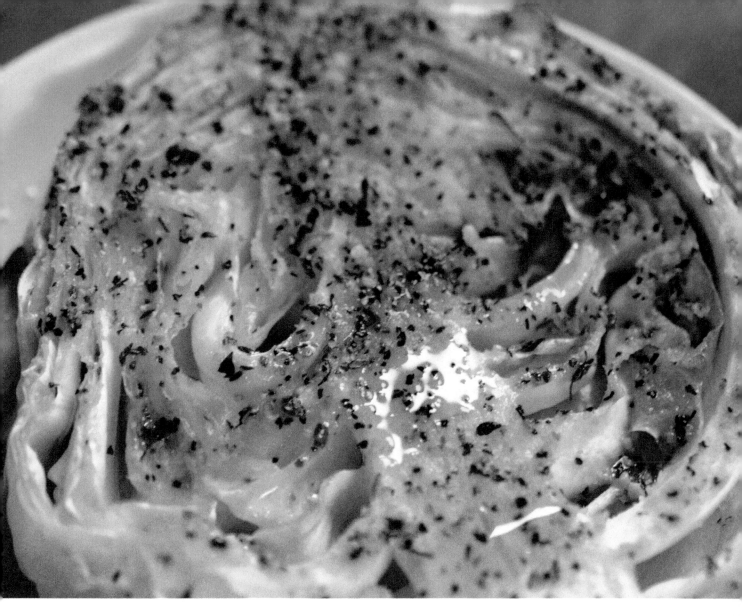

Roasted Cabbage

....

4-6 servings

- 6 half-inch slices of green cabbage (8 ounces total)
- 2 teaspoons extra-virgin coconut oil
- 2 teaspoons garlic powder
- ½-1 teaspoon Nature's Sunshine® sea salt
- ½ teaspoon ground black pepper
- ½ teaspoon Italian seasoning OR dash cayenne pepper

Directions:

1) Select a small green cabbage. Slice 6 half-inch slices and place in a 9x13x2 inch glass baking dish coated with non-stick grapeseed oil spray.

2) In a small bowl, combine the coconut oil, garlic powder, sea salt, pepper and your choice of Italian seasoning or cayenne pepper. Mix well. Using a pastry brush, coat the cabbage with the oil and seasonings. Bake in preheated 350 degree oven for 40 minutes until slightly golden. Serve immediately.

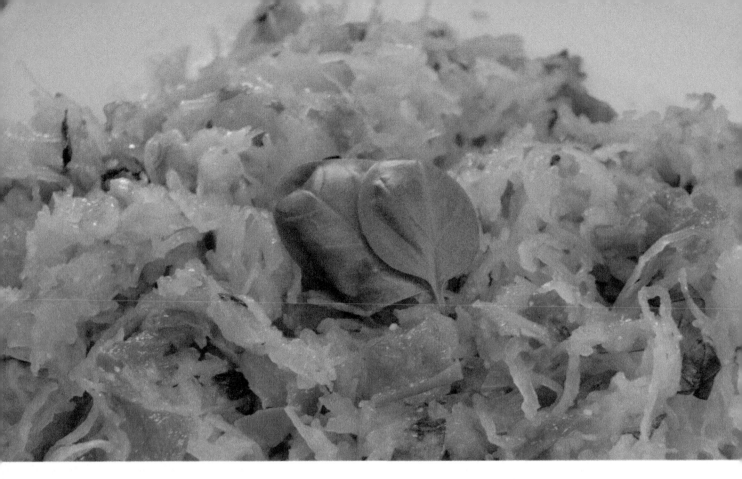

Mild Comforting Spaghetti Squash

6-8 servings

- 2 ½ pound spaghetti squash
- 1 Tablespoons extra-virgin olive oil
- 2 Tablespoons fresh basil, minced
- 1 teaspoon garlic powder

- ½ teaspoon Nature's Sunshine® sea salt
- Dash cayenne pepper
- 2 Tablespoons oil from sundried tomatoes
- ½ cup sundried tomatoes in extra-virgin olive oil, chopped
- ¼ cup walnuts, chopped

Directions:

1) Cut the squash into 4-6 chunks and arrange the squash pieces upside down on a steamer basket over boiling water in a large pot. Cook on medium-high for 15-20 minutes.

2) Remove squash from the boiling pot and let cool slightly on a plate. Scoop out the flesh (noodles) with a fork. The squash should flake out of the rind easily. Scoop all the way to the rind. Place the noodles in a serving bowl.

3) In a measuring cup, combine the olive oil, basil, garlic powder, sea salt, cayenne pepper and oil from the sundried tomatoes. Stir well to combine. Pour over the spaghetti squash noodles and toss to coat. Add the sundried tomatoes and walnuts. Serve warm.

Tip: The spaghetti squash noodles have a tendency to get cold quickly. You might want to warm your plates in the oven before plating. It would help keep the dish warmer longer while eating it. However, chilled leftovers are surprisingly delicious with grilled chicken.

How to make Steamed Spaghetti Squash

1 spaghetti squash

Tools: Cutting board, large sharp knife, steamer basket, large pot, a fork and a plate

Directions:

1) Wash the outside of the spaghetti squash and lightly dry it. Place on a cutting board. Make sure your hands are dry because when you cut into the squash, it is hard and dense and you don't want your hand to slip and cut yourself!

2) Slice it in half then cut each half into four pieces.

3) Fill the large pot with one inch of water and place the steamer basket inside the pot. Cover pot with a lid and bring to a boil. Arrange the squash pieces upside down on the steamer basket over boiling water. Cook on medium-high for 15-20 minutes.

4) Remove squash from the boiling pot and let cool slightly on a plate. Scoop out the flesh (noodles) with a fork. The squash should flake out of the rind easily. Scoop all the way to the rind.

Use spaghetti squash noodles in place of pasta. If you have a little plain spaghetti squash noodles left over, refrigerate and then reheat with a little butter, sea salt and ground black pepper. It's simple and delicious.

Recipes to try: Caul-it-Fredo, Chicken Pomodoro, Flavorful Spaghetti Squash Lasagna, Panzetti, classic Spaghetti and Meatballs and Savory Seeds.

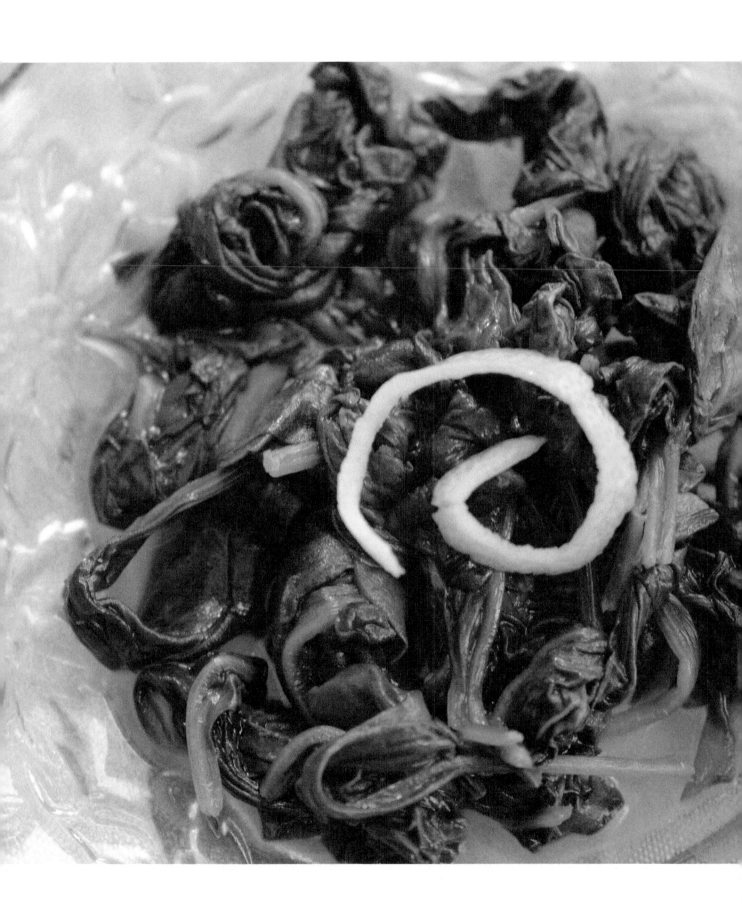

Superb Spinach

Gluten Free
Grain Free
Dairy Free

2-4 servings

- ⅓ cup chicken broth
- 8 cups fresh spinach
- 1 teaspoon extra-virgin coconut oil
- ¼ teaspoon garlic powder
- ¼ teaspoon Nature's Sunshine® sea salt
- Organic Lemon rind, for serving (optional)

Directions:

1) Warm broth in a stainless steel skillet for 2 minutes on medium heat. Add the spinach and cover with a lid. Cook for 3-5 minutes until wilted.

2) Turn off heat and add the coconut oil, garlic powder and sea salt. Toss to coat and serve immediately. Garnish with lemon rind or lemon zest, if desired.

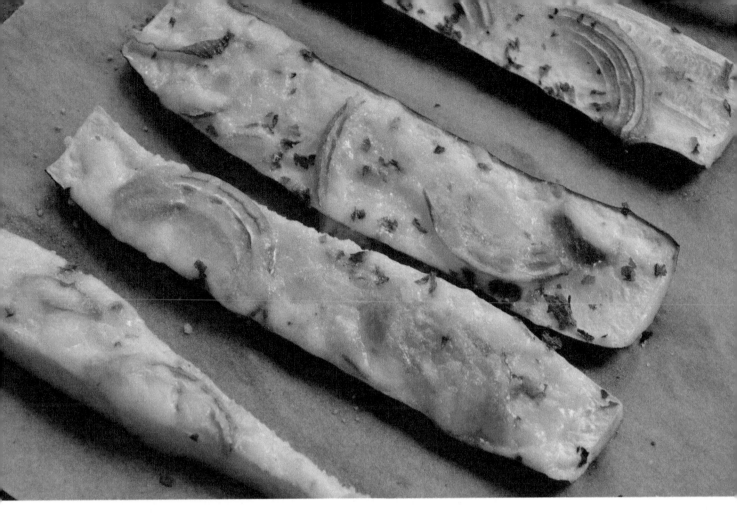

Zucchini Garlic Bake

Gluten Free

Grain Free

4 servings

- 1 medium zucchini (approximately 8 inches x 2 inches)
- 1 teaspoon grapeseed oil
- ½-1 teaspoon garlic powder
- ½-1 teaspoon dried parsley
- ¼ - ½ teaspoon Nature's Sunshine® sea salt, to taste
- Sliced red onion, as desired
- ¼ cup mozzarella cheese, shredded, optional

When served with an Italian dish it tastes like garlic bread. For dairy free, omit cheese.

Directions:

1) Slice the zucchini in ¼ inch slices and massage them really well with the grapeseed oil. Place in a glass baking dish or on a stoneware baking pan.

2) Season each slice with the garlic powder, parsley flakes and sea salt.

3) Top with the desired amount of sliced red onion and cheese, if desired.

4) Place in preheated 350 degree oven for 15-20 minutes. Serve immediately.

A cheerful heart is good medicine...

Her vibrant personality and invaluable help in the kitchen made some of my cooking and proofing days more enjoyable! Ruthie and I have had precious times traveling together to a Nature's Sunshine Convention, grocery shopping, going to estate sales for dishes and she was one of my stellar IN.FORM™ participants.

This saying is true; a friend knows everything about you and loves you anyway.

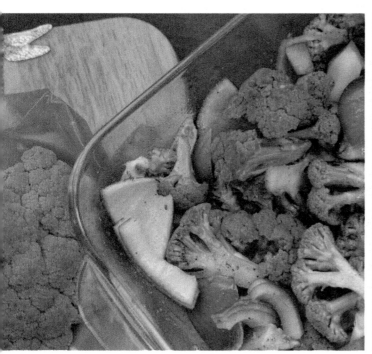
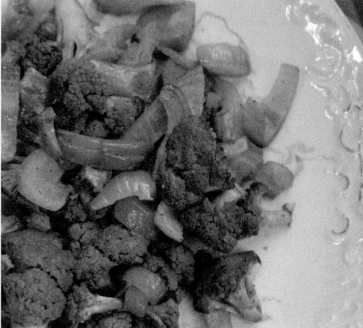

Vibrant Violet Veggies

Gluten Free
Grain Free
Dairy Free

2-4 servings

- **3 cups purple cauliflower florets**
- **1 cup red onion, chopped**
- **½ Tablespoon grapeseed oil**

- **½ teaspoon garlic powder**
- **¼ teaspoon Nature's Sunshine® sea salt**
- **Dash ground black pepper**

Directions:

1) In a 9x9x2inch glass baking dish combine all ingredients.

2) Mix well to coat. Bake in preheated 375 degree oven for 25-30 minutes, stirring once during baking.

These are amazingly delicious! Roasting makes all the difference in the taste!

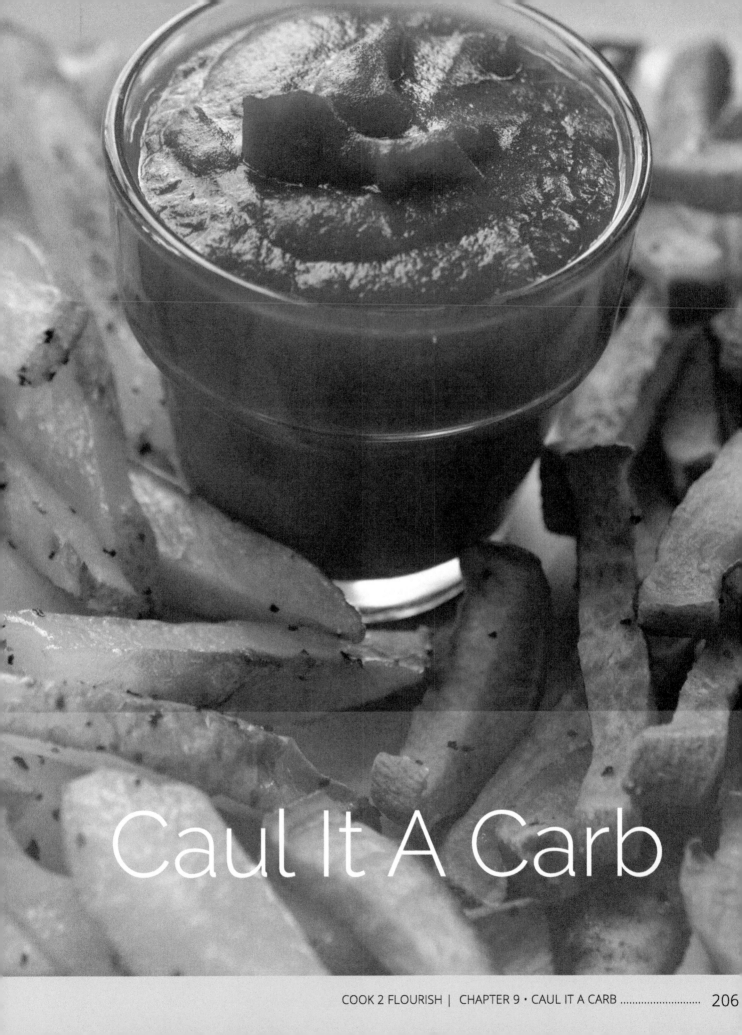

Caul It A Carb

Baked Fries

Gluten Free
Grain Free
Dairy Free

4 servings

- **3-4 medium large organic potatoes with skin, cut length wise into fries**
- **1- 1 ½ Tablespoons grapeseed oil**
- **1 teaspoon Nature's Sunshine® sea salt, to taste**
- **½ teaspoon ground black pepper, to taste**
- **½ teaspoon garlic powder, optional**

Directions:

1) Toss potatoes with grapeseed oil in a large bowl. Place a single layer on an unbleached parchment paper lined stainless steel baking sheet. Season with sea salt, pepper and garlic powder (if desired). Bake in preheated 350 degree oven for 25-30 minutes until golden brown. Serve immediately.

Sweet Fries

Gluten Free
Grain Free
Dairy Free

4 servings

- **2-3 medium sweet potatoes OR 1 (1½ pound) butternut squash**
- **1- 1 ½ Tablespoons grapeseed oil**
- **Nature's Sunshine® sea salt**
- **Ground black pepper**

> *Tip: Select a butternut squash that is less curvaceous. It will peel easily with a vegetable peeler and it will cut easier in lengthwise fries.*

Directions:

1) Sweet Potato – with skin cut lengthwise into fries.

2) Butternut Squash – peeled, seeded and cut lengthwise into fries.

3) Toss sweet fries with grapeseed oil in a large bowl. Place a single layer on an unbleached parchment paper lined stainless steel baking sheet. Season with sea salt and ground black pepper to taste. Bake in preheated 350 degree oven for 25-30 minutes until golden brown. Serve immediately with or without ketchup (page 251)

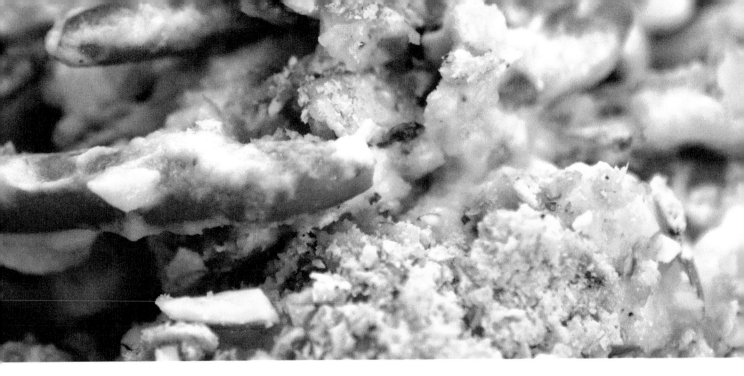

Green Bean Casserole

6-8 servings

- 8 cups green beans, fresh or frozen
- 1 ½ cups mushrooms, sliced or chopped
- ½ cup onion, diced
- 2 Tablespoon grapeseed oil
- ½ Tablespoon garlic powder
- ½ teaspoon Nature's Sunshine® sea salt
- ¼ teaspoon ground black pepper
- 8 cups cauliflower florets

- ⅔ cup unsweetened almond milk
- ½ teaspoon Nature's Sunshine® sea salt
- ¼ teaspoon ground black pepper
- ¼ teaspoon garlic powder
- 1 ½ Tablespoons organic butter
- ½ cup (3 ounces) uncured organic turkey bacon, diced
- ½ cup Crunchmaster® cracker crumbs
- ¼ cup almonds, coarsely chopped

Directions:

1) Rinse green beans if they have frost on them and snap into bite size pieces. In a large mixing bowl toss the green beans, mushrooms and onion with the oil, garlic powder, sea salt and pepper. Mix well to coat. Place in a 9x13x2 inch glass baking dish and bake in preheated 350 degree oven for 25 minutes. (Keep mixing bowl to use in step 5).

2) Meanwhile, bring water to a boil in a 2 quart saucepan with steamer basket in it. Steam the cauliflower over boiling water for 10-12 minutes. Drain the water.

3) Puree the cauliflower, almond milk, sea salt, pepper, garlic powder and butter in a high speed blender on high. Keep a firm hand on the lid since the contents are hot. Clean the sides of the blender once or twice if needed, then blend again. This makes 4 cups.

4) Pour the green beans, mushrooms and onions into the large mixing bowl and pour the cauliflower mixture over the vegetables, add in the turkey bacon. Mix well to combine.

5) Pour the casserole mixture back into a 9x13x2 inch glass baking dish coated with non-stick grapeseed oil spray.

6) Using a food processor, process approximately 22 crackers until they are fine crumbs.

7) Using a food processor, process ¼ cup whole almonds, until coarsely chopped.

8) Combine the crackers and almonds. Mix well. Sprinkle on top of the casserole. Bake in preheated 350 degree oven for 20-30 minutes until hot and bubbly and topping is lightly browned. Serve immediately.

Garlic Pasta

4 servings

Eat In Moderation

- 1 Tablespoon garlic powder
- 2 ½ cups Jovial® 100% Organic Einkorn whole wheat pasta, cooked and drained
- 1 ½ Tablespoons extra-virgin olive oil
- 1 ½ Tablespoons dried parsley
- 1 ½ Tablespoons grated parmesan cheese
- ¼ - ½ teaspoon Nature's Sunshine® sea salt, to taste
- 2 cups broccoli florets, steamed
- 1 ½ cups carrots, sliced, steamed

Directions:

1) Add to the warm pasta in the saucepan: the oil, parsley, parmesan cheese, garlic powder and sea salt. Toss to coat.

2) Add the steamed broccoli and carrots and toss again. Serve immediately.

Tip: This is a quick side dish to a piece of fish or chicken breast. If you have leftover pasta from another meal, warm the pasta in ¼ cup chicken broth and proceed with the recipe. Substitute spaghetti squash or spiralized zucchini for the pasta if you desire. Frozen peas are also a good compliment to the broccoli and carrots.

Mexican Pasta

4 servings

Dairy Free

- 1 garlic clove, minced
- ½ onion, finely chopped
- 1 ½ cups of cooked Jovial® 100% Organic Einkorn whole wheat spaghetti pasta
- ⅓ cup salsa OR Muir Glen® fire roasted tomatoes
- ⅓ cup red bell pepper, diced OR organic frozen corn, optional
- 1 teaspoon ground cumin
- 1 teaspoon taco spice (page 237)
- ¼ cup fresh organic cilantro, finely chopped OR 1 teaspoon dried cilantro

Directions:

1) When the pasta is nearly done, pour the frozen corn (if using) into the hot water for 5 minutes. Drain the pot and turn the heat to low.

2) Add the garlic, onions, your choice of salsa or fire roasted tomatoes, red bell pepper (if using) cumin, taco spice and cilantro to the pasta. Stir to mix and serve warm.

Tip: Before boiling the pasta, break into 2 inch pieces for easier eating. Substitute spaghetti squash for the spaghetti noodles. Serve with tacos.

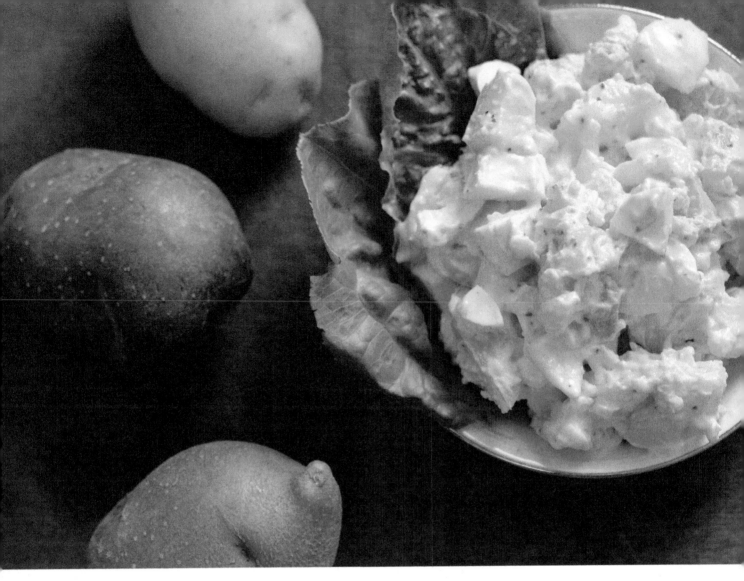

Mom's Potato Salad

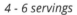

Gluten Free
Grain Free

4 - 6 servings

- 4 large boiled eggs, chopped
- 4 large potatoes, baked OR boiled, chopped
- ¾ cup organic Greek yogurt, plain whole milk
- ¾ cup Vegenaise®
- 2 Tablespoons prepared yellow mustard
- 1 teaspoon dried onion flakes
- ½ teaspoon Nature's Sunshine® sea salt
- ½ teaspoon paprika
- ½ teaspoon celery seeds
- ⅛ teaspoon ground black pepper

Directions:

1) Place the eggs and potatoes in a salad bowl along with the yogurt and Vegenaise®.

2) Add in the yellow mustard, onion flakes, sea salt, paprika, celery seeds and pepper. Stir all together until well combined. Refrigerate until ready to serve.

Note: Some traditional potato salad recipes call for pickle relish which contains sugar, vinegar and food colorings. IF you must have this in your potato salad, find a jar of kosher pickles without sugar or coloring added. Finely dice then stir into your salad.

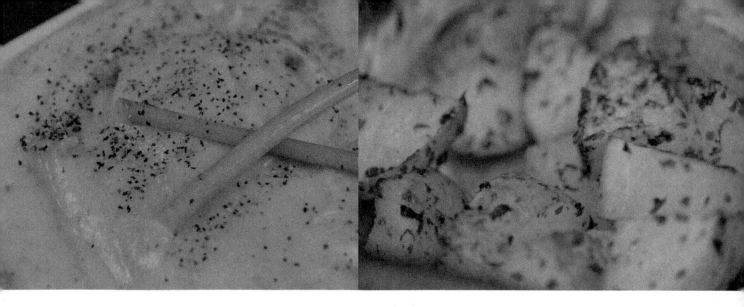

Caul-it-Tatoes

Gluten Free
Grain Free

4 servings

- 6 cups cauliflower florets
- 2 Tablespoon organic butter
- ½ teaspoon Nature's Sunshine® sea salt
- ¼ teaspoon ground black pepper

Directions:

1) Bring water to a boil in a 2 quart saucepan with steamer basket in it.

2) Steam the cauliflower over boiling water for 10-12 minutes. Drain the water.

3) Puree the cauliflower, butter, sea salt and pepper in a high speed blender on high. Keep a firm hand on the lid since the contents are hot. Clean the sides of the blender once or twice if needed, then blend again.

4) Pour into a glass baking dish and keep warm in the oven until ready to serve. More butter may be added if desired. These are best when served hot right out of the oven.

Note: If the blender is having trouble mixing the cauliflower, you may add 2 Tablespoons to ¼ cup of unsweetened almond milk to get the cauliflower to puree.

Garlic Spud Caul-it-Tatoes: Add 2 small organic potatoes with skin, russet or Yukon, ½ Tablespoon roasted garlic and ¼ cup unsweetened almond milk.

Herbed Roasted Potatoes

Gluten Free
Grain Free
Dairy Free

4 - 6 servings

- 4-6 organic potatoes, with skin
- 2-3 Tablespoons grapeseed oil
- 2 garlic cloves, minced
- ½ medium onion, chopped
- ¼ teaspoon ground black pepper
- ½ teaspoon Nature's Sunshine® sea salt
- ½ Tablespoon dried parsley
- ½ Tablespoon dried thyme
- 1 Tablespoon dried whole rosemary

Directions:

1) Cut up the potatoes into small chunks and place in a 9x13x2 inch glass baking dish coated with non-stick grapeseed oil spray. Pour the oil over the potatoes and stir to coat.

2) Combine the garlic and herbs together in a measuring cup then shake over the potatoes and toss to coat. Bake in preheated 350 degree oven for 40-50 minutes.

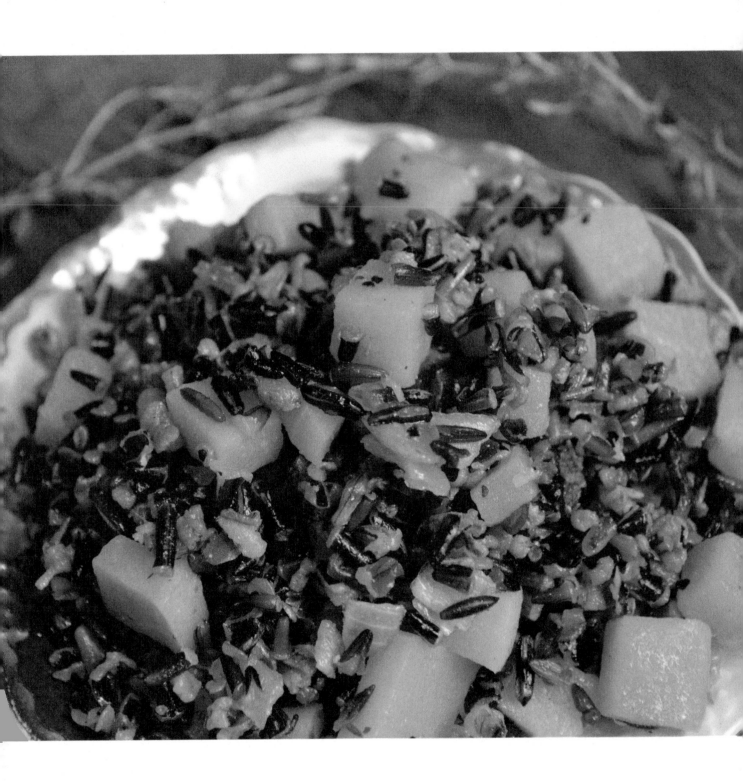

Wild Rice Butternut Pilaf

6 servings

- 2 cups of organic wild rice, cooked
- 2 cups butternut squash, diced
- ½ cup onion, diced
- ½ Tablespoon extra-virgin coconut oil
- ¼ teaspoon Nature's Sunshine® sea salt
- Dash ground black pepper

Dressing:
- 2 Tablespoons fresh squeezed organic orange juice
- ¼ teaspoon organic orange zest
- 1 Tablespoon extra-virgin olive oil
- 1 teaspoon orange thyme leaves, minced
- 1 teaspoon fresh sage, minced
- ⅛ teaspoon Nature's Sunshine® sea salt
- Dash ground nutmeg
- 4 drops liquid stevia

Directions:

1) Remember to soak the wild rice before cooking. Use approximately 2/3 cup dry to become the 2 cups cooked measurement. Keep warm.

2) In a large bowl, toss the butternut squash and onion in coconut oil, sea salt and pepper. Place on a baking sheet lined with unbleached parchment paper and bake in preheated 350 degree oven for 25-30 minutes or until fork tender.

3) In a measuring cup, whisk together the dressing ingredients. Pour dressing over the cooked wild rice. Then add in the roasted butternut squash and toss to combine. Simmer on low for 10 minutes and serve warm.

Tasty additions to the above recipe: ½ cup pecans and ½ cup organic apple, unpeeled, chopped.

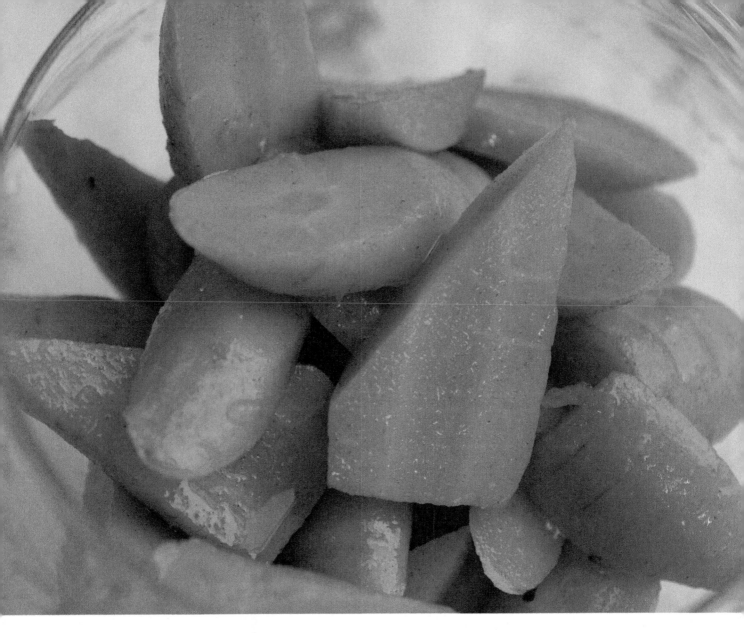

Cinnamon Carrots

....

4 - 6 servings

- 4-6 organic carrots, sliced
- 2 Tablespoons organic butter OR extra-virgin coconut oil
- 2 teaspoons raw honey
- 1 teaspoon fresh squeezed orange juice
- ¼ teaspoon cinnamon, to taste

Directions:

1) Steam carrots in a saucepan or cook with ½ inch water until tender, about 8 to 10 minutes. Drain.

2) Add your choice of butter or coconut oil, honey, juice and cinnamon. Stir to combine and heat until warm. Serve immediately.

For dairy free, omit the butter and use extra-virgin coconut oil instead.

Spotlight: Carrots

• •

Did you know that carrots are cousins of cumin, parsley, and parsnips? Furthermore, it is noteworthy that carrots come in a myriad of vibrant colors- purple, yellow, reddish pink, and orange. In fact, the orange variety is more recently popular whereas the other colors were eaten exclusively prior to the 1500-1600s. A true "eye candy," carrots are sweet and the beta carotene brimming within them nourishes the eyes. When eaten in tandem with healthy fats, the beta carotene is more absorbable, and it enhances the flavor (who wouldn't enjoy some organic butter on steamed carrots?).

Carrots can be helpful in supporting: the immune system, healthy eyesight, and cardiovascular health. Gratefully, even steaming carrots can provide beneficial amounts of beta carotene. In addition to their antioxidants, carrots offer a cascade of nutrients such as fiber, biotin, vitamin C, potassium, vitamin K, and molybdenum.

How to cook Quinoa

2 (½ cup) servings

• **½ cup quinoa**
• **½ cup chicken OR vegetable broth**

Directions:

1) Place the dry quinoa in a glass jar. Cover with 1 ½ cups filtered water. Let soak on the counter for 8 hours. Pour off the water and rinse well. Drain.

2) In a sauce pan, bring broth to a boil.

3) Add drained quinoa to the broth and stir to combine then cover with a lid and simmer on low for 6 minutes.

4) Look to see if the broth is absorbed. If yes, continue with your recipe. If the broth is not absorbed, then keep the lid on it and set it aside for 5-10 minutes. It should be absorbed and you should have nice fluffy quinoa.

> **Suggestion:** Use the quinoa in the Parade of Flavors Salad & in the Berry Kissed Quinoa Salad. (pages 108, 97)
>
> Benefits of soaking the quinoa: Quicker to cook, easier to digest and the nutrients are easier to be absorbed. If you didn't soak the quinoa, cook according to package directions (page 25).

Breakfast Quinoa:

Early morning rush hour: Bring ½ cup unsweetened almond milk to a boil then add the drained and soaked quinoa, stir to combine then cover with a lid and cook on medium high.

Cook for 3 minutes then remove from heat. Look and see if the milk is absorbed. If the milk is not absorbed, then keep the lid on it and set it aside for 3 more minutes. It should be absorbed and you should have nice fluffy quinoa.

If yes, then proceed with making your breakfast quinoa by adding in a dash of cinnamon and pumpkin puree with a touch of sweetness such as stevia, coconut sugar or raw honey. Stir in protein powder for added protein and sprinkle a few nuts on top.

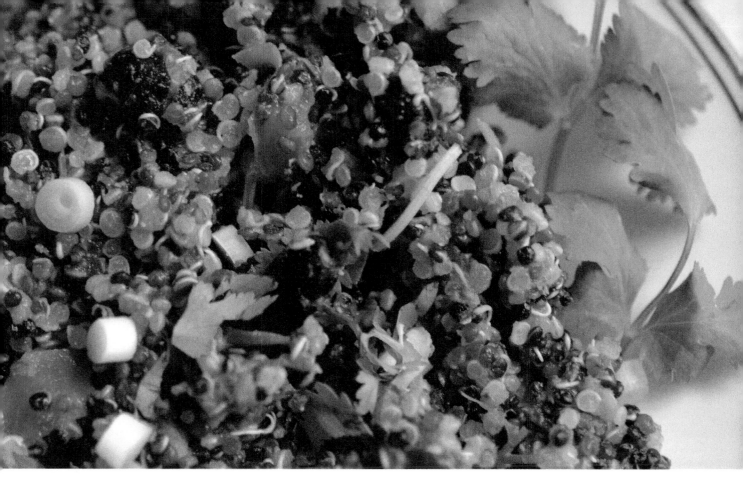

Fiesta Quinoa
. . . .

4 servings

- ½ cup soaked quinoa
- 1 cup chicken OR vegetable broth
- ½ teaspoon Nature's Sunshine® sea salt
- Pinch ground turmeric
- Pinch cayenne pepper
- ½ teaspoon smoked paprika
- ½ teaspoon garlic powder

- ½ teaspoon ground cumin
- ½ teaspoon fresh squeezed lime juice
- ½ teaspoon extra-virgin coconut oil
- 2 Tablespoons fresh organic cilantro
- 2 Tablespoons green scallions OR sweet onion, diced
- ¼ cup black beans
- ¼ cup red OR yellow bell pepper, diced
- ¼ cup Muir Glen® crushed fire roasted tomatoes

Directions:

1) Place the dry quinoa in a glass jar. Cover with filtered water. Let soak on the counter for 30 minutes. Pour off the water and rinse well. Drain.

2) In a sauce pan, bring the chicken broth to a boil. Add in the sea salt, turmeric, cayenne pepper, paprika, garlic powder, and cumin. Add in the quinoa and cover with a lid. Cook on medium heat for approximately 18 minutes or until the broth is absorbed.

3) Add remaining ingredients and heat through. Serve immediately.

Tip: If you soaked the quinoa overnight, reduce cooking time by 8-10 minutes and reduce the broth to about ¾ cup. If you find that after the quinoa is cooked and you have too much broth in it, just drain off the broth.

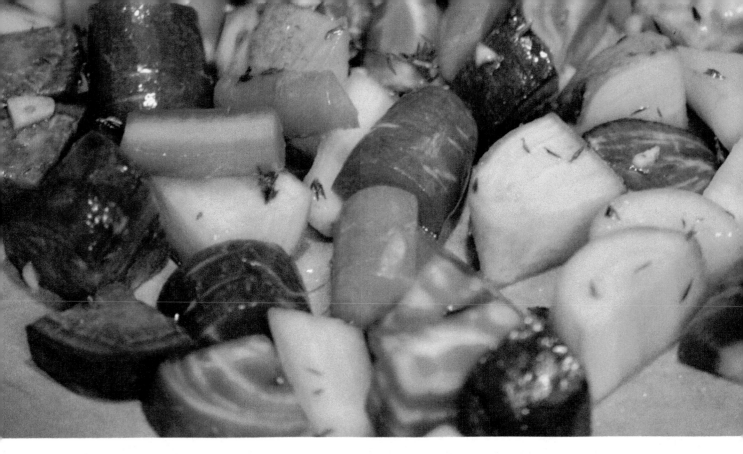

Getting to the Root of It - Roasted Root Vegetables

4-6 servings

- 4 cups rainbow carrots, golden beets and or purple sweet potatoes
- 1 Tablespoon grapeseed oil
- 2 garlic cloves, minced
- ¼ teaspoon Nature's Sunshine® sea salt
- ½ teaspoon fresh lemon thyme leaves only, no twig

Directions:

1) In a large 9x13x2inch glass baking dish combine all ingredients. Mix well to coat.

2) Bake in preheated 350 degree oven for 40-45 minutes, stirring once during baking.

"As you therefore have received Christ Jesus the Lord, so walk in Him, rooted and built up in Him and established in the faith, as you have been taught, abounding in it with thanksgiving. Beware lest anyone cheat you through philosophy and empty deceit, according to the tradition of men, according to the basic principles of the world, and not according to Christ. For in Him dwells all the fullness of the Godhead bodily; and you are complete in Him, who is the head of all principality and power." Colossians 2:6-10 NKJV

To be rooted is to be strong, but our roots must be deep and secured in the right soil. Just like a plant would not grow well in infertile or toxic soil, so we must be rooted in Jesus, abiding in the "true vine" (John 15:1). As a result, our lives will be fruitful and effective, as our roots deepen and tap into the Living Water (John 4).

Delectable Turkey Dressing

Eat in Moderation

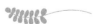

Serves 8

- 1 cup 100% whole grain dry bread, chunks
  OR dry leftover cornbread, crumbled (page 267)
- 1 ¾ cup organic long grain brown rice, cooked in broth
- 2 Tablespoons grapeseed oil OR organic butter, melted
- 2 cups organic celery, chopped
- 2 Tablespoons dried parsley
- 1 teaspoon ground garlic powder
- ½ teaspoon ground sage

- 1 Tablespoon vegetable herb seasoning (page 237)
- Nature's Sunshine® sea salt, to taste
- Ground black pepper, to taste
- 1 large onion, chopped
- 2 cups turkey meat, cooked
- ½ cup turkey broth
- 2 organic eggs, beaten
- 3 cups turkey broth, set aside

Directions:

1) Coat a 9x13x2 inch glass baking dish with 1 teaspoon of grapeseed oil.

2) Mix all of the ingredients in a bowl and pour into the glass baking dish.

3) Pour the 3 cups of turkey broth over the dressing mixture.

4) Bake uncovered in preheated 350 degree oven for 1 hour until the top is lightly browned.

Note: If several dishes are cooking in the oven at one time, this recipe may need more time to bake. Add more broth if the rice is getting too dry.

How to cook Brown Rice

Gluten Free
Dairy Free

4 servings

- 1 cup organic long grain brown rice
- 1 cup chicken broth

- ¼ teaspoon Nature's Sunshine® sea salt

Directions:

1) In a glass bowl or large glass measuring cup, combine 1 cup dry organic long grain brown rice and enough water to cover the rice by two inches (2-3 cups water). Soak for 8 hours or overnight. Drain and rinse the brown rice.

2) In a medium sauce pan, bring the broth and sea salt to a boil over medium heat for 3 to 5 minutes.

3) Add the soaked rice and cover with a lid, then let the broth come up to a boil again.

4) Keep covered and reduce heat to medium low, let simmer for 15-20 minutes or until broth is absorbed. Rice should be soft but not mushy.

Tip: If rice was not soaked, increase the broth to 2 ½ to 3 cups of broth or filtered water.

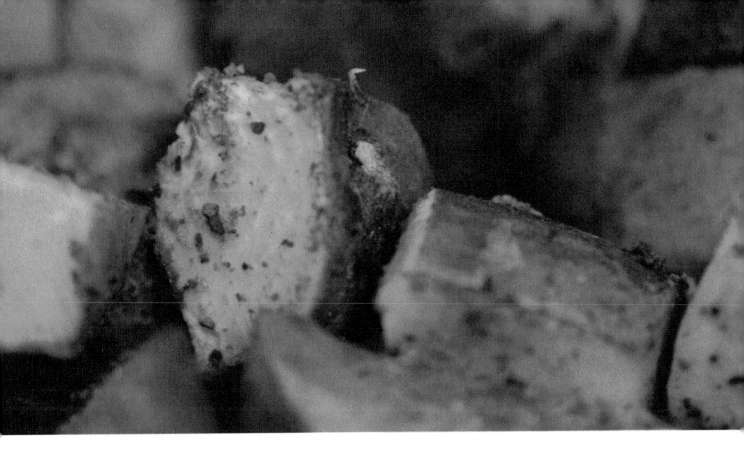

Coconut Baked Sweet Potatoes

4 servings

- 1 ½ Tablespoons extra-virgin coconut oil, melted
- 1 ½ Tablespoons unsweetened, shredded coconut flakes, optional
- 2-3 medium sweet potatoes with skin cut into cubes OR ¼ inch slices
- ½ Tablespoon cinnamon
- 1 Tablespoon raw honey, optional

Directions:

1) Cut up the potatoes into a mixing bowl. Coat a glass baking dish with ½ teaspoon of the melted coconut oil then pour the rest of the oil over the sweet potatoes. Toss to coat.

2) Sprinkle them with the cinnamon and add the honey (if desired). Toss to coat.

3) Pour the sweet potatoes into the baking dish and sprinkle with the coconut flakes (if using). Cover the dish with foil and bake for 20 minutes. Then remove the foil and continue to bake 10-15 minutes longer. Serve immediately.

Tip: If you're short on time, steam the cubed potatoes for 10 minutes over boiling water then bake uncovered for 12 minutes.

Fun snack for kids: Curly-Q Shoe Lace Potatoes: Spiralize sweet potatoes and follow the directions above. Omit the coconut. Bake 20-25 minutes total. Toss once during baking.

Did you know that cravings for sugar may decrease by eating more sweet vegetables such as sweet potatoes, butternut squash, onions and carrots? The naturally sweet taste and minerals they provide allow the body to be more satisfied and less apt to crave refined sugary foods.

Whipped Sweet Potatoes

4 servings

- **4 ½ cups sweet potato, with skin, chopped**
- **3 Tablespoons unsweetened almond milk**
- **½ Tablespoon organic orange zest**
- **3 Tablespoons fresh squeezed orange juice**

- **1 Tablespoon organic butter**
- **½ Tablespoon cinnamon**
- **½ teaspoon almond extract**
- **2 Tablespoons almonds, chopped**
- **1 Tablespoon unsweetened coconut flakes**

Directions:

1) Place steamer basket in saucepan with 1 inch of water and cover with a lid. Turn on medium heat and bring water to a boil. Meanwhile, wash and chop the sweet potato. Add potatoes to steamer basket and steam for 10 minutes. Potatoes should be soft.

2) Pour the sweet potatoes into a food processor and process until smooth with almond milk.

3) Add in the organic orange zest, orange juice, butter, cinnamon and almond extract. Process for 45 seconds.

4) Pour into a small glass baking dish coated with non-stick grapeseed oil spray.

5) Top with the chopped almonds and coconut flakes. Bake in preheated 350 degree oven for 20 minutes. Serve immediately.

This is a great accompaniment to fish, chicken or turkey.

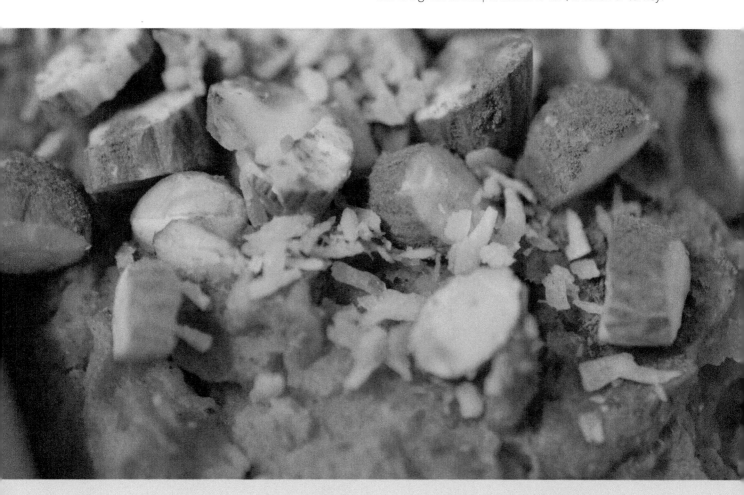

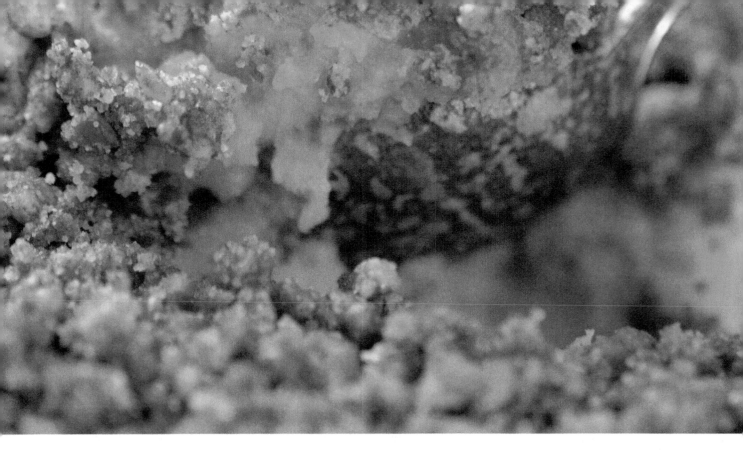

Butternut Pecan Crumble

4 servings

- 4 cups butternut squash, peeled, chopped
- 3 Tablespoons unsweetened almond milk
- 2 Tablespoons organic butter
- 1 Tablespoon raw honey
- ½-1 teaspoon cinnamon, to taste
- ⅛ teaspoon stevia

Crumble Topping:
- ½ cup pecans
- 1 ½ Tablespoons sweetener: raw honey, coconut sugar OR pure maple syrup grade B
- ½ Tablespoon fresh squeezed orange juice
- 2 teaspoons coconut flour
- 1 ½ teaspoons cinnamon
- 1 teaspoon extra-virgin coconut oil
- ¼ teaspoon organic pure vanilla extract

Directions:

1) Place steamer basket in saucepan with 1 inch of water and cover with a lid. Turn on medium heat and bring water to a boil. Meanwhile, peel and chop the butternut squash. Add squash to steamer basket and steam for 10-12 minutes. Squash pieces should be soft, when fork inserted comes out clean.

2) Pour the squash into a food processor and process until smooth with almond milk.

3) Add in the butter, honey, cinnamon and stevia. Process for 45 seconds.

4) Pour into a small glass baking dish coated with non-stick grapeseed oil spray.

5) Into the food processor add the pecans, your choice of sweetener, orange juice, flour, cinnamon, oil and vanilla. Process until coarse and well combined. Pour this crumble topping over the butternut squash puree then bake in preheated 350 degree oven for 20 minutes. Serve immediately. Refrigerate any leftovers.

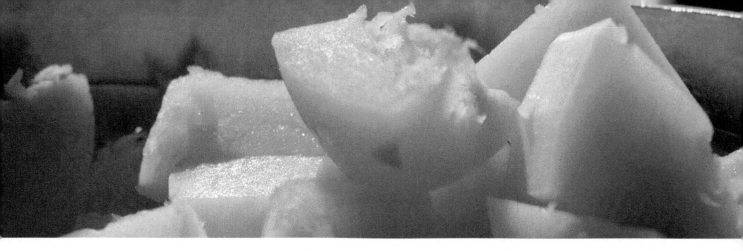

Squash for Dessert

4 servings

- ½ butternut squash, washed, seeded
- 1-2 Tablespoons grapeseed oil
- ¼ teaspoon stevia
- ¼ teaspoon organic pure almond OR vanilla extract
- ½ Tablespoon cinnamon
- 2 Tablespoons raw honey OR pure maple syrup grade B
- ¼ cup slivered almonds OR chopped pecans, to serve

Directions:

1) Coat an 8x8x2 inch glass baking dish with non-stick grapeseed oil spray.

2) Cut the butternut squash into ½ inch chunks then place into the dish and toss with the grapeseed oil.

3) Combine the stevia, your choice of extract, cinnamon and your choice of honey or maple syrup. Mix well and drizzle over the squash. Toss together to coat the squash.

4) Bake in preheated 350 degree oven for 30-45 minutes or until soft. Check after 30 minutes.

5) Five minutes before the dish is done, sprinkle with your choice of nuts and bake for 5 minutes. Serve with a main dish or as a dessert.

Refried Black Beans

4 servings

- 2 cups Crock-Pot® prepared black beans, cooked and drained (page 224)
- 1 teaspoon garlic powder
- ½ teaspoon onion granules
- ½ teaspoon chili powder
- ¼ teaspoon Nature's Sunshine® sea salt
- 1 teaspoon olive oil

Directions:

1) In a bowl, mash the beans with a potato masher.

2) Combine the beans, garlic powder, onion granules, chili powder, sea salt and oil.

3) Place the beans in an approved Green® non-stick skillet and cover with a lid. Cook on medium-low until warm.

Tip: Serve as a side dish to Mexican food or use in place of canned refried beans.

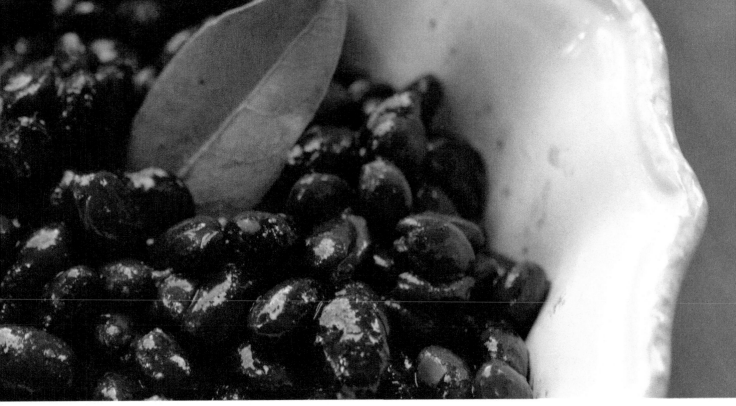

How to make Crock-Pot® Black Beans

*Makes *5-6 cups*

- **2 cups dry black beans, rinsed**
- **Filtered water**
- **1 teaspoon Nature's Sunshine® sea salt**

- **1 teaspoon dulse flakes (seaweed), optional**
- **3-4 bay leaves**
- **6 cups chicken broth and or filtered water**

Directions:

1) Place the dry black beans in a glass jar or bowl and fill with enough filtered water to cover by two inches. Let set on the counter over night. If using high alkaline water, you can soak the beans for 4 ½ hours and they will be ready to cook. (see Ratio below).

2) Drain and rinse the beans then place in the pot with sea salt, dulse flakes (if using) and bay leaves.

3) Pour in the chicken broth, water or a combination of broth and water to equal 6 cups.

4) Set Crock-Pot® to low and cook for 4 hours. If you cooked the beans in chicken broth, the beans and the broth will be delicious!

* 1 ½ cups dry beans became 5 cups after soaking overnight in high alkaline water. The 5 cups of soaked beans became 6 cups of beans after cooking in the Crock-Pot®.

* 2 cups dry beans became 4 cups after soaking 4 ½ hours in high alkaline water. The 4 cups of soaked beans became 5 cups of beans after cooking in the Crock-Pot®.

Note: It's best to cook the beans in a Crock-Pot® because they are considered to have more protein if cooked on low. If they are boiled and cooked at a higher temperature, they are more of a carbohydrate.

Tip: If you do not have homemade beans, simply add ½ teaspoon of ground cumin to the beans for added flavor and digestion benefits.

Caul-it-Rice

2 servings

• 2 ½ cups cauliflower, diced
• ¼ cup broth
• ¼ teaspoon Nature's Sunshine® sea salt, to taste
• Dash ground black pepper, to taste

Directions:

1) Dice the cauliflower into tiny pieces. Cook the cauliflower in a saucepan in the broth over medium heat for 6 or 7 minutes until crunchy tender or 8 or 9 minutes tender soft.

2) Season with the sea salt and pepper to taste. Serve immediately.

Caul-it-Rice can be served instead of a starch in your meal. Serve it instead of rice in a stir-fry or with chicken and vegetables. Tastes great when seasoned with Bragg® liquid aminos or coconut aminos.

Tabouli

2-4 servings

• 2 cups cauliflower, finely diced
• ½ cup black olives, sliced
• ½ cup onion, diced
• ¼ cup sundried tomatoes in extra-virgin olive oil, drained and chopped
• ½ cup fresh parsley, chopped
• 2 Tablespoons extra-virgin olive oil
• 1 Tablespoon Persian Lime flavor olive oil
• 2 Tablespoons fresh squeezed lemon juice
• ⅛ teaspoon Nature's Sunshine® sea salt, to taste
• ⅛ teaspoon ground black pepper, to taste
• Dash ground cumin

Directions:

1) Dice the cauliflower into tiny pieces. Place in a serving bowl along with the olives, onion, tomatoes, parsley, olive oil, lemon juice, sea salt, pepper and cumin. Mix well and refrigerate before serving.

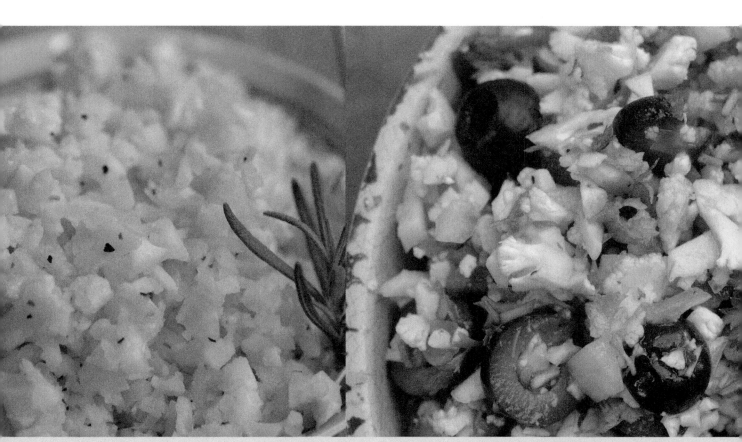

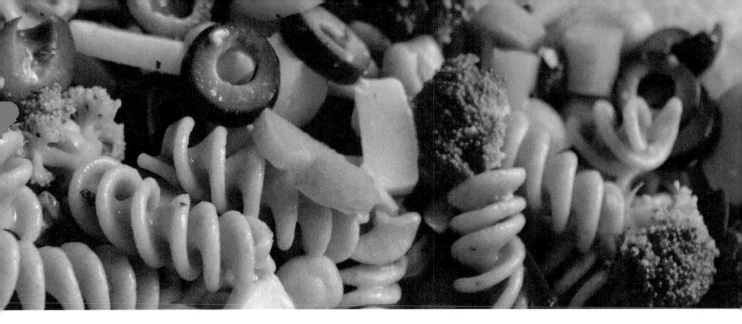

Make It Again Salad

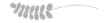

4-6 servings (serve warm or chilled)

Italian Vinaigrette Dressing:
- ¼ cup fresh squeezed lemon juice
- ¼ cup extra-virgin olive oil
- ¼ cup filtered water
- ½ Tablespoon Vegenaise® OR ripe avocado, mashed
- 1 garlic clove, minced
- 1 teaspoon dried Italian seasoning (page 240)
- ⅛ teaspoon ground black pepper
- ¼ teaspoon Nature's Sunshine® sea salt
- ¼ teaspoon stevia (21 drops liquid stevia)

Salad:
- 1 ½ cups dry pasta = 2 cups cooked
- 1 cup organic carrot, sliced
- 1 ½ cups broccoli florets
- 1 cup red bell pepper, diced
- 1 cup garbanzo beans, drained and rinsed
- 1 cup black olives, sliced (30 olives)
- ½ cup organic pepper jack cheese, diced

Directions:

1) Blend all ingredients for the dressing on high for 30 seconds until thoroughly mixed.

2) Cook pasta according to package directions. Scoop out of the hot water and place in a large salad bowl.

3) Blanch the carrots in the hot pasta water for 3 minutes, covered with a lid.

4) Blanch the broccoli in the hot pasta water for 1 minute, covered with a lid.

5) Remove the carrots and broccoli and place in the salad bowl.

6) Add the bell pepper, garbanzo beans, black olives and the cheese to the salad bowl.

7) Pour the Italian vinaigrette over the salad and toss to coat.

Tip: You could substitute spiralized zucchini for the pasta or omit the pasta all together.

If using pasta use: Jovial® 100% Einkorn whole wheat pasta or Jovial® gluten free 100% organic brown rice pasta. The salad is really good even without the cheese.

Refreshing Rice

4 servings

Gluten Free
Dairy Free

- ½ teaspoon garlic powder
- 1 teaspoon ground cumin
- Pinch cayenne pepper
- 2 cups organic long grain brown rice, cooked in chicken broth
- ½ teaspoon Nature's Sunshine® sea salt
- 1 Tablespoon fresh squeezed lime juice
- 2 Tablespoons fresh organic cilantro, finely chopped OR 1 teaspoon dried cilantro

Directions:

1) Add sea salt, garlic powder, cumin, cayenne, lime juice and cilantro to warm rice and stir. Serve immediately.

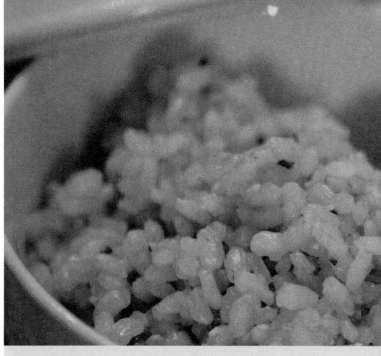

Refreshing Rice

Herbed Rice Pilaf

6 servings

Gluten Free
Dairy Free

- 1 cup organic celery, chopped
- ¾ cup onion, chopped
- 1 cup of organic long grain brown rice, dry (1 ½ cups soaked)
- 2 ½ Tablespoons grapeseed oil
- 2 cups broth
- 1 ¼ cups filtered water, divided
- 1 Tablespoon dried parsley
- ½ teaspoon dried thyme
- ¼ teaspoon rubbed sage
- ¼ teaspoon ground black pepper
- 1 teaspoon Nature's Sunshine® sea salt, to taste

Directions:

1) In a large stainless steel skillet, sauté the soaked rice, celery and onion in the oil over medium heat, stirring constantly for 5-7 minutes. Add in the broth, ½ cup of water, parsley, thyme, sage, pepper and sea salt. Cover and bring to a boil for 25 minutes. Add ½ cup more water and cook covered for 15 more minutes. Test to see if rice is tender. If not, add ¼ cup more water and cook 10 more minutes. When it is done, remove from the heat and let stand, covered, for 10 minutes. Serve immediately.

Scrumptious Spanish Rice

4 servings

Gluten Free
Dairy Free

- 1 ½ teaspoons grapeseed oil
- 1 garlic clove, minced
- ¼ cup onion, finely chopped
- 1 cup of organic long grain brown rice, rinsed and soaked overnight*
- 1 ½ cups chicken broth OR filtered water
- 1 teaspoon taco spice (page 237)
- ½ teaspoon ground cumin
- ¼ cup fresh organic cilantro, finely chopped OR 1 teaspoon dried cilantro
- ¼ cup salsa

Directions:

1) Sauté garlic, onion, and brown rice in oil over medium heat for 3 minutes.

2) Add the broth, taco spice, cumin and cilantro. Let simmer for at least 30 minutes. Add more broth or water if necessary until rice is fluffy and done.

3) Stir in salsa and serve immediately.

*Tip: if the rice was not soaked overnight, increase the broth or water to 3 cups.

Simple Scalloped Sweet Potatoes

2 servings

- **1 large sweet potato, with skin**
- **5 Tablespoons unsweetened almond milk**
- **½ Tablespoon organic orange zest, to taste**

- **2 Tablespoons organic butter**
- **1 Tablespoon cinnamon**
- **2 Tablespoons almonds, chopped**

Directions:

1) Place steamer basket in saucepan with 1 inch of water and cover with a lid. Turn on medium heat and bring water to a boil. Meanwhile, wash and slice the sweet potato into ¼ inch slices. Add potatoes to steamer basket and steam for 10 minutes. (Potatoes will continue to cook in the oven.)

2) Arrange layers of the sweet potatoes, almond milk, zest, butter and cinnamon in a small glass loaf pan coated with non-stick grapeseed oil spray.

3) Top with the chopped almonds and bake in preheated 350 degree oven for 20 minutes uncovered. Serve immediately.

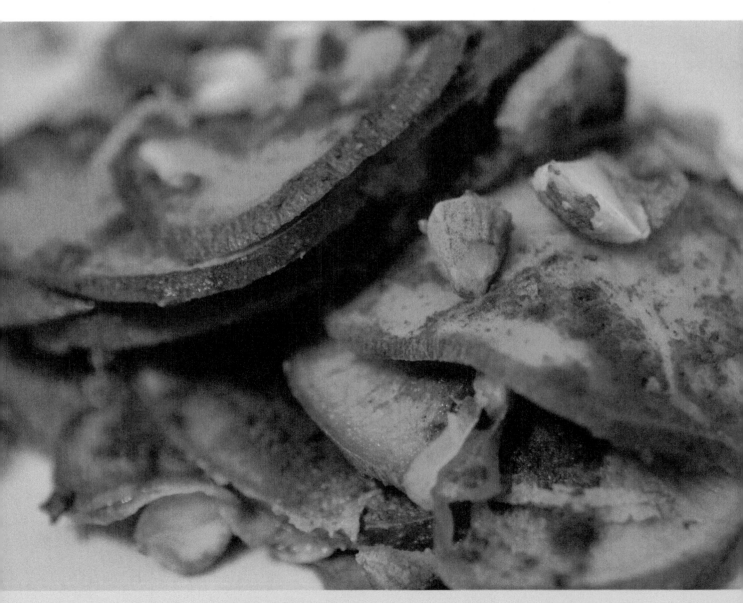

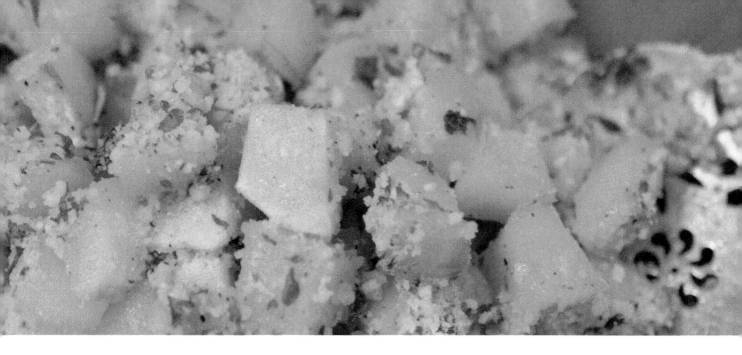

Butternut Bake

4 servings

Roasted Butternut Squash:
- 4 cups butternut squash
- ½ Tablespoon grapeseed oil
- ½ teaspoon Nature's Sunshine® sea salt
- ½ teaspoon ground black pepper
- 1 teaspoon fresh sage, minced
- ½ teaspoon garlic, minced

Almond Parmesan Topping:
- 2 Tablespoons almond flour
- 2 Tablespoons grated parmesan cheese
- 1 Tablespoon dried parsley
- ½ teaspoon garlic, minced
- ¼ teaspoon Nature's Sunshine® sea salt
- ¼ teaspoon ground black pepper

Directions:

1) Peel and cut the butternut squash into ½ inch chunks. In a mixing bowl combine the squash, oil, sea salt, pepper, sage and garlic. Toss to coat.

2) Place in a 9x13x2 inch glass baking dish coated with non-stick grapeseed oil spray.

3) Bake in preheated 350 degree oven for 25 minutes until the squash is tender.

4) Meanwhile, in a small bowl, combine the topping ingredients and stir well.

5) Remove butternut from oven and top with the almond parmesan topping then bake for 15-20 minutes, but be careful to not let it burn.

For dairy free, omit parmesan cheese and use 2 Tablespoons more of almond flour. Enjoy this topping on chicken, fish, broccoli, green beans or zucchini.

Butternut benefits: With its mildly sweet and satisfying texture, butternut squash provides a great alternative to sweet potatoes by only packing approximately 22 grams of carbs per cup. With a stellar nutrient line up starring Vitamin E, Vitamin B6, Magnesium, Manganese, and Potassium, butternut squash is certainly one of my favorite foods! For easiest peeling, select a squash that is as uniformly shaped as possible and the least curvaceous. Enjoy!

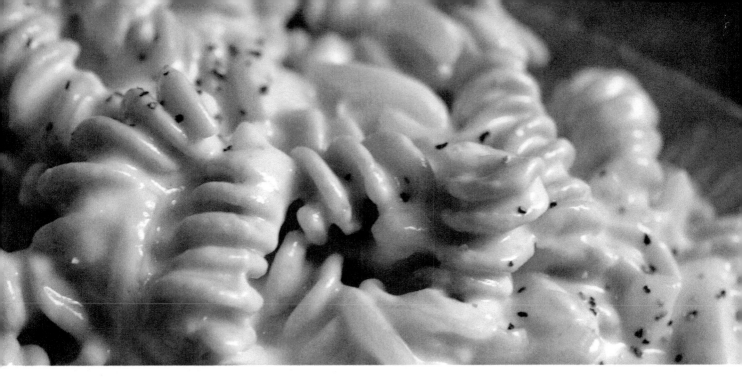

Mac N Cheese

. . . .

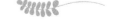

4 - 6 servings

- **4 cups cauliflower florets**
- **½ cup unsweetened almond milk**
- **2 ½ cups Jovial® 100% Organic Einkorn whole wheat spiral pasta, dry**
- **1 cup zucchini, peeled and spiralized**
- **3 ounces Applegate® Organics® organic cheddar cheese, mild**

- **3 ounces Organic Valley® Raw Jack style cheese**
- **⅛ teaspoon Nature's Sunshine® Curcumin BP™ capsule contents (for color)**
- **¼-½ teaspoon Nature's Sunshine® sea salt, to taste**
- **¼ teaspoon ground black pepper, optional**

Directions:

1) Bring water to a boil in a 2 quart saucepan with steamer basket in it. Steam the cauliflower over boiling water for 10-12 minutes. Drain the water.

2) Bring water to a boil in another saucepan and cook pasta according to package directions. Reserve the water for zucchini (if using).

3) Zucchini (if using), peel off the peeling with a vegetable peeler so there is no green showing. Place on a spiralizer and spiralize as though it were macaroni. You may need to trim the spirals to look like macaroni curls. Blanch the zucchini in the reserved pasta water for 4 minutes. Drain the water and add the pasta back into the saucepan and keep warm.

4) Puree the cauliflower, almond milk, cheddar cheese, Jack cheese, Curcumin, sea salt and pepper (if using) in a high speed blender on high. Keep a firm hand on the lid since the contents are hot. Clean the sides of the blender once or twice if needed, then blend again. This makes 2 cups.

5) Pour cheese sauce over the pasta and stir to combine. Simmer on low until ready to serve. Serve warm.

For a gluten free option, simply replace the whole wheat pasta with spaghetti squash or spiralized zucchini.

Tender Potato and Green Bean Dish

2 servings

- **2 cups green beans, frozen**
- **1 organic potato, with skin, diced**
- **⅓ cup chicken broth**
- **Dash Nature's Sunshine® sea salt**

- **Dash ground black pepper**
- **½ teaspoon Our Favorite Seasoning (page 238)**
- **1 teaspoon extra-virgin olive oil**

Directions:

1) Rinse green beans if they have frost on them and place in a small to medium stainless steel skillet. Snap the green beans into bite size pieces and add the broth. Add the potato. Cover with a lid and cook on medium heat for 10-15 minutes or until tender.

2) Season with sea salt, pepper, seasoning and olive oil. Toss to coat. Serve immediately.

> Tip: Use this same recipe for fresh garden vegetables when they are in season. Omit the green beans and potatoes and use yellow squash, broccoli, carrots, zucchini and onions.

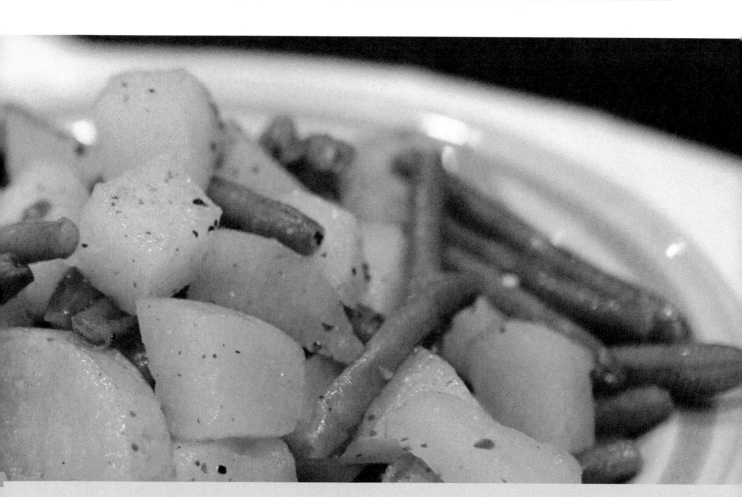

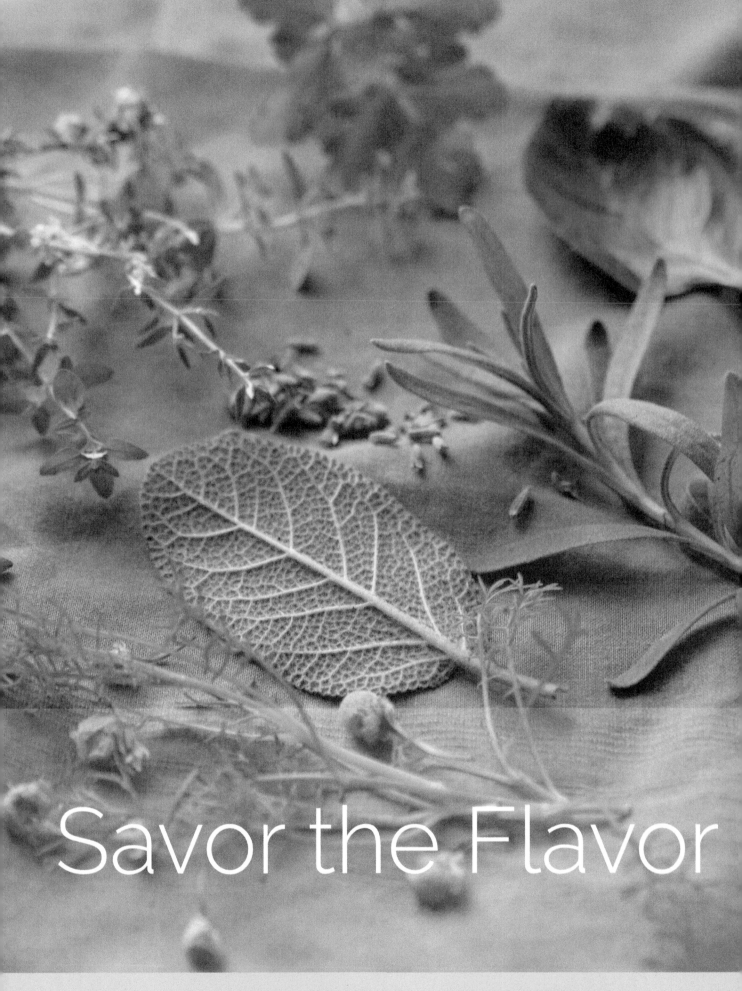

Savor the Flavor

Herbs for the Healing of the Nations...

....

"Fruit trees of all kinds will grow on both banks of the river. Their leaves will not wither, nor will their fruit fail. Every month they will bear fruit, because the water from the sanctuary flows to them.

Their fruit will serve for food and their leaves for healing."

Ezekiel 47:12 NIV

Flavor 2 Flourish

For maximum flavor and benefits, select herbs that are non-irradiated (if dried) or organic if fresh (or from the farmer's market). Dry herbs should last for 6 months to a year and some fresh herbs such as basil, mint, parsley, sage, and thyme can be frozen. Here are some notes and potential benefits of herbs and spices:

Basil

related to mint, great for digestion, stomach cramps, supports the immune system, and strengthens the lungs.

Garlic

has been shown to strengthen the immune system, has antifungal qualities even against candida, supports the heart and circulation, aids in detoxifying the body of heavy metals, supports the liver, and has been used to help with blood sugar balance, bronchitis, joint pain and more.

*Garlic retains more of its beneficial compounds when smashed and allowed to sit 10 minutes before cooking.

Cayenne

circulation, digestion, antispasmodic, metabolism, decongestant, repels the bacteria that causes stomach ulcers.

Cinnamon

blood sugar, circulation support, helps relieve intestinal gas and indigestion, inhibits candida proliferation, warming effect in the body, supports the heart, lungs and kidneys, and has an array of phytochemicals.

Ginger

cholesterol, circulation, anti-nausea, indigestion, anti-parasitic, anti-inflammatory, and may help diminish a fever.

Cumin

enhances digestion and discourages gas, may help headaches, and supplies antioxidants.

Mint

Cooling effect, helps soothe an upset stomach, calms nerves, and improves digestion of fats.

Oregano

decongestant, may help the skin, has been used to support digestion and relieve diarrhea, antioxidant, enhances the efficiency of insulin, antifungal, and antiviral.

Sage

antioxidants, enhances the efficiency of insulin, and has been used as a gargle for sore throats.

Paprika

anti-inflammatory, has been shown to provide phytochemicals, and may boost the immune system.

Tarragon

related to dandelion and daisies, supplies antioxidants, anti-inflammatory, antiviral, supports the liver, and boosts immunity.

Parsley

rich in Vitamin C, immunity, masks garlic breath, prevents carcinogins from forming on cooked meat, supports digestion, has a diuretic effect and aids kidney function, promotes detoxification, and encourages thyroid and adrenal health.

Thyme

(we all need more!)
has been used to ease sore throats and laryngitis, chest congestion, support digestion, anti-fungal, antioxidant, anti-inflammatory, and more.

Rosemary

circulation, memory, potent antioxidant, supports digestion, may help intestinal cramping, anti-fungal, and may reduce respiratory congestion.

Tumeric

related to ginger, anti-inflammatory, antibacterial, circulation, may reduce cholesterol levels, supports digestion, it has been used to help eczema, may ease carpal tunnel, may aid endometriosis, and its curcumin compound may diminish swelling and arthritis symptoms.

Nature's Sunshine® Sea Salt

Nature's Sunshine® Capsicum (cayenne pepper)

Throughout this book we use Nature's Sunshine sea salt and cayenne pepper to bring flavor and added nutrition to our dishes.

Nature's Sunshine® sea salt provides at least 50 trace minerals, including iodine which helps to balance out the sodium content of salt. The salt is sourced from Utah and is unbleached and unheated. It is combined with celery seed for extra flavor and benefits, and we were astonished when we began using it how much better flavor it imparts to dishes (Package of 2 shaker bottles).

Nature's Sunshine® Capsicum is thoughtfully sourced in regions that allow the pepper to develop its full spectrum of benefits and attain 35,000- 45,000 heat units (just the right amount). It comes in a package of 2 shaker bottles.

If you want to shake into action, www.n2flourish.mynsp.com is where you can get them!

Blackened Seasoning

Makes < ½ cup

Gluten Free
Grain Free
Dairy Free

- 1 teaspoon Hungarian paprika
- 1 teaspoon ground black pepper
- 2 teaspoons Nature's Sunshine® sea salt
- 2 teaspoons cayenne pepper
- 2 ½ Tablespoons garlic powder
- 2 ½ Tablespoons dried parsley

Directions:

1) Combine all the spices together and pour into a spice shaker.

Use: Season to taste. Sprinkle ½ teaspoon on a piece of fish. (If you use smoked paprika in this seasoning mix, it might taste like barbeque.)

Taco Seasoning

Makes 1/3 cup

Gluten Free
Grain Free
Dairy Free

- ½ Tablespoon chili powder
- ½ Tablespoon coriander
- 1 teaspoon onion granules
- 1 ½ Tablespoons Hungarian paprika
- 1 ½ Tablespoons ground cumin
- 1 ½ Tablespoons garlic powder
- ½ Tablespoon Nature's Sunshine® sea salt, to taste
- ¼ teaspoon cayenne pepper

Directions:

1) Combine all the spices together in a bowl and stir well. Pour into a spice container.

Use: Season to taste. Sprinkle 1 Tablespoon on 1 pound of ground beef.

Vegetable Herb Seasoning – Salt Free

Makes ½ cup

Gluten Free
Grain Free
Dairy Free

- 2 Tablespoons whole rosemary
- 2 Tablespoons onion granules
- 1 Tablespoon garlic granules
- 1 cup dehydrated soup vegetables blend

Directions:

1) Combine all the spices together in a high speed blender. Cover the opening of the blender with wax paper and put the lid on it. Pulse 3 or 4 times. Pour into a spice shaker.

Dehydrated soup vegetables blend is a blend of dehydrated carrots, peas, tomatoes, bell pepper, green beans, etc. but with NO added herbs, spices or flavorings that could contain gluten. Check the ingredient list! Dehydrated soup vegetables blend is available in the bulk spice and herb section of local health food stores.

Breakfast Sausage Seasoning

Makes ¼ cup

- 2 teaspoons smoked paprika
- 1 ½ teaspoons garlic powder
- 1 teaspoon ground cumin
- 1 teaspoon rubbed sage
- 1 teaspoon fennel seeds
- 1 teaspoon dried thyme
- ½ teaspoon onion granules
- ½ teaspoon Nature's Sunshine® sea salt
- ⅛ teaspoon ground black pepper
- ⅛ teaspoon ground nutmeg

- ⅛ teaspoon cayenne pepper
- ¼ teaspoon red pepper flakes

Directions:

1) Combine all the spices together in a high speed blender. Cover the opening of the blender with wax paper and put the lid on it. Pulse 3 or 4 times. Pour into a spice shaker.

Season to taste. Use 2 ½ teaspoons or more to your taste, of seasoning mix to ½ pound of ground meat.
½ pound makes 4 small patties.

Our Favorite Seasoning

Makes < ½ cup

- 3 Tablespoons dried whole rosemary
- 2 teaspoons dried parsley
- ½ teaspoon smoked paprika
- 1 Tablespoon dried red bell pepper
  (not hot peppers)
- ½ Tablespoon garlic granules
- ½ Tablespoon onion granules
- ½ Tablespoon basil
- ½ Tablespoon black, white and red peppercorns
- 1 teaspoon Nature's Sunshine® sea salt

- ½ teaspoon marjoram leaves
- ¼ teaspoon cayenne pepper

Directions:

1) Combine all the spices together in a high speed blender. Cover the opening of the blender with wax paper and put the lid on it. Pulse 3 or 4 times. Pour into a spice shaker.

Use: Season to taste. Season baked chicken, baked salmon or any fish, steamed vegetables, roasted potatoes, baked turkey or a pasta and vegetable stir-fry.

"Fruit trees of all kinds will grow on both banks of the river. Their leaves will not wither, nor will their fruit fail. Every month they will bear fruit, because the water from the sanctuary flows to them. Their fruit will serve for food and their leaves for healing."

Ezekiel 47:12 (NIV)

. . . .

Barbecue Seasoning - Spicy

Gluten Free
Grain Free
Dairy Free

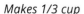

Makes < ½ cup

- 1 ½ Tablespoon smoked paprika
- ½ Tablespoon chili powder
- ½ Tablespoon ground cumin
- ½ Tablespoon garlic powder
- 1 Tablespoon coconut sugar
- 1 teaspoon onion granules
- ½ teaspoon ground coriander
- ½ teaspoon Nature's Sunshine® sea salt

- ¼ teaspoon ground turmeric
- Dash cinnamon

Directions:

1) Combine all the spices together in a bowl and stir well. Pour into a spice container.

Use: Season chicken pieces with desired amount of barbecue seasoning then bake or grill.

Barbecue Seasoning - Sweet

Gluten Free
Grain Free
Dairy Free

Makes 1/3 cup

- 1 ½ Tablespoon smoked paprika
- ½ Tablespoon ground cumin
- ½ Tablespoon garlic powder
- 1 Tablespoon coconut sugar
- 1 teaspoon onion granules
- ½ teaspoon ground coriander

- ½ teaspoon Nature's Sunshine® sea salt
- Dash cinnamon

Directions:

1) Combine all the spices together in a bowl and stir well. Pour into a spice container.

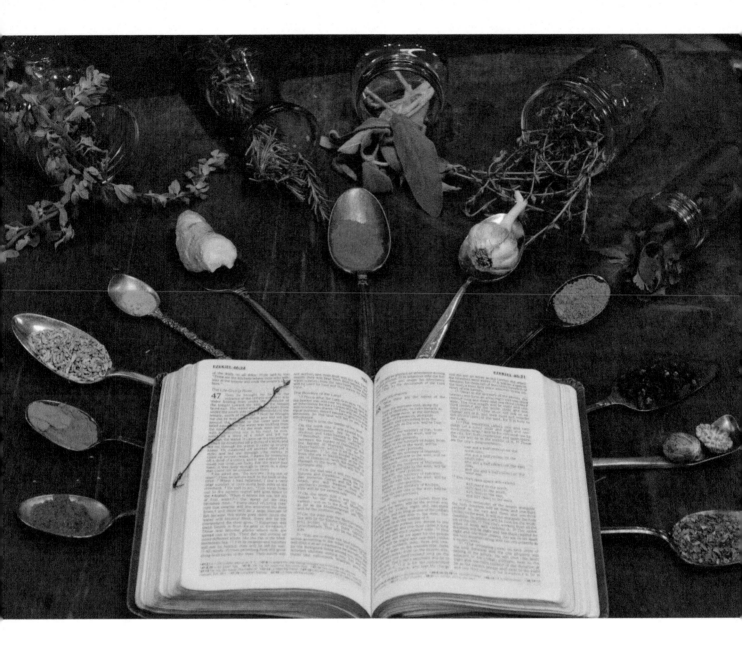

Italian Seasoning

Makes < ½ cup

- **2 Tablespoons dried whole rosemary**
- **2 Tablespoons dried oregano**
- **1 Tablespoon dried sweet basil**
- **1 Tablespoon dried thyme**
- **1 Tablespoon dried parsley**

Directions:

1) Combine all the herbs together in a bowl and stir well. Pour into a spice container.

Mesquite Seasoning

Makes 1/3 cup

- 1 Tablespoon + ½ teaspoon smoked paprika
- ½ Tablespoon garlic granules
- ½ Tablespoon onion granules
- 2 teaspoons ground cumin
- 1 teaspoon ground coriander
- ½ teaspoon Nature's Sunshine® sea salt
- ¼ teaspoon coconut sugar

- ¼ teaspoon ground turmeric
- Dash cayenne pepper

Directions:

1) Combine all the spices together in a bowl and stir well. Pour into a spice shaker.

Use: Season to taste. Sprinkle on chicken, burgers, beef with desired amount of mesquite seasoning then bake or grill.

Chicken Seasoning

Makes ½ cup

- 2 Tablespoons dried whole rosemary
- 2 Tablespoons dried parsley
- 2 Tablespoons garlic powder
- 1 Tablespoon Hungarian paprika
- 1 Tablespoon Nature's Sunshine® sea salt
- 2 teaspoons ground black pepper
- ½ teaspoon cayenne pepper

Directions:

1) Combine all the spices together in a high speed blender. Cover the opening of the blender with wax paper and put the lid on it. Pulse 3 or 4 times. Pour into a spice shaker.

Use:

Season to taste. Sprinkle on any chicken.
Bake it, fry it or grill it!

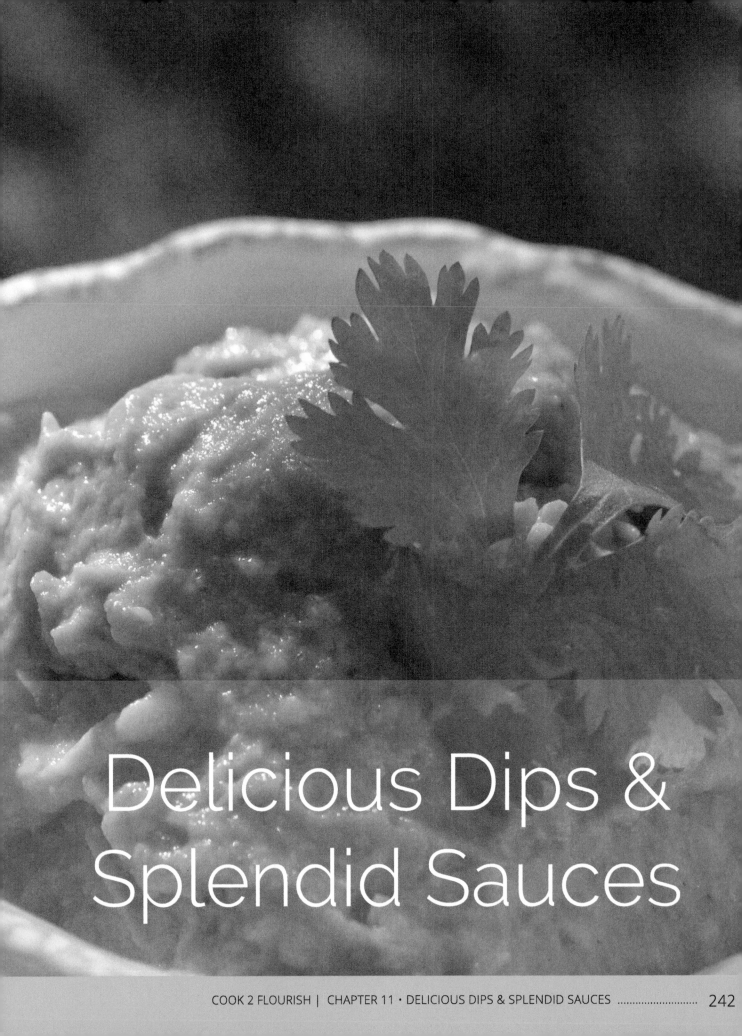

Delicious Dips & Splendid Sauces

Guacamole
. . . .

Gluten Free
Grain Free
Dairy Free

Shortcut Guacamole
. . . .

4 servings

• 1 ½ ripe avocados, pit removed and peeled
• ¼ cup salsa, homemade OR one without natural flavoring or sugar added

Directions:

1) Mash the avocado in a small bowl until creamy. Add in the salsa and stir to combine.

Tasty Guacamole
. . . .

4-6 servings

• 2 ripe avocados, pit removed and peeled
• 1 teaspoon fresh squeezed lime juice
• ¼ teaspoon Nature's Sunshine® sea salt
• ¼-½ teaspoon garlic powder
• 1-3 Tablespoons fresh organic cilantro, to taste

Directions:

1) Mash the avocado in a small bowl until creamy. Add in the lime juice, sea salt and garlic powder. Chop the cilantro and stir to combine. Serve immediately.

Jono's Authentic Guacamole
. . . .

6-8 servings

• 2 ½ avocados, pit removed and peeled
• ¼ cup onion, chopped
• 2 Tablespoons jalapeno pepper, seeded and diced
• ⅓ cup organic cilantro, finely minced
• ½ cup fresh organic tomato, diced
• the juice from ½ of a fresh lime
• ½ teaspoon Nature's Sunshine® sea salt, to taste
• ⅛ teaspoon ground black pepper

Directions:

1) Mash the avocado in a medium sized bowl until creamy. Add in the onion, jalapeno pepper, cilantro, tomato, fresh lime juice, sea salt and pepper. Stir to mix well. Serve immediately. Keep the pit of one avocado to put in the guacamole to help keep it from turning brown.

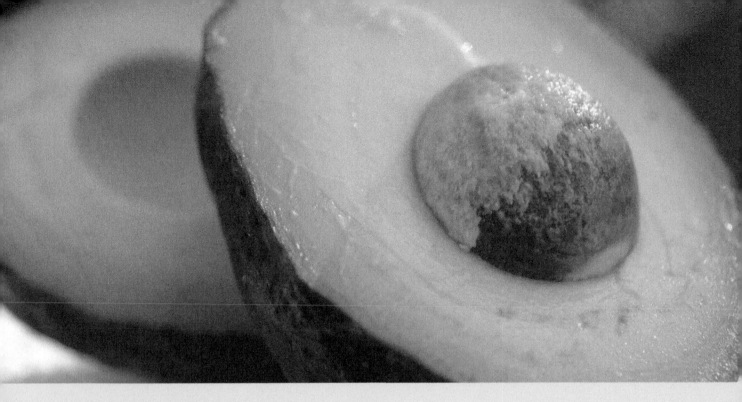

Spotlight: Avocados
....

One of my favorite foods since eating healthier is definitely the avocado! It is a food with an array of functions and nutrients; I often use it as my mayo, in place of cheese, and to give smoothies a delectable creaminess... and it hides under cover in pudding too. Shhh... don't tell anyone. Although avocados have been grown for thousands of years, they did not enter the scene in North America until the 1900's- they were missing out! When you add a few slices to your lunch wrap, on top of a salad, or a dollop of guac on your organic tortilla chip, here is what you are scooping up:

• Being a stellar source of fiber and healthy fats, avocados encourage a healthy blood sugar balance.
• Brimming with an array of antioxidants, avocados can help prevent excess inflammation and even provide vitamin E!

What's better than an avocado by itself? An avocado with leafy greens- the combination of the healthy fats in avocados paired with the beta-carotene in greens such as spinach is a dynamic duo for nutrient absorption!

Jono's Authentic Salsa Verde

Gluten Free
Grain Free
Dairy Free

Makes 2 ½ cups

- **6 green tomatillos, outer paper-thin skin removed, washed and quartered**
- **1 medium-large onion, chopped**
- **3 garlic cloves**
- **2-4 jalapeno peppers, halved and seeded**
- **1 Tablespoon grapeseed oil**
- **½ teaspoon Nature's Sunshine® sea salt, to taste**
- **1 cup fresh organic cilantro, loosely packed**
- **2 teaspoons fresh squeezed lime juice, to taste**

Directions:

1) Place the tomatillos, onion, garlic and jalapeno peppers in a glass baking dish and toss with the grapeseed oil. Roast in preheated 350 degree oven for 25 minutes.

2) Remove from oven and allow to cool for 10 minutes. Place the tomatillos, onion and garlic in a high speed blender along with the sea salt, cilantro and lime juice. Add in one or two jalapeno peppers at a time if they are hot and spicy. You might not use all of them.

3) Pulse 12 times for chunky salsa or blend on high 20 seconds for a creamy consistency. Taste first, and then add more jalapeno peppers, if desired. Serve immediately or chilled.

Taco Tuesdays

Jono, our jeweler, has expertise at the jewelry bench as well as making authentic Mexican cuisine handed down from his mother and grandmother. We love tacos and have come to enjoy our own "Taco Tuesday" in the back of our family jewelry store. Jono makes his guacamole and salsa verde and mom makes the tacos. What a delicious fiesta we enjoy!

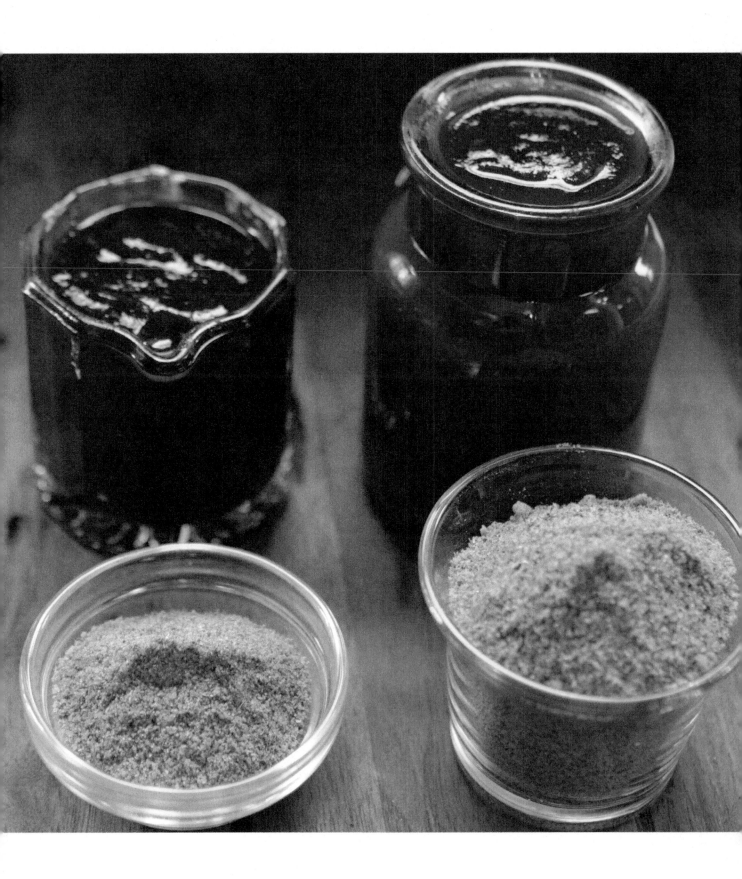

Barbecue Sauce - SWEET

Makes 1¼ cup

Eat in Moderation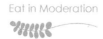

To make ½ cup Ketchup:
- **1 (8 ounce) can tomato puree OR sauce**
- **¼ teaspoon garlic powder**
- **¼ teaspoon onion granules**
- **¼ teaspoon Nature's Sunshine® sea salt**
- **1 teaspoon lemon juice**
- **2 Tablespoons coconut sugar OR raw honey**

The rest of the ingredients:
- **½ cup tomato puree OR sauce**
- **½ Tablespoon organic butter**
- **½ Tablespoon Bragg® liquid aminos**
- **1 Tablespoon Barbecue Seasoning - SWEET (page 239)**
- **2 Tablespoons apple flavored vinegar**
- **2 Tablespoons molasses**
- **2 Tablespoons lemon juice**
- **¼ cup coconut sugar**
- **½ teaspoon smoked paprika**
- **¼ teaspoon garlic powder**
- **¼ teaspoon liquid smoke, mesquite flavor**
- **Dash cayenne pepper**

Directions:

1) Combine all the ingredients for the ketchup in a small saucepan over medium heat. Bring to a boil, stirring constantly. Let boil for 2 minutes while stirring.

2) Reduce heat to low-simmer and cover just slightly with a piece of foil or parchment paper so that steam can escape. Let simmer for 20 minutes.

3) Uncover and stir. Reduce heat to low while adding in all the rest of the ingredients in order given. Bring heat back up to medium and stir constantly for 10 minutes.

4) Pour into a glass serving bowl. Serve immediately or refrigerate until ready to use.

Tip: If you don't have apple flavored vinegar, you could substitute a balsamic vinegar or apple cider vinegar.

Barbecue Sauce - SPICY

Makes 1¼ cup

Eat in Moderation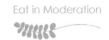

To make ½ cup Ketchup:
- **1 (8 ounce) can tomato puree OR sauce**
- **¼ teaspoon garlic powder**
- **¼ teaspoon onion granules**
- **¼ teaspoon Nature's Sunshine® sea salt**
- **1 teaspoon lemon juice**
- **2 Tablespoons coconut sugar OR raw honey**

The rest of the ingredients:
- **½ cup tomato puree OR sauce**
- **½ Tablespoon organic butter**
- **½ Tablespoon Bragg® liquid aminos**
- **1 Tablespoon Barbecue Seasoning - SPICY (page 239)**
- **1 Tablespoon molasses**
- **1 Tablespoon lemon juice**
- **2 Tablespoons Bragg® apple cider vinegar**
- **¼ cup coconut sugar**
- **½ teaspoon smoked paprika**
- **¼ teaspoon garlic powder**
- **¼ teaspoon liquid smoke, mesquite flavor**
- **⅛ teaspoon cayenne pepper**

Directions:

1) Combine all the ingredients for the ketchup in a small saucepan over medium heat. Bring to a boil, stirring constantly. Let boil for 2 minutes while stirring.

2) Reduce heat to low-simmer and cover just slightly with a piece of foil or parchment paper so that steam can escape. Let simmer for 20 minutes.

3) Uncover and stir. Reduce heat to low while adding in all the rest of the ingredients in order given. Bring heat back up to medium and stir constantly for 10 minutes.

4) Pour into a glass serving bowl. Serve immediately or refrigerate until ready to use.

This is really simple and quick to make!

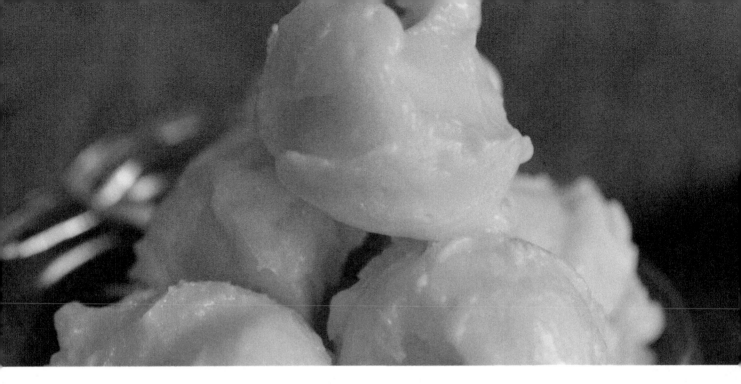

Better Butter

Makes 1 cup

- ½ cup extra-virgin olive oil
- ½ cup organic butter

Directions:

1) Place the oil and butter in a food processor and blend until smooth. Pour into a glass dish, cover and refrigerate until hardened. Use a melon baller to make butter balls for serving.

To make Garlic Herb Butter, simply add:

- ¼ teaspoon garlic powder
- ¼ teaspoon Nature's Sunshine® sea salt

- ground black pepper, to taste
- ½ teaspoon Italian herb seasoning (page 240)

Emerald Pesto

Makes 1 cup

- 4 cups fresh parsley OR basil
- ¼ cup filtered water
- 2 Tablespoons extra-virgin olive oil
- 4-5 garlic cloves

- ½ teaspoon Nature's Sunshine® sea salt
- ¼ cup feta OR goat cheese
- ¼ cup walnuts
- ½ teaspoon ground black pepper

Directions:

1) Place all ingredients into a food processor and blend until smooth.

Enjoy on top of soup for extra zing; on crackers, pizza, pasta or on spaghetti squash.

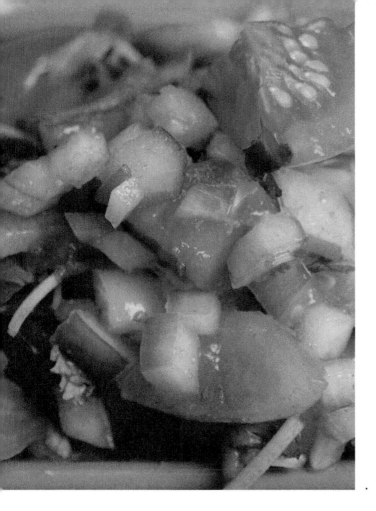

Garden Salsa

4 servings

- 1 small garlic clove, minced
- ½ red bell pepper, diced
- ½ green bell pepper, diced
- 1 large ripe tomato, diced
- ½ teaspoon ground cumin
- ¼ cup organic corn, optional
- ¼ cup onion, diced, optional
- 2 Tablespoons fresh organic cilantro, minced

Directions:

1) In a small mixing bowl add the garlic, bell peppers, tomato, cilantro and cumin. If desired, add the corn and onion. Mix well to combine.

2) Refrigerate or serve immediately.

Quick Pico de Gallo

4-6 servings

- ½ cup onion, diced
- ⅛ teaspoon ground black pepper
- ¼ cup fresh organic cilantro, minced
- ½ -1 jalapeno pepper, seeded and diced
- 2 Tablespoons fresh squeezed lime juice
- ¼ - ½ teaspoon Nature's Sunshine® sea salt, to taste
- ½ teaspoon garlic powder, optional
- 1 large ripe organic tomato, diced (½ - ¾ cup)

Directions:

1) Mix ingredients well to combine. Serve immediately or refrigerate until ready to serve.

Salsa Bravo

Makes 1 1/4 cups

- ¼ cup onion
- 2 garlic cloves
- 1 ½ cups organic tomato, diced OR 1 (14.5 ounce) can Muir Glen® Fire Roasted • tomatoes 1/2 cup fresh organic cilantro, loosely packed
- ⅛ teaspoon cayenne pepper
- 1 teaspoon ground cumin
- ½-1 teaspoon Nature's Sunshine® sea salt, to taste
- 1 teaspoon fresh squeezed lime juice, optional

Directions:

1) In a small mixing bowl add the garlic, bell peppers, tomato, cilantro and cumin. If desired, add the corn and onion. Mix well to combine.

2) Refrigerate or serve immediately.

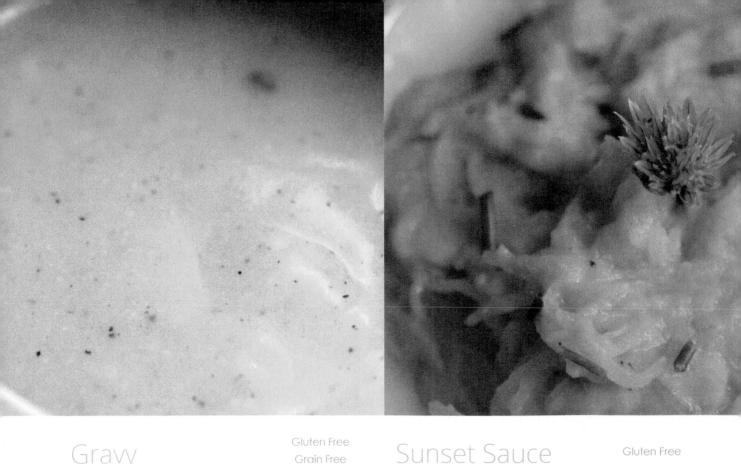

Gravy

Makes 1 cup

- 1 Tablespoon organic butter, no substitutes
- 1 ½ Tablespoons garbanzo bean flour
- 1 cup broth
- 1 Tablespoon arrowroot powder

Directions:

1) In a stainless steel skillet over medium heat, sauté the butter and garbanzo flour together to make a roux. Use a whisk or a fork.

2) Pour in the broth while stirring the roux, stir together for 2 minutes.

3) Remove ¼ cup of the roux mixture and sift the arrowroot into it and stir well to combine. Then pour the roux back into the skillet and continue stirring for 1 or 2 minutes or until thick. Serve immediately.

Tip: The more flavorful the broth, the more flavorful your gravy will be. If your broth is not flavorful then you may want to add Nature's Sunshine® sea salt and ground black pepper to taste.

Sunset Sauce

Makes 1 cup

- 8 roasted garlic cloves
- ½ cup roasted onion
- ⅔ cup roasted carrots
- 1 Tablespoon avocado OR grapeseed oil
- 1 cup unsweetened almond milk
- ½ teaspoon Nature's Sunshine® sea salt
- Dash ground black pepper
- ½ teaspoon fresh sage
- ½ teaspoon fresh chives, optional

Directions:

1) Toss the garlic, onion and carrots in the oil and roast in a glass baking dish for 45 minutes.

2) Remove from the oven and cool for a few minutes then place in a high speed blender along with the almond milk, sea salt, pepper, sage and chives (if desired). Process until smooth and creamy.

Suggestions:

Serve over spaghetti squash or Einkorn pasta.

Ketchup

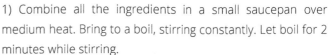

Makes ½ cup

- 1 (8 ounce) can tomato puree OR sauce
- ¼ teaspoon garlic powder
- ¼ teaspoon onion granules
- ¼ teaspoon Nature's Sunshine® sea salt
- 1 teaspoon fresh squeezed lemon juice
- 2 Tablespoons coconut sugar OR raw honey

Directions:

1) Combine all the ingredients in a small saucepan over medium heat. Bring to a boil, stirring constantly. Let boil for 2 minutes while stirring.

2) Reduce heat to low simmer and cover slightly with a piece of foil or parchment paper so that steam can escape. Let simmer for 20 minutes. Uncover and stir, cover slightly again and simmer for 10 more minutes. Pour into a glass serving bowl. Serve immediately or refrigerate until ready to use.
This is really simple and quick to make!

Mexican Dip

Makes ½ cup

- ¼ cup Vegenaise®
- ¼ cup organic Greek yogurt, plain whole milk
- ¼ teaspoon cayenne pepper
- ½ teaspoon taco seasoning (page 237)
- ½ teaspoon dried onion flakes
- ½ teaspoon dried cilantro or 1 Tablespoon fresh
- ½ teaspoon ground ginger

Directions:

1) Mix all ingredients together and serve with veggies or organic blue corn chips.

> The ginger adds an additional kick and is very good in this dip. See page 234 for nutritional benefits of ginger. Also try Marvelous Mexican Dip (Satisfying Snacks page 86-87)

Tuna Salad

4-6 servings

- ¾ cup garbanzo beans, drained, rinsed and mashed
- 2 (3 ounce) cans skip jack chunk light tuna in water, drained
- ¼ cup organic celery, diced
- ¼ cup Vegenaise®
- ¼ cup organic Greek yogurt, plain whole milk
- 1 teaspoon celery seeds
- ½ Tablespoon sesame seeds, optional
- 1 Tablespoon dried onion flakes
- Dash Nature's Sunshine® sea salt
- Dash cayenne pepper, optional

Directions:

1) Stir all ingredients until combined. Refrigerate or serve immediately.

Tip: Serve as a sandwich, lettuce wrap or as a dip with vegetables sticks or Crunchmaster® multi-grain crackers. Two boiled eggs could also be added to the recipe.

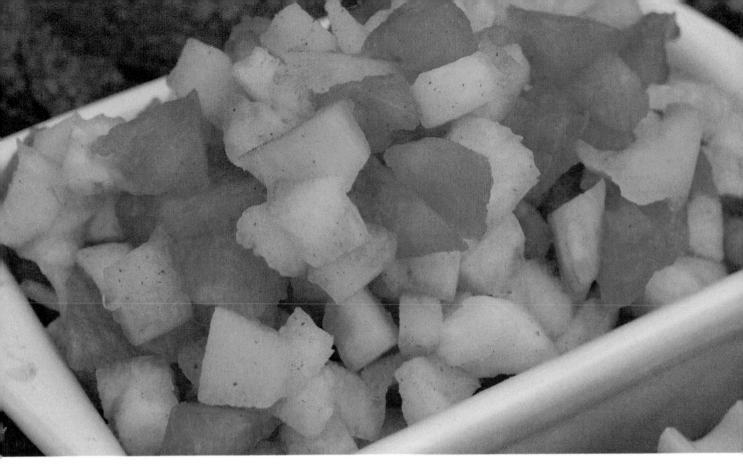

Melon Salsa

4-6 servings

- 1 cup watermelon
- 1 cup cantaloupe
- 1 cup fresh pineapple
- ¼ teaspoon cinnamon

Directions:

1) Dice the watermelon, cantaloupe and pineapple into a small mixing bowl. Add the cinnamon and mix well to combine. Serve immediately or refrigerate until ready to serve. Serve with sliced cucumber, sliced raw sweet potato, celery or organic blue corn chips.

Fiesta Fruit Salsa

6-8 servings

- 2 ½ cups organic apples with peeling
- 1 cup fresh pineapple
- 4 fresh strawberries, diced
- ½ teaspoon cinnamon

Directions:

1) Wash, core and dice the apples into a small mixing bowl. Dice the pineapple and strawberries. Add the cinnamon and mix well to combine. Serve immediately or refrigerate until ready to serve.

Tip: Substitute 2 Kiwis, peeled and diced for the pineapple.

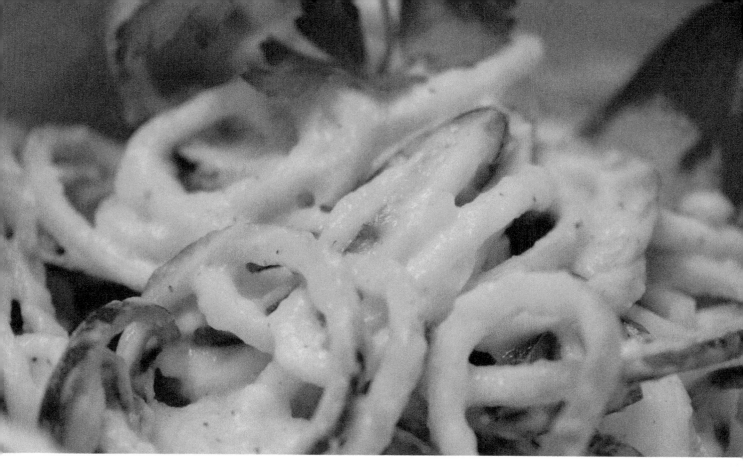

Caul-it-Fredo Sauce – Parmesan Cheese

Gluten Free
Grain Free

Makes 2 ½ cups

- **4 cups cauliflower florets**
- **½ cup unsweetened almond milk**
- **½ - ¾ cup grated parmesan cheese**

- **3 ounces Organic Valley® Raw Jack style cheese**
- **¼-½ teaspoon Nature's Sunshine® sea salt, to taste**
- **¼ teaspoon ground black pepper**

Directions:

1) Bring water to a boil in a 2 quart saucepan with steamer basket in it. Steam the cauliflower over boiling water for 10-12 minutes. Drain the water.

2) Puree the cauliflower, almond milk, parmesan cheese, Jack cheese, sea salt and pepper in a high speed blender on high. Keep a firm hand on the lid since the contents are hot. Clean the sides of the blender once or twice if needed, then blend again.

3) Simmer on low until ready to serve. Serve warm.

Serve over Jovial® 100% organic whole wheat pasta with chicken and steamed broccoli. Serve over steamed spiralized zucchini. Use in any casserole recipe that requires a creamy cheese base and season as desired.

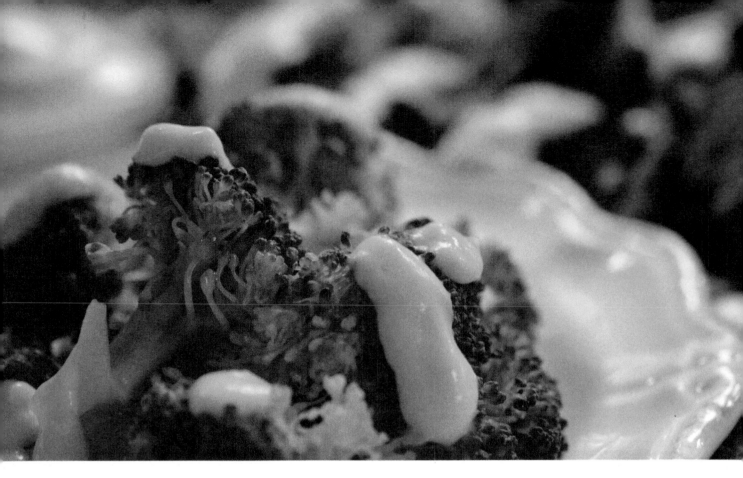

Cheese Dip/Sauce

Makes 2 ½ cups

- **4 cups cauliflower florets**
- **½ cup unsweetened almond milk**
- **3 ounces Organic Valley® Raw Jack style cheese**

- **3 ounces Applegate® Organics® organic cheddar cheese, mild**
- **¼ teaspoon garlic powder**
- **⅛ teaspoon Nature's Sunshine® CurcuminBP™ capsule contents (for color)**
- **¼-½ teaspoon Nature's Sunshine® sea salt, to taste**

Directions:

1) Bring water to a boil in a 2 quart saucepan with steamer basket in it. Steam the cauliflower over boiling water for 10-12 minutes. Drain the water.

2) Puree the cauliflower, almond milk, cheddar cheese, Jack cheese, CurcuminBP™, sea salt and garlic powder in a high speed blender on high for 30-40 seconds. Keep a firm hand on the lid since the contents are hot. Clean the sides of the blender once or twice if needed, then blend again.

3) Simmer on low until ready to serve or place in a mini Crock-Pot®. Serve warm.

Uses: Drizzle over organic corn chips for nachos. Drizzle over enchiladas. Serve on steamed broccoli or steamed veggies. Use in any casserole recipe that requires a creamy cheese base and season as desired.

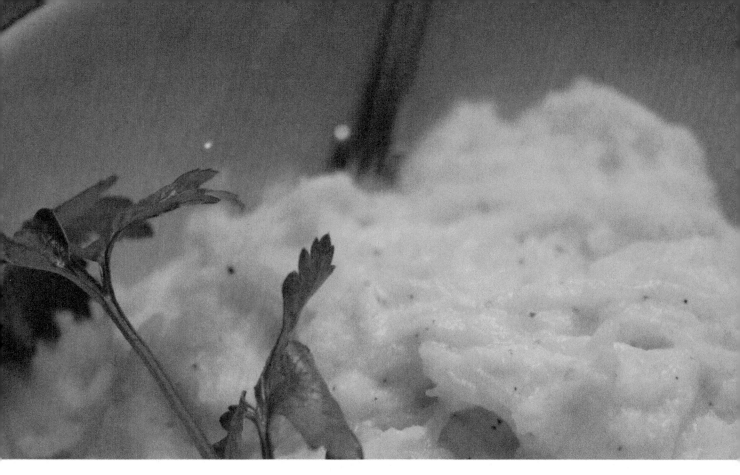

Caul-it-Fredo Sauce

Gluten Free

Grain Free

Makes 2 cups

- 4 cups cauliflower florets
- 4 garlic cloves, minced
- 2 Tablespoon organic butter

- ½ cup unsweetened almond milk
- ½ teaspoon Nature's Sunshine® sea salt
- ½ teaspoon ground black pepper

Directions:

1) Bring water to a boil in a 2 quart saucepan with steamer basket in it.

2) Steam the cauliflower for 12 minutes. Drain the water.

3) In a small saucepan over medium-low heat, sauté the garlic and butter together for 2 or 3 minutes.

4) Puree the cauliflower, garlic and butter, milk, sea salt and pepper in a high speed blender on high. Keep a firm hand on the lid since the contents are hot. Clean the sides of the blender once or twice if needed, then blend again.

5) Pour back into the saucepan and keep warm until ready to serve.

Caul-it-Fredo Sauce is great over spaghetti squash, in chicken pot pie, a cream sauce over new potatoes and garden peas, or in recipes that call for mushroom soup.

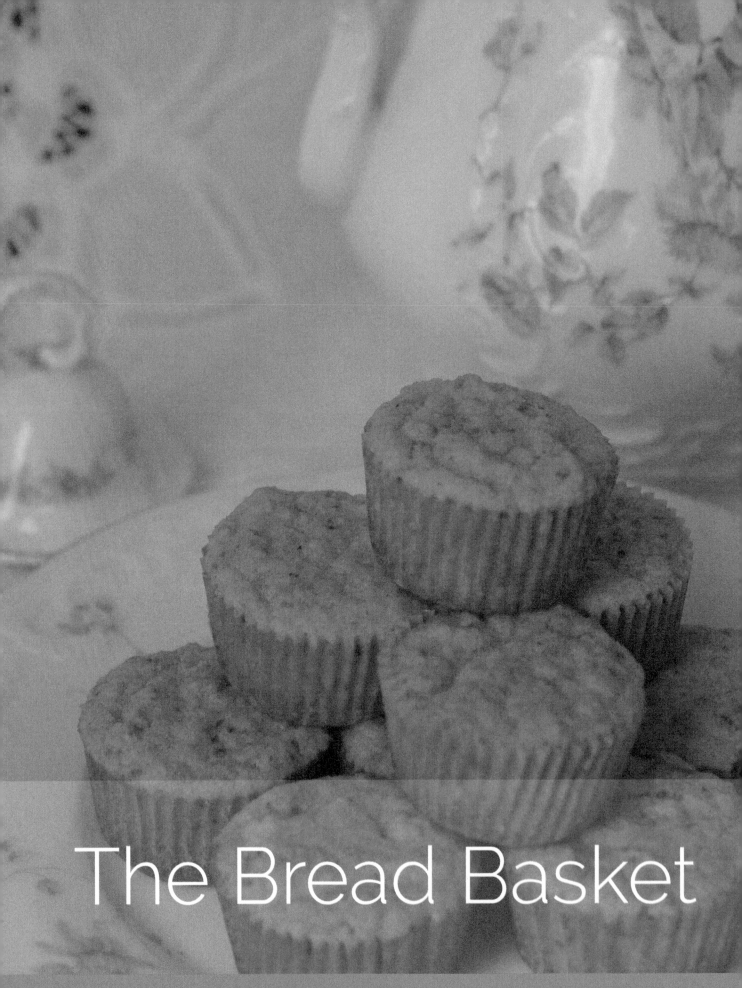

The Bread Basket

Lemon Chia Seed Muffins

. . . .

Makes 3 dozen mini muffins

- ¾ cup yellow squash, steamed (1 small squash)
- ¼ cup coconut oil, melted
- 4 organic eggs
- 1 Tablespoon fresh squeezed lemon juice
- 1 teaspoon organic pure lemon extract
- 1 teaspoon organic pure vanilla extract
- 2 Tablespoons raw coconut nectar OR raw honey

- 1 cup unsweetened almond milk, divided
- ½ cup coconut flour
- ⅔ cup Love and Peas® protein powder
- 2 Tablespoons chia seeds
- 1 teaspoon baking powder
- ½ teaspoon Nature's Sunshine® sea salt
- ½ teaspoon stevia
- ¼ teaspoon baking soda

Directions:

1) After steaming the squash in a steamer basket, place it in the food processor along with ¼ cup of the almond milk. Puree for 45 seconds. Measure out 1 cup of the puree for this recipe.

2) To the food processor, add the 1 cup of squash puree, melted coconut oil, eggs, lemon juice, lemon extract, vanilla extract, your choice of raw coconut nectar or raw honey and the remaining ¾ cup of almond milk. Process for 30 seconds.

3) Add in the coconut flour, protein powder, chia seeds, baking powder, sea salt, stevia and baking soda.
Process 30 seconds.

4) Pour into unbleached mini muffin liners in a stainless steel muffin pan or use a stoneware muffin pan only! Bake in preheated 350 degree oven for 20-25 minutes or until toothpick inserted comes out clean. Refrigerate any leftovers.

My family has no idea these have yellow squash in them! They are delicious!
If you want these to be more like a dessert, add 2 more Tablespoons of raw coconut nectar or raw honey for sweetness.

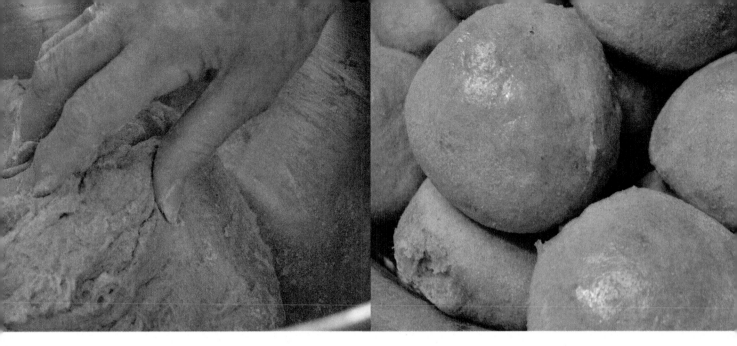

Grandma's Wonderful Rolls

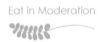

Makes 2 ½ dozen rolls

- 1 ½ Tablespoons active dry yeast
- 1 cup warm filtered water
- 1 ½ Tablespoons raw honey
- 7 cups whole sprouted spelt flour, sifted, and divided
- 1 ½ teaspoons Nature's Sunshine® sea salt

- ⅓ cup grapeseed oil
- 1 Tablespoon molasses
- 2 eggs, beaten
- ¾ cup warm filtered water (110-115 degrees)
- Non-stick grapeseed oil spray
- 1 Tablespoon organic butter, no substitutes

Directions:

1) In a very large mixing bowl combine the yeast, 1 cup warm water and honey together. Set aside and let it double in size.

2) Sift the flour in a large bowl and remove ½ cup for kneading later. Add the sea salt to the 6 ½ cups and set aside.

3) To the yeast mixture add oil, molasses, eggs and ¾ cup warm water. Stir to combine.

4) Add the flour one cup at a time, stirring constantly with a sturdy spatula. Continue stirring in the same direction folding the dough over itself. This will take approximately 5 minutes.

5) Let the dough rest in its bowl for 40 minutes. It should have doubled in size after that time.

6) If the dough is sticky, sift the remaining ½ cup flour onto the dough and knead it for 2 to 3 minutes.

7) Pre-heat the oven to 375 degrees.

8) Pinch off golf ball size dough balls and tuck the pinched side under then place in a 9x13x2 inch glass pan coated with non-stick grapeseed oil spray or place on a baking sheet lined with unbleached parchment paper. Spray the dough balls with grapeseed oil so as they rise, they are able to expand and not crack. Let them rise 30 minutes.

9) Carefully place in the oven and bake for 20 minutes. Remove from oven and butter the tops of the hot rolls with butter.

Tip: This recipe is easily doubled. Let rolls cool completely before storing in tightly sealed container. These freeze well in BPA free Ziploc® freezer bags.

It is easier to stir and knead the dough on a surface no higher than your waist.

Grandma's Rolls

I can honestly say that I grew up in the kitchen; as a toddler, my grandma would set me on her "bread board" as she kneaded her dough. When I began learning about whole grains years later, I encouraged my grandma to swap out the all purpose flour for whole spelt flour in her famous rolls. Admittedly, they still have gluten, but when Thanksgiving and Christmas roll around, these are a healthier alternative to the traditional white rolls.

Garlic Bread

Eat in Moderation

1 serving

- 1 slice Ezekiel 4:9 bread®
- 1 teaspoon organic butter, no substitutes
- ½ teaspoon garlic granules OR garlic powder
- Dash Nature's Sunshine® sea salt
- ¼ teaspoon dried parsley
- ½ teaspoon grated parmesan cheese
- 1 Tablespoon goat cheese, crumbled, optional

Directions:

1) Spread the butter on the slice of bread.
2) Sprinkle with your choice of garlic granules or garlic powder (not garlic salt).
3) Season with sea salt, parsley flakes and parmesan cheese.
4) Top with goat cheese, (if desired).
5) Bake in preheated 300 degree oven for 10 minutes on a baking sheet lined with parchment paper.

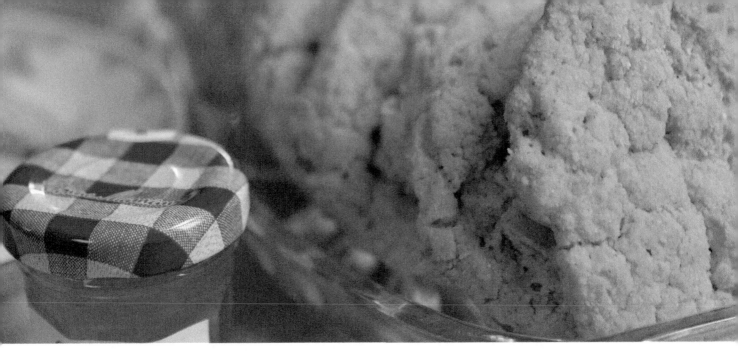

Oatmeal Biscuits

10-12 biscuits

- 1 ½ cups organic gluten free oatmeal flour, sifted, divided
- 1 cup garbanzo bean flour, sifted
- ¼ teaspoon Nature's Sunshine® sea salt
- 3 teaspoons baking powder
- ¾ cup organic butter, cold
- ¾ cup unsweetened almond milk

Directions:

1) Make your own oatmeal flour, see below. Place 1 cup oatmeal flour and garbanzo bean flour, sea salt and baking powder in a mixing bowl. Stir well to combine.

2) Cut in the butter using a pastry blender or a fork until mixture resembles coarse crumbs.

3) Stir in the milk just until moistened. Do not over mix.

4) Dust the counter with additional oatmeal flour and pour the dough out onto the floured surface. Dust the top with additional oatmeal flour and pat it lightly shaping it to ½ inch or ¾ inch thickness.

5) Take a 2 ½ inch biscuit cutter or juice glass dipped in flour and cut the biscuits. The dough will be light and sticky. Do your best to pick them up with a spatula and place on a baking sheet one inch apart. Lightly coat the baking sheet with non-stick grapeseed oil spray. Bake in preheated 375 degree oven for 20-25 minutes or until slightly golden brown.

These are really good! They are light and crispy on the outside and tender on the inside.

How to make Oatmeal Flour

Makes 2 cups

- 2 cups organic gluten free old fashioned rolled oats

Directions:

1) Place the dry old fashioned rolled oats in a high speed blender with "Food Processing" "Grains" setting. (Blendtec® or similar brand). Process one 47 second session. Sift the flour into your favorite recipe. Store in a BPA free Ziploc® style bag in refrigerator.

This also works for millet, buckwheat and spelt berries. If you process flax seeds for flax meal, be sure to store in the freezer as it becomes rancid quickly.

Sweet Carrot Zucchini Muffins

Makes 2 ½ dozen mini muffins

- ½ cup coconut flour
- ¼ cup Love and Peas® protein powder
- ½ cup coconut sugar
- ½ teaspoon stevia
- 1 Tablespoon cinnamon
- ⅛ teaspoon ground nutmeg
- ¼ teaspoon ground ginger
- ¼ teaspoon ground cloves
- 1 ½ teaspoons baking soda
- ¼ teaspoon Nature's Sunshine® sea salt

- 3 organic eggs
- ½ cup melted coconut oil
- ¼ cup canned pumpkin puree
- 1 teaspoon organic pure vanilla extract
- 2 teaspoons organic orange zest
- 2 cups carrot, shredded
- 1 cup zucchini, shredded and well drained
- ½ cup organic apple, with peeling, shredded
- ½ cup pecans, chopped

Directions:

1) In a small bowl, combine the dry ingredients and stir to mix well.

2) In a large mixing bowl, beat the eggs then add in the coconut oil, pumpkin and vanilla and mix until creamy. Add in the dry ingredients and mix well.

3) Next, add in the orange zest, carrots, zucchini and apple. Fold in the pecans.

4) Drop batter by spoonfuls into unbleached mini muffin liners in a stainless steel muffin pan or use a stoneware muffin pan only! Bake in preheated 350 degree oven for 20-25 minutes. Place on wire rack to cool. Store uncovered slightly.

> These are delicious warm muffins; however,
> they are wonderful as a dessert with Vanilla Cream Cheese Frosting (page 294)

Mulegrain Cornbread

6 servings

- 1 ½ cup organic yellow corn meal
- ½ cup garbanzo bean flour
- ½ cup millet flour
- 1 teaspoon Nature's Sunshine® sea salt
- 1 teaspoon baking soda

- 2 teaspoons baking powder
- 1 ½ cups unsweetened almond milk
- 2 organic eggs, slightly beaten
- 5 Tablespoons organic butter, softened
- ¼ cup unsweetened canned pumpkin puree
OR unsweetened applesauce
- 2 Tablespoons raw honey

Directions:

1) In a medium size mixing bowl add corn meal, flour, sea salt, baking soda and baking powder. Stir to combine.

2) Pour in the milk, eggs, butter, your choice of pumpkin or applesauce and honey. Mix with a fork just until all ingredients are mixed together. Do not over mix.

3) Bake in preheated 375 degree oven in a glass 9x9x2 or 9x13x2 inch baking dish coated with non-stick grapeseed oil spray for 30-35 minutes or until golden brown and knife inserted comes out clean.

Why Mulegrain? There is no such thing as Mulegrain, but Timo just called this recipe that when he first tried it. It was more hearty than we had been used to, but it was a hit.

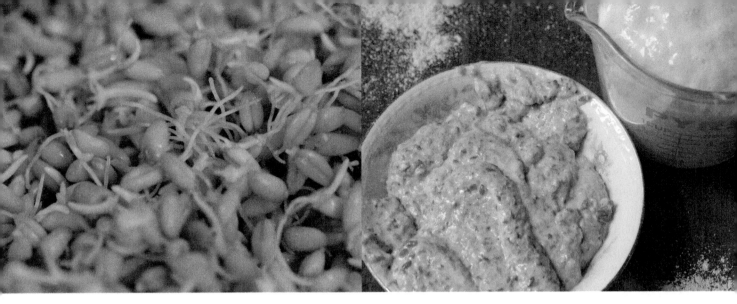

Sprout 2 Flourish Spelt Bread

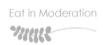

Makes 1 loaf

- ⅓ cup organic dry whole spelt berries
- 2 Tablespoons flax seeds
- 2 Tablespoons fresh squeezed orange juice
- ⅓ cup filtered water
- 1 Tablespoon active dry yeast
- ⅓ cup warm filtered water (110-115 degrees)
- ½ teaspoon raw honey
- 3 cups whole sprouted spelt flour
- 2 Tablespoons grapeseed oil OR coconut oil, melted
- 1 Tablespoon molasses
- 1 Tablespoon raw honey
- 1 teaspoon Nature's Sunshine® sea salt

- 2 teaspoons grapeseed oil, divided
- 1 pint glass jar
- 1 large mesh strainer to rinse the spelt berries in
- 1 large shallow bowl to sprout the spelt berries in and for the spelt berry mixture
- 1 small glass bowl for yeast
- 1 (3 or 4 cup) measuring cup
- 1 food processor with sharp blade and dough blade
- 1 large mixing bowl for dough
- BPA free plastic wrap
- 1 loaf pan
- Non-stick grapeseed oil spray

Directions:

1) Begin the night before: Soak the dry whole spelt berries in the pint jar filled with filtered water. Soak overnight.

2) *Sprouting Day Morning:* Rinse the spelt berries well. Drain very well through a mesh strainer. Place a double layer of paper towels in a large shallow bowl and pour the spelt berries into the paper towel lined bowl. Place a paper towel over the top of the bowl and set it aside on the counter to continue draining and sprouting.

Sprouting Day Evening: Rinse the spelt berries again. Drain very well through the mesh strainer. Place a new double layer of paper towels in the same bowl. Pour in the spelt berries and cover with a new paper towel. Set aside for overnight.

3) *Time to Bake, Morning of Day Two:* Rinse the spelt berries. Now they are ready to use for bread. Prepare the spelt berries by placing them in a food processor with the sharp blade. Add to the sprouted berries flax seeds, orange juice and water. Process 3-4 minutes pausing each minute to scrape the sides of the processor bowl down. The mixture will be milky and have a slightly gritty texture. With a spatula, pour out the spelt berry mixture into the shallow bowl while removing the sharp blade and installing the dough blade. Do not wash the processor bowl because you will pour the flour directly into it in a minute.

4) In a small bowl add the warm water to the yeast and stir in the honey. Set aside to rise while getting the flour together.

5) Sift 3 cups of whole sprouted spelt flour into the large measuring cup. Now sift half of this flour into the food processor bowl.

6) To the food processor bowl add the spelt berry mixture, yeast, oil, molasses, honey and sea salt. Turn on the food processor using the dough setting. Now add the rest of the whole sprouted spelt flour a spoon full at a time and continue processing until the dough cleans the side walls. (Sometimes you need one or two more Tablespoons of flour to get the dough to clean the sides of the processor bowl.) Once the dough has cleaned the sides of the bowl, while processor is still on, let it continue to knead the dough for approximately 30 more seconds. Hold the machine firmly on the counter.

7) Remove dough and place on a work surface coated with 1 teaspoon of grapeseed oil. Let rest 5 minutes. Lightly oil your hands and knead 2 minutes. Cover with a large bowl that is big enough for it to rise inside of and will not allow any air into the bowl when upside down on the work surface. After 10 minutes, knead for 10 seconds then cover. After 10 minutes, knead for 10 seconds then cover. After 10 minutes, knead for 10 seconds and then place the dough in the bowl coated with 1 more teaspoon of grapeseed oil. Now cover the bowl tightly with BPA free plastic wrap. Let rise 1 hour.

8) Punch dough down and shape the dough into a loaf and place in glass or stoneware loaf pan coated with non-stick grapeseed oil spray. Let rise another 40 minutes to 1 hour then place in preheated 350 degree oven for 40-50 minutes.

Once you have done this a couple of times, you will get the hang of it. It's not as hard as it looks.

Filling for cinnamon rolls:
- 1 Tablespoon extra-virgin coconut oil
- ⅓ cup pecans, chopped
- ½ Tablespoon cinnamon
- 2 Tablespoons raw honey

Frosting for cinnamon rolls:
- 1 Tablespoon organic butter, no substitutes, melted
- ½ scoop Love and Peas® protein powder (Sugar Free)
- ½ Tablespoon raw honey OR raw coconut nectar
- 2 ½ Tablespoons unsweetened almond milk

Stir together and spread on top of warm rolls.

- Stir together and spread out on dough. Roll up and slice into 12 cinnamon rolls. Bake in preheated 350 degree oven in a 9x13x2 inch glass baking dish coated with non-stick grapeseed oil spray.

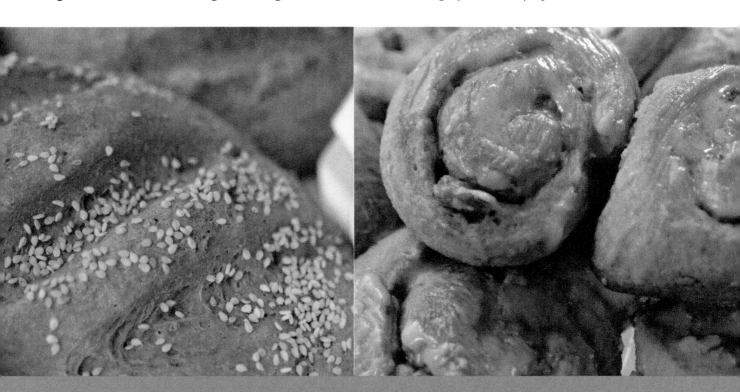

Pumpkin Rolls

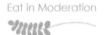

Makes 2 dozen

- ½ Tablespoon active dry yeast
- ½ Tablespoon raw honey
- ¼ cup warm filtered water (110-115 degrees)
- 1 cup unsweetened almond milk
- ¼ teaspoon stevia
- ¼ cup raw honey
- ¼ cup grapeseed oil
- 2 Tablespoons extra-virgin coconut oil, melted

- 1 cup unsweetened canned pumpkin puree
- 2 teaspoons organic orange zest
- 2-3 Tablespoons fresh squeezed orange juice
- 1 teaspoon Nature's Sunshine® sea salt
- 4 ¼ - 5 cups whole sprouted spelt flour, sifted
- ½ Tablespoon grapeseed oil
  OR extra-virgin coconut oil, melted for rising

Directions:

1) Combine yeast, honey, and ¼ cup warm water in a small bowl; stir to combine. Let stand for 5 minutes, mixture should double in size.

2) In a food processor with dough blade, pour the milk, stevia, honey, oil, pumpkin, orange zest, orange juice and the yeast mixture. Process for 25 seconds.

3) Add sea salt and 2 cups of flour. Process 10 seconds. Add 2 more cups of flour and process on "dough" setting, adding flour by the spoonfuls through the spout until dough forms a ball and cleans the sides of the food processor bowl.

4) Dough should be a little sticky and elastic. Remove from mixer and knead briefly in a bowl drizzled with grapeseed oil or coconut oil. Form into a ball and cover bowl with a clean towel. Allow dough to rise in a warm place until doubled, about 1 hour.

5) Punch down dough. Turn onto a lightly floured surface; knead 1 minute until smooth and elastic. Pinch off 24 golf ball size pieces of dough and shape into balls. Place 2 inches apart on an unbleached parchment paper lined stainless steel or stoneware baking sheet or 9x13x2 inch glass baking dish coated with non-stick grapeseed oil spray. Allow dough to rise in a warm place until doubled, about 30 minutes. Bake in preheated 375 degree oven for 15 -18 minutes or until golden brown. Remove from oven and cool on wire rack.

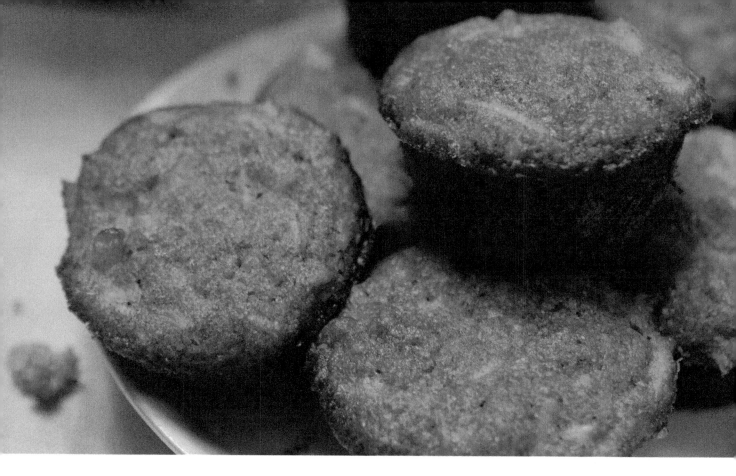

Orange Carrot Muffins

Gluten Free
Grain Free

24 mini muffins

- 2 organic eggs, beaten
- ¼ teaspoon stevia
- ⅓ cup coconut sugar OR raw honey
- 1 Tablespoon grated organic orange peel
- ½ cup fresh squeezed organic orange juice
- 6 Tablespoons organic butter, no substitutes
- 1 teaspoon organic pure vanilla extract
- 2 cups organic carrots, shredded

- 2 Tablespoons coconut flour
- ½ cup garbanzo bean flour
- ½ cup almond flour
- 1 teaspoon baking powder
- 1 teaspoon baking soda
- 1 ½ teaspoons cinnamon
- ⅛ teaspoon ground cloves
- ⅛ teaspoon ground ginger
- ½ cup walnuts, chopped, optional

Directions:

1) In a large mixing bowl, beat the eggs until fluffy. Add in the stevia, your choice of coconut sugar or honey, orange peel, orange juice, butter and vanilla. Mix well.

2) Combine flour, baking powder, baking soda, cinnamon, cloves and ginger. Stir together and slowly add to the wet ingredients in the mixing bowl.

3) Fold in the carrots and the walnuts (if using) and mix well.

4) Pour into unbleached mini muffin liners in a stainless steel muffin pan or use a stoneware muffin pan only! Bake in preheated 350 degree oven for 20-25 minutes.

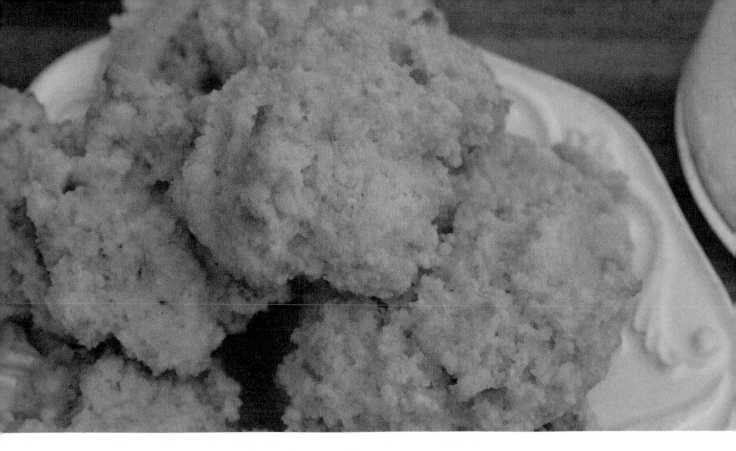

Coconut Biscuits

Gluten Free
Grain Free

8-10 biscuits

- ½ cup coconut flour, sifted
- ¼ teaspoon Nature's Sunshine® sea salt
- ½ teaspoon baking soda
- 1 Tablespoon raw honey OR coconut sugar

- 4 Tablespoons organic butter, cold
- ½ cup canned pumpkin puree
- 2 organic eggs, separated
- 1 Tablespoon unsweetened almond milk

Directions:

1) Place the coconut flour, sea salt, baking soda and your choice of honey or coconut sugar in a mixing bowl. Stir well to combine.

2) Cut in the butter using a pastry blender or a fork until mixture resembles coarse crumbs.

3) Stir in the pumpkin puree.

4) Separate the eggs in two small bowls. Beat the egg whites with a mixer until frothy and doubled in size. Add in the yolks while mixer is going and mix 20-30 seconds.

5) Fold into the batter and add in the almond milk. Continue folding with a spoon until all mixed in.

6) Scoop out 2 Tablespoons at a time and shape into a ½ inch to ¾ inch thick round biscuit. Place on an unbleached parchment paper lined stainless steel or stoneware baking sheet and bake in preheated 375 degree oven for 22 minutes. Serve immediately.

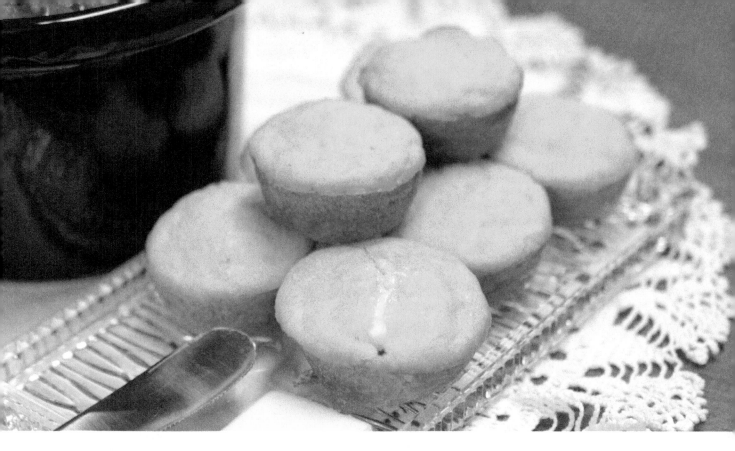

Faux Cornbread

6 servings or 24 mini muffins

- ½ cup garbanzo bean flour
- 1 ½ cups millet flour
- ½ teaspoon Nature's Sunshine® sea salt
- 1 teaspoon baking soda
- 2 teaspoons baking powder
- 1 cup unsweetened almond milk
- 2 organic eggs, slightly beaten

- ½ cup organic Greek yogurt, plain whole milk
- ¼ cup unsweetened canned pumpkin puree OR unsweetened applesauce
- ¼ cup grapeseed oil
- ¼ teaspoon stevia

Directions:

1) Fluff the garbanzo bean and millet flours to measure them. No need to sift. Place the flour in a medium size mixing bowl with the sea salt, baking soda and baking powder. Stir to combine.

2) Pour in the milk, eggs, yogurt, your choice of pumpkin or applesauce, oil and stevia. Mix with a fork just until all ingredients are mixed together. Do not over mix.

3) Pour into a glass 9x9x2 inch baking dish coated with non-stick grapeseed oil spray and bake in preheated 375 degree oven for 30-35 minutes or until golden brown and knife inserted comes out clean OR Pour into unbleached mini muffin liners in a stainless steel muffin pan or use a stoneware muffin pan only! Bake in preheated 350 degree oven for 12-15 minutes or until toothpick inserted comes out clean.

This is really good! It is very light, tall and fluffy. It is not grainy like the Mulegrain Cornbread recipe.

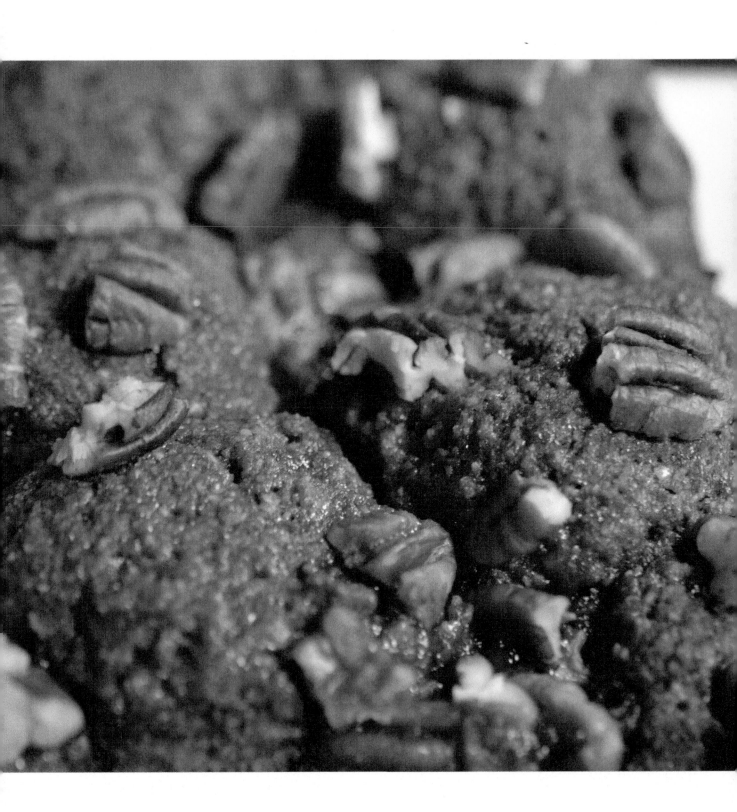

Kan't Believe It's Not Bread - Cinnamon

Gluten Free

Grain Free

Makes 18 small rolls

- ⅓ cup organic Greek yogurt, plain whole milk
- 2 ½ Tablespoons fresh squeezed orange juice
- ½ cup unsweetened almond milk
- ¾ cup almond flour, fluffed
- ¼ cup coconut flour, fluffed
- 5 Tablespoons psyllium husk powder, no substitutes
- 1 teaspoon baking soda
- ½ teaspoon Nature's Sunshine® sea salt
- 3 Tablespoons coconut sugar
- ¼ teaspoon stevia
- 1 Tablespoon cinnamon

- 1 teaspoon organic pure vanilla extract
- 3 organic eggs
- 2 Tablespoons extra-virgin coconut oil
- ½ cup pecans, coarsely chopped

Sauce:
- 3 Tablespoons raw honey
- 2 Tablespoons coconut oil
- 2 ½ teaspoons cinnamon
- 1 Tablespoon coconut sugar

Directions:

1) In a small bowl, combine the yogurt and orange juice. Stir well and set aside.

2) In a small saucepan over medium heat, bring almond milk to a boil.

3) Meanwhile, in a mixing bowl, stir together almond flour, coconut flour, psyllium husk powder, baking soda, sea salt, coconut sugar, stevia and cinnamon. Stir well with a fork.

4) Add the yogurt mixture, vanilla, eggs and coconut oil to the mixing bowl and stir well with a fork to combine until it becomes a stiff dough.

5) Add the hot almond milk to the dough and stir quickly to combine until liquid is absorbed.

6) Place the coconut oil for the sauce in the warm saucepan until melted. Then add the honey, cinnamon and coconut sugar. Mix well to combine.

7) Shape the dough into 1 inch balls and dip into the cinnamon sauce. Coat a 9 inch glass loaf pan with non-stick grapeseed oil spray. Place one layer of dough balls on bottom then sprinkle some pecans on top then layer the rest of the dough balls and sprinkle the remaining pecans on top. Bake in preheated 350 degree oven for 45-50 minutes.

Tip: Make sure to purchase finely ground psyllium husk powder and NOT psyllium seed powder; otherwise the rolls will turn bluish-purple while baking.

Dairy Free: Omit yogurt. Use a total of ¾ cup + 2 Tablespoons almond milk in the recipe.

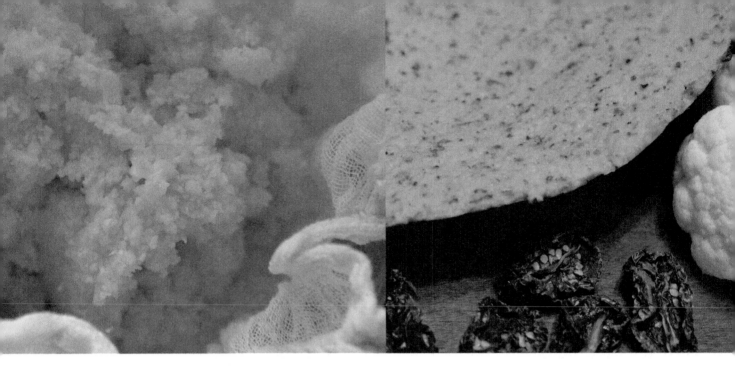

Cauliflower Flat Bread

4-6 servings

- 4 cups cauliflower, bite size florets (14 ounces)
- 3 large organic eggs
- 2 Tablespoons coconut flour
- 1 teaspoon garlic powder

- 1 teaspoon Italian herb seasoning
- ½ teaspoon Nature's Sunshine® sea salt
- ⅛ teaspoon ground black pepper
- ¼ cup sundried tomatoes in extra-virgin olive oil, drained

Directions:

1) Process the cauliflower florets in a food processor until fine granules that look like snow. Pour the cauliflower granules into the cheese cloth. Gather the four corners of the cheese cloth and gently twist and continue twisting the cauliflower granules to release excess water. Twist and squeeze as much water out as possible! You may drain as much as a ½ cup of water out of the cauliflower. This is important, otherwise the dough will not be able to be picked up and eaten.

2) Place the cauliflower granules back into the blender along with the eggs, coconut flour, garlic powder, Italian herb seasoning, sea salt and pepper. Drain the sundried tomatoes. Add in only the tomatoes. Process 40 seconds or until well combined.

3) Line a stainless steel or stoneware baking sheet with unbleached parchment paper and pour the batter onto the parchment paper. The batter should be creamy and cohesive. If grainy and crumbly, it needs one more egg. (3 large eggs should work, 3 small-medium wasn't always enough to hold it together). Smooth out with a spatula to about 1/8 of an inch thickness evenly across the parchment paper.

4) Bake in preheated 400 degree oven for 15-20 minutes until golden brown. Some thin areas may brown first or burn a little.

5) Remove from oven and test to see if the dough is able to hold together when lifted up off edge of parchment paper. Immediately slide the dough off of the parchment paper onto a cooling rack. Do not let it sweat! Otherwise it will get soggy. Looks hard, but it's not!

Suggestions: Enjoy as a wrap, as a garlic bread with spaghetti, use as bread for a sandwich, eat with an egg or alongside a salad. Makes a great pizza crust!

Spotlight: Cauliflower

Have you heard of the "cruciferous" vegetable clan? These stellar vegetables include: cauliflower, cabbage, broccoli, bok choy, Brussels sprouts and kohlrabi. They are unique in that their flowering petals resemble a cross, thus the name "cruciferous." I don't know about you, but I see the Lord's design in this: to remind us of His sacrifice on the cross and also to point to their protective properties.

Cauliflower provides versatility in the kitchen with a fork full of nutrition. Cauliflower supports the body by providing antioxidants, influencing the body's inflammation response, and promoting detoxification. Believe it or not, cauliflower packs a powerful vitamin C punch, provides manganese, and adrenal nourishing pantothenic acid. Want to change your cauliflower color palette? Try green, orange, or purple cauliflower such as in our Vibrant Violet Veggies (page 205)!

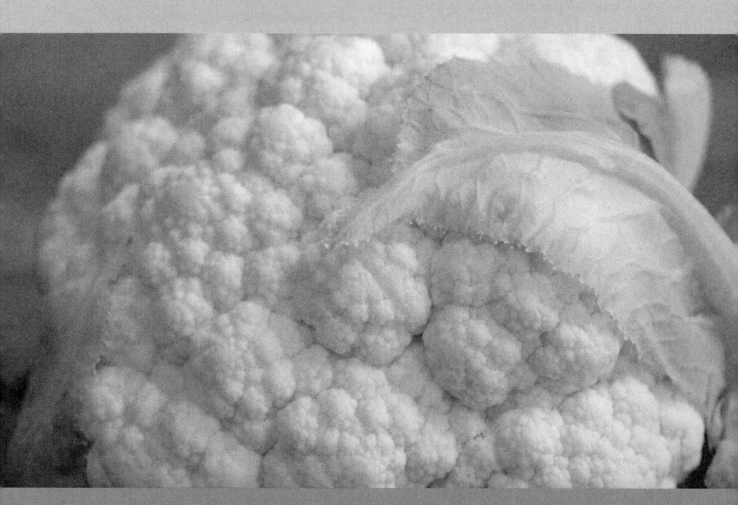

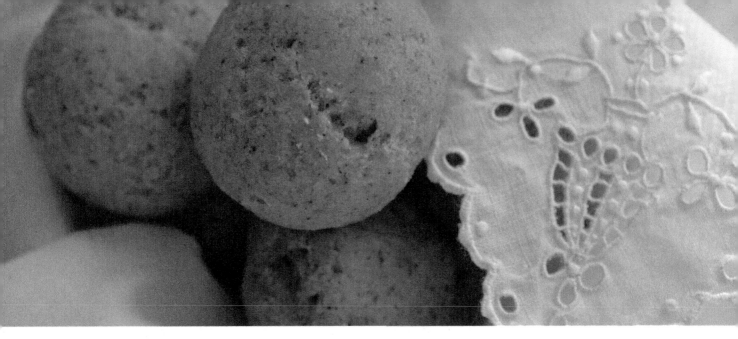

Kan't Believe It's Not Bread

Gluten Free
Grain Free

Makes 18 small rolls

- ⅓ cup organic Greek yogurt, plain whole milk
- 2 ½ Tablespoons fresh squeezed lemon juice
- ½ cup unsweetened almond milk
- ¾ cup almond flour, fluffed
- ¼ cup coconut flour, fluffed

- 5 Tablespoons psyllium husk powder, no substitutes
- 1 teaspoon baking soda
- ½ Tablespoon Nature's Sunshine® sea salt
- 1 Tablespoon coconut sugar OR raw honey
- 3 organic eggs
- 1 Tablespoon extra-virgin coconut oil, melted

Directions:

1) In a small bowl, combine the yogurt and lemon juice. Stir well and set aside.

2) In a small saucepan over medium heat, bring almond milk to a boil.

3) Meanwhile, in a mixing bowl, stir together almond flour, coconut flour, psyllium husk powder, baking soda, sea salt and your choice of coconut sugar or honey. Stir well.

4) Add the yogurt mixture, eggs and coconut oil to the mixing bowl and stir well with a fork to combine until it becomes a stiff dough.

5) Add the hot almond milk to the dough and stir quickly to combine until liquid is absorbed.

6) Shape the dough into 1 inch balls then place on a stainless steel or stoneware baking sheet lined with unbleached parchment paper allowing 2 inches of space between each roll.

7) Bake in preheated 350 degree oven for 25-35 minutes.

Tip: Make sure to purchase finely ground psyllium husk powder and NOT psyllium seed powder; otherwise the rolls will turn bluish-purple while baking.

Dairy Free: Omit yogurt. Use a total of ¾ cup + 2 Tablespoons almond milk in the recipe.

Kan't Believe It's Not Bread - Italian

Gluten Free

Grain Free

Makes 18 small rolls

- ⅓ cup organic Greek yogurt, plain whole milk
- 2 ½ Tablespoons fresh squeezed lemon juice
- ½ cup unsweetened almond milk
- ¾ cup almond flour, fluffed
- ¼ cup coconut flour, fluffed
- 5 Tablespoons psyllium husk powder, no substitutes
- 1 teaspoon baking soda
- ½ Tablespoon Nature's Sunshine® sea salt

- 1 teaspoon raw honey
- ½ teaspoon onion granules
- 2 teaspoons garlic powder
- 1 teaspoon Italian seasoning (page 240)
- ½ Tablespoon fresh basil, chopped
  OR ½ teaspoon, dried
- 2 Tablespoons sundried tomatoes
  in extra-virgin olive oil, drained and chopped
- 3 organic eggs

Directions:

1) In a small bowl, combine the yogurt and lemon juice. Stir well and set aside.

2) In a small saucepan over medium heat, bring almond milk to a boil.

3) Meanwhile, in a mixing bowl, stir together almond flour, coconut flour, psyllium husk powder, baking soda, sea salt, honey, onion granules, garlic powder, Italian seasoning and basil. Stir well with a fork.

4) Add the yogurt mixture, sundried tomatoes and eggs to the mixing bowl and stir well with a fork to combine until it becomes a stiff dough.

5) Add the hot almond milk to the dough and stir quickly to combine until liquid is absorbed.

6) Shape the dough into 1 inch balls then place on a stainless steel or stoneware baking sheet lined with unbleached parchment paper allowing 2 inches of space between each roll.

7) Bake in preheated 350 degree oven for 25-35 minutes.

Tip: Make sure to purchase finely ground psyllium husk powder and NOT psyllium seed powder; otherwise the rolls will turn bluish-purple while baking.

Encourage 2 Flourish: One Cup Short

Sometimes it feels as if we are scraping the bottom of the barrel, so to speak, or that we just have enough to get by. In these times, it is easy to get discouraged and be fearful, but God reminds us of His faithfulness in His Word. Psalm 34:9-10 encourages us "Fear the LORD, you his holy people, for those who fear him lack nothing. The lions may grow weak and hungry, but those who seek the LORD lack no good thing." Trusting God to provide what we need can be challenging, but so rewarding and relieving because He has enabled us to have peace. The widow in 1 Kings 17 was posed with a predicament- her flour and oil were running out and the prophet Elijah asked her for some bread. She hesitated, but he told her that God would provide. She stepped out in faith to make the bread, and God provided. She went away and did as Elijah had told her. "So there was food every day for Elijah and for the woman and her family. For the jar of flour was not used up and the jug of oil did not run dry, in keeping with the word of the LORD spoken by Elijah." We may think we are one cup short, but when we surrender our resources to God, He can do far more than we can imagine. You may just be one cup away from a miracle...

1 Kings 17:15-16 NIV

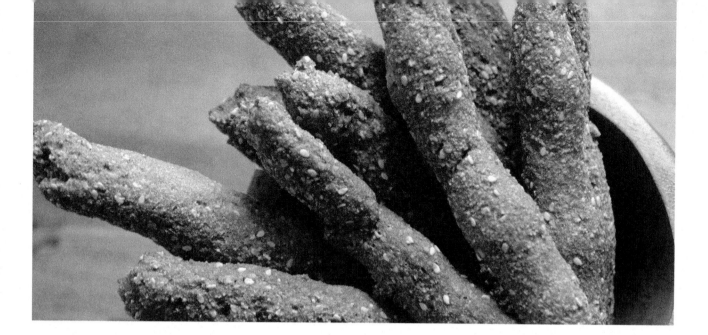

Kan't Believe It's Not Bread - RYE

Makes 18 small rolls

- ⅓ cup organic Greek yogurt, plain whole milk
- 1 Tablespoon fresh squeezed lemon juice
- ½ cup unsweetened almond milk
- ¾ cup almond flour, fluffed
- ¼ cup coconut flour, fluffed
- 3 organic eggs

- 5 Tablespoons psyllium husk powder, no substitutes
- 1 Tablespoon caraway seeds
- 1 teaspoon baking soda
- 1 ¼ teaspoons Nature's Sunshine® sea salt
- 1 Tablespoon molasses
- 1 Tablespoon extra-virgin coconut oil, melted

Directions:

1) In a small bowl, combine the yogurt and lemon juice. Stir well and set aside.

2) In a small saucepan over medium heat, bring almond milk to a boil.

3) Meanwhile, in a mixing bowl, stir together almond flour, coconut flour, psyllium husk powder, caraway seeds, baking soda, sea salt and molasses. Stir well with a fork.

4) Add the yogurt mixture, eggs and coconut oil to the mixing bowl and stir well with a fork to combine until it becomes a stiff dough.

5) Add the hot almond milk to the dough and stir quickly to combine until liquid is absorbed.

6) Shape the dough into 1 inch balls then place on a stainless steel or stoneware baking sheet lined with unbleached parchment paper allowing 2 inches of space between each roll.

7) Bake in preheated 350 degree oven for 25-35 minutes.

Tip: Make sure to purchase finely ground psyllium husk powder and NOT psyllium seed powder; otherwise the rolls will turn bluish-purple while baking.

Dairy Free: Omit yogurt and use a total of ¾ cup + 2 Tablespoons unsweetened almond milk in the recipe.

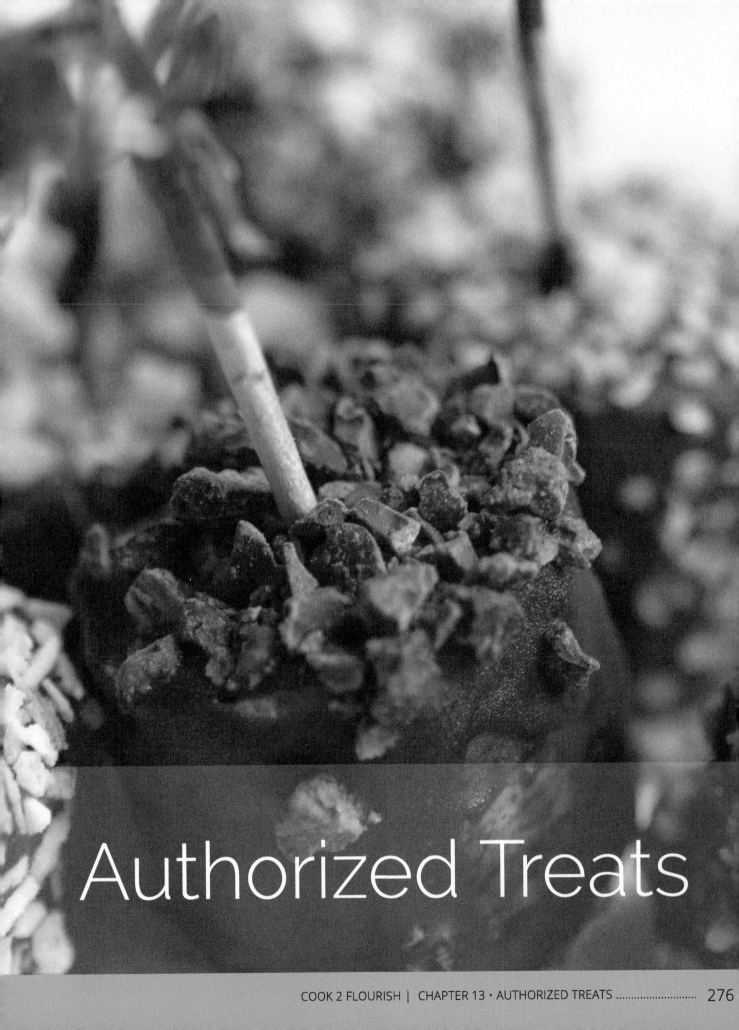

Authorized Treats

Banana Pops

· · · · · · · · · · · · · · · · · · ·

Makes 15

- 3 medium, firm, ripe bananas
- 2 ounces 70% or higher dark chocolate, melted
- ⅛ teaspoon stevia
- ⅛ teaspoon cinnamon
- ½ Tablespoon coconut oil

Your Choice of Toppings:
- Unsweetened coconut flakes
- Cacao nibs, chopped in a food processor
- Hemp seeds
- Sesame seeds
- Walnuts, pecans or almonds, chopped

Directions:

1) Peel the bananas and cut each banana into 5 (1 ½ inch) chunks.
Poke a toothpick in each chunk and place on waxed paper.

2) Combine the melted chocolate with the stevia, cinnamon and coconut oil in a small bowl.

3) Dip the banana into the chocolate then roll it in or sprinkle on the topping of choice. Place on the waxed paper. When all the bananas are coated with chocolate and topping, place in the freezer for at least 2 hours. Store covered in the freezer.

Note: Depending on what dark chocolate you use, some of these treats can also be dairy free.

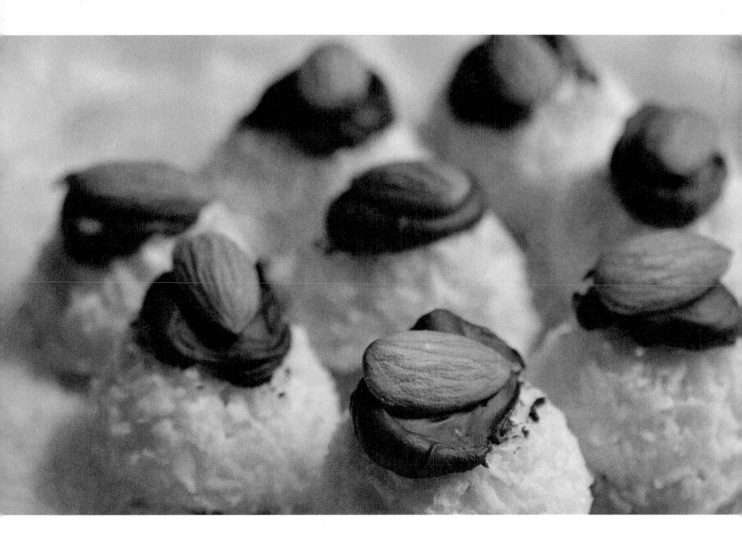

Almond Coconut Macaroons

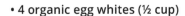

Gluten Free
Grain Free

Makes 2 ½ dozen

- 4 organic egg whites (½ cup)
- ⅓ cup raw honey OR coconut sugar
- ¼ teaspoon organic pure almond extract
- ¼ teaspoon organic pure vanilla extract

- 2 ¼ cups unsweetened coconut flakes
- 1 Tablespoon coconut flour
- ¼ cup almonds
- 2 ½ ounces 70% or higher dark chocolate, melted

Directions:

1) In a mixer, beat the egg whites until soft peaks form, approximately 1 minute.

2) Gradually add in your choice of honey or coconut sugar and continue beating on high speed for 5 minutes. Continue beating 1 more minute while adding in the extracts.

3) Combine the coconut flour and the coconut flakes. Fold the coconut into the egg whites until thoroughly combined.

4) Take a rounded 1 Tablespoon measuring spoon and drop batter onto a lightly greased stainless steel baking sheet or stoneware. Space is not required between the macaroons.

5) Bake in preheated 325 degree oven for 20 minutes. Cool on wire rack.

6) Place a dab of melted chocolate in the center of the macaroon and top with 1 almond.

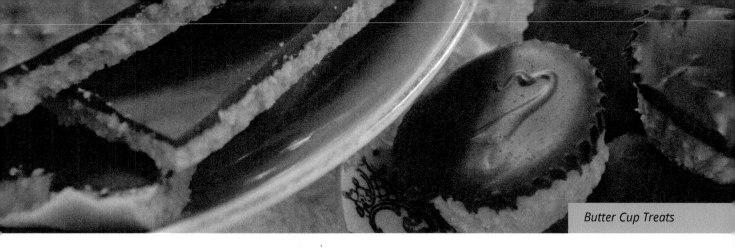

Cashew Frosting - Chocolate

Gluten Free
Dairy Free

Makes 1 ½ cups

- 1 cup cashews, soaked
- ¼ cup extra-virgin coconut oil
- ¼ cup canned pumpkin puree
- 3 Tablespoons unsweetened almond milk
- 12-18 drops liquid stevia
- 3 Tablespoons raw honey OR coconut sugar
- 1 ½ Tablespoons arrowroot powder
- ½ teaspoon organic pure vanilla extract
- ½ teaspoon organic pure almond extract
- 2 Tablespoons carob powder

Directions:

1) Place the cashews in a cup and fill with enough water to cover by one inch. Soak the cashews for 2 hours. Drain and roll up in a towel to soak up any excess liquid.

2) Pour cashews into a high speed blender along with coconut oil, pumpkin puree, almond milk, stevia, your choice of honey or coconut sugar, arrowroot powder, extracts and carob powder. Blend on high until smooth and creamy.

3) Frost onto a completely cooled cake and store in the refrigerator up to one week.

This is so good! Our taste testers all really liked it and couldn't believe it was cashews!

Butter Cup Treats

Eat in Moderation

Makes 36 treats

- 4 cups Love Grown® Power O's™ original cereal
- 1 cup organic oat bran
- 1 teaspoon powdered stevia, no substitutes
- ½ cup organic butter, no substitutes, melted
- 1 cup organic peanut butter, no sugar added
- 8-10 ounces 70% or higher dark chocolate
- 12 drops of liquid stevia (chocolate flavored, optional)

Directions:

1) In a food processor, process the cereal until fine.

2) Add in the oat bran, powdered stevia, melted butter and peanut butter. Process until well combined.

3) In a double boiler, melt the chocolate and stevia.

Mini muffin cup treats: Drop peanut butter mixture by spoonfuls into unbleached mini muffin paper liners in a stainless steel or stoneware mini muffin pan. Press the mixture down with a spoon to flatten. Spoon the melted chocolate into the muffin cups to cover the peanut butter crust. Refrigerate at least 30 minutes to 1 hour to harden. Cover and store in the refrigerator.

Easy one dish treats: Pour all the peanut butter mixture into a 9x13x2 inch glass pan and press into the bottom like a flat smooth crust. Pour all the melted chocolate over the peanut butter crust until smooth and completely covered to the edge of the glass pan.

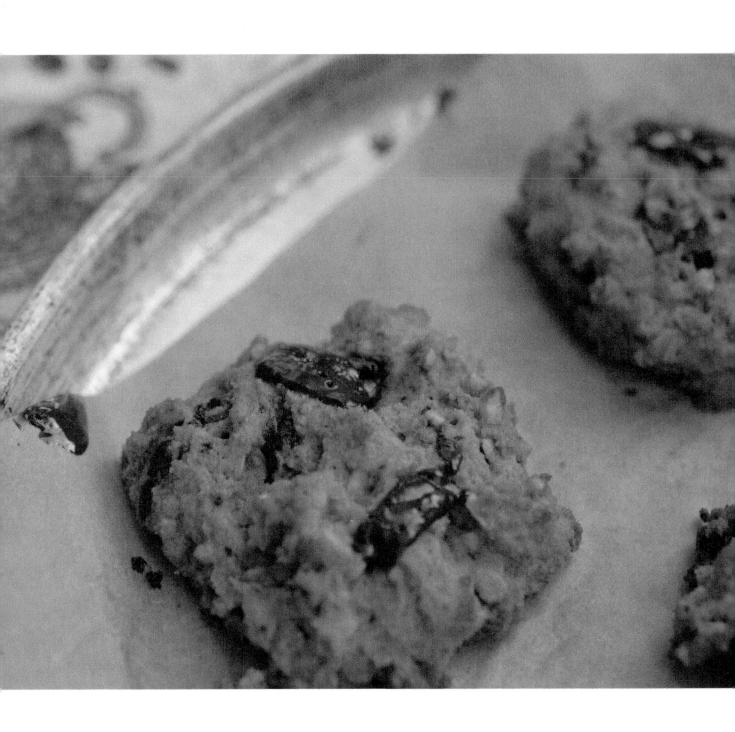

Endurance Sports Cookies

Makes 4 dozen

- 2 organic eggs
- 1 cup organic butter, no substitutes, softened
- ¼ cup extra-virgin coconut oil
- ½ cup unsweetened canned pumpkin puree
  OR baked sweet potato
- 1 cup coconut sugar
- ¼ teaspoon powdered stevia
- 1 Tablespoon organic pure vanilla extract
- 1 ½ cups whole sprouted spelt flour, sifted
- 1 cup millet flour, sifted
- ½ teaspoon Nature's Sunshine® sea salt

- 1 teaspoon cream of tartar
- 1 teaspoon baking soda
- 1 cup organic old fashioned rolled oats, dry
- 1 cup Love & Peas® protein powder (Sugar Free)
- 1 cup whole grain buckwheat, dry
- ¼ cup cashews, chopped
- ¼ cup walnuts, chopped
- ½ cup pecans, chopped
- 1 cup (5 ounces) 70% or higher dark chocolate,
  chopped

Directions:

1) In a mixing bowl, beat the eggs on high for 3 to 4 minutes until fluffy. Pour out into a bowl and set aside.

2) In the same mixing bowl, whip the butter and oil on high for 1 minute.

3) Add your choice of pumpkin or sweet potato and coconut sugar to the butter and then mix well. Pour in the eggs and the vanilla and mix well about 1 minute.

4) Combine the spelt flour, millet flour, sea salt, cream of tartar, baking soda, oats, protein powder, and buckwheat in a bowl and mix to combine. Add into the batter in the mixing bowl one big spoonful at a time until all combined. Fold in the nuts and chocolate.

5) Drop batter by spoonfuls and flatten down onto unbleached parchment paper lined stainless steel cookie sheet or use a stoneware baking pan. Bake in preheated 350 degree oven for 12-14 minutes for small cookies. Remove from cookie sheet to wire racks to cool. Store uncovered for 24 hours, then cover very lightly or they will get soggy.

This recipe has several ingredients because I am trying to diversify the flour and sugar. Athletes expend a lot of energy. This cookie will satisfy and give them nourishment to keep going.

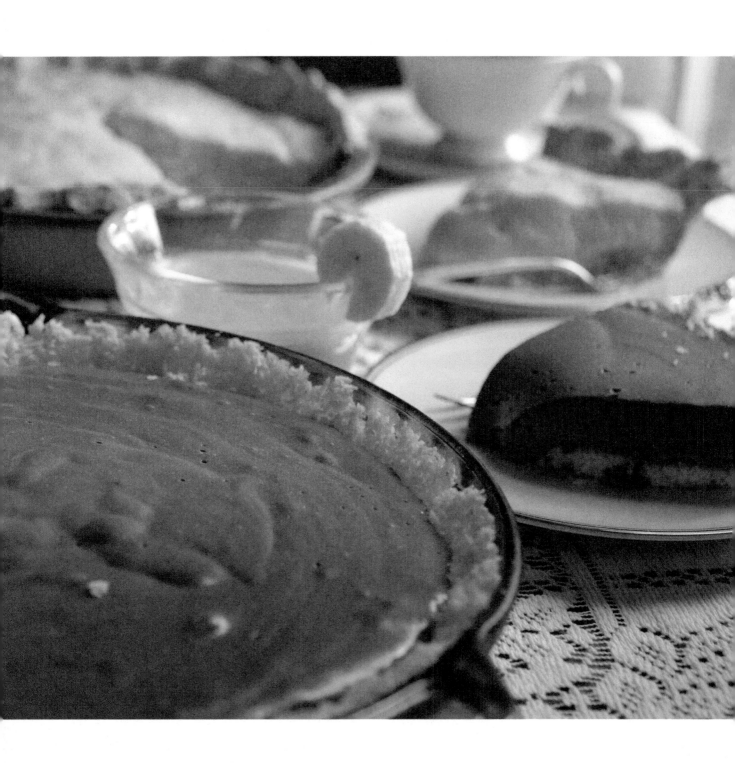

Chocolate Cream Pie Filling

1 (9 inch) pie

- 1 Tablespoon raw honey
- ½ Tablespoon Pomona's Universal Pectin®
- 2 cups unsweetened almond milk
- ¾ cup minus 1 Tablespoon coconut sugar
- ⅛ teaspoon Nature's Sunshine® sea salt
- 3 organic egg yolks, lightly beaten
- ⅓ cup Love and Peas® protein powder (Sugar Free)

- 2 Tablespoons organic butter, no substitutes
- 1 teaspoon organic pure vanilla extract
- 1 Tablespoon arrowroot
- 1 teaspoon guar gum
- 2 Tablespoons carob powder
- 1 coconut pie shell, baked, page 297

Directions:

1) In a small mixing bowl, mix together the honey and the pectin until well combined. Set aside.

2) Pour the almond milk into a 2 quart saucepan and bring to a boil over medium high heat, stirring constantly with a wire whisk. Just before it comes to a boil, add the coconut sugar and sea salt. Stir constantly.

3) Just as it begins to boil, pour in all the honey and pectin, stirring vigorously for 1 minute.

4) Remove saucepan from the heat and reduce heat to medium.

5) Add 5 Tablespoons of hot liquid one at a time slowly into the yolks, stirring constantly. Pour the eggs into the milk and stir constantly over the burner for 2 minutes. Turn off burner and remove from heat.

6) Stir in the protein powder, butter and vanilla and continue stirring for 1 minute.

7) Place the saucepan in a cool water bath for 10 minutes.

8) Cover saucepan and place in the refrigerator for 30 minutes.

9) Scoop ½ cup of filling out of the saucepan and into a round mixing bowl. Sift the arrowroot and guar gum into the filling. Stir to combine. It will be clumpy. Add in the carob powder and stir to combine.

10) Pour all the filling from saucepan and mixing bowl into a high speed blender and blend for 20-30 seconds on high.

11) Pour into prepared coconut pie shell and refrigerate at least 2 hours before serving.

This pie is light and amazing! It will keep 3 days in the refrigerator.

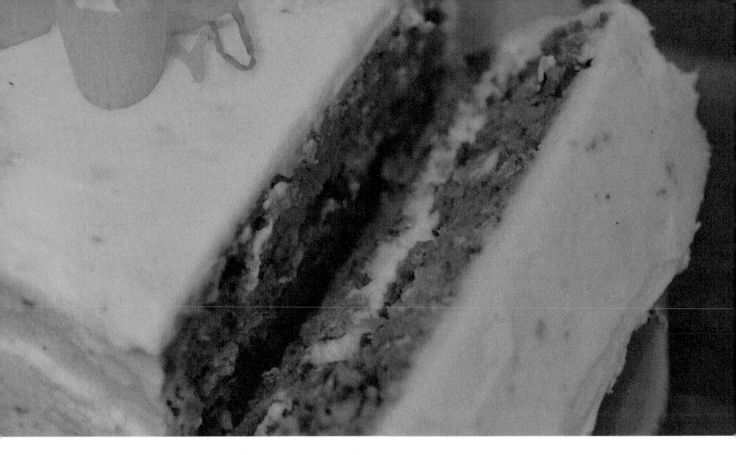

Healthy Carrot Cake

1 loaf cake or 24 mini muffins

- **2 organic eggs, beaten**
- **¼ teaspoon stevia**
- **⅓ cup coconut sugar OR raw honey**
- **1 Tablespoon grated organic orange peel**
- **½ cup fresh squeezed organic orange juice**
- **6 Tablespoons organic butter, no substitutes**
- **1 teaspoon organic pure vanilla extract**
- **2 cups organic carrots, shredded**

- **2 Tablespoons coconut flour**
- **½ cup garbanzo bean flour**
- **½ cup almond flour**
- **1 teaspoon baking powder**
- **1 teaspoon baking soda**
- **1 ½ teaspoons cinnamon**
- **⅛ teaspoon ground cloves**
- **⅛ teaspoon ground ginger**
- **½ cup walnuts, chopped, optional**

Directions:

1) In a large mixing bowl, beat the eggs until fluffy.

2) Add in the stevia, your choice of coconut sugar or honey, orange peel, orange juice, butter and vanilla. Mix well.

3) Combine flour, baking powder, baking soda, cinnamon, cloves and ginger. Stir together and slowly add to the wet ingredients in the mixing bowl.

4) Fold in the carrots and the walnuts (if using) and mix well.

5) For loaf cake: Pour the batter into two 5.25x9x3 inch glass or stoneware loaf pans coated with non-stick grapeseed oil spray. Bake in preheated 350 degree oven for 35-40 minutes or until knife inserted comes out clean. Frost cooled cake with Lemon Cream Cheese Frosting (page 294).

For mini muffins: Pour into unbleached mini muffin liners in a stainless steel muffin pan or use a stoneware muffin pan only! Bake in preheated 350 degree oven for 20-25 minutes.

Ingredients

. . . .

Heavy hearted – home from church and after lunch, I went to my bedroom to pray and hear from the Lord. TeTe (grandma) was asleep in her hospital bed, Robin was doing homework on her floor, Timo was watching sports with PaPa and my parents were supposed to arrive sometime this afternoon to help me care for TeTe.

I prayed "Oh, Dear Jesus, I know you are holding me, but I just need to hear from you! This is too much! Del is so weary in his soul from the store and TeTe is near death. I must be strong and I don't know what is up ahead. I don't know what our future is and I am just trusting you. Speak to my heart Lord, I need peace! ......"
This is what He spoke to my heart....
"Oh, my child, every good thing has a process -
I take ingredients and stir them well and prepare to bake as though making a delicious cake. Before it can be served or divided out, it must go through the fire to bake. But after the fire, there is a time to cool before removing from the pan, then the dressing and preparation of decoration comes, then it's time to serve:

A portion of the ingredients
A portion of the process
A portion of the fire
A portion of the cooling - the calm
A portion of the decoration - the restoration
is given out to every person that partakes of the cake, which is the ministry.

"I Am" is with you – I haven't left you. I am here. Life is a process, life all sums up to experiences, lessons, wisdom and testimonies that can be used for the Kingdom of God.
The most important ingredient of all of life is Me, God Almighty! Nothing much else matters. My plan, My vision, the people I want you to touch matter.

Do not fear during this time – Declare with your words every moment of the Day, WHO I AM. This will build your strength – your spiritual strength! Your mental strength, your emotional strength.

When I'm done with the cake – there is a celebration, as in a birthday, a wedding ..."

(interrupted...... TeTe is calling for me downstairs)
Wow! Thank you, Lord. I needed this.

Julie

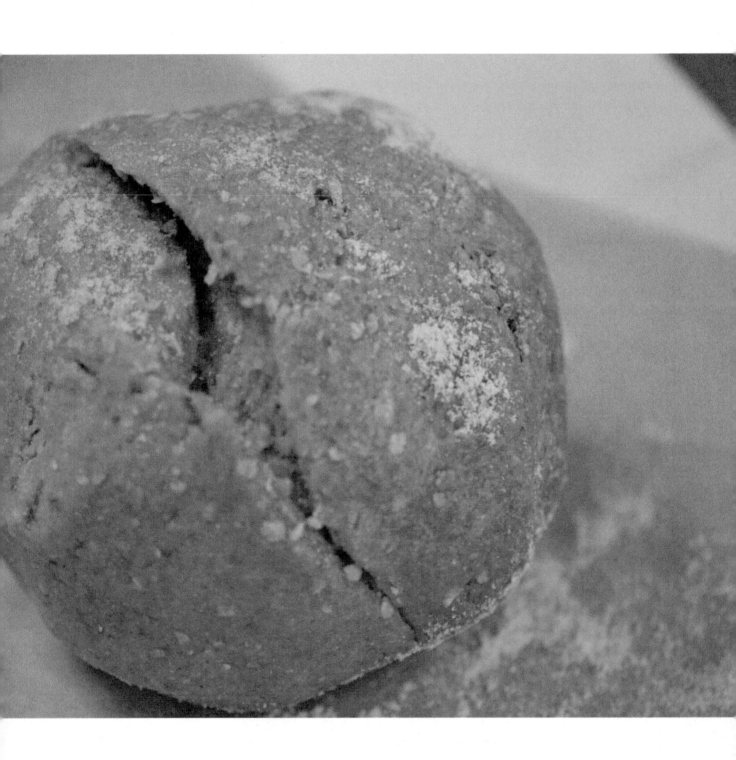

Buttery Spelt Pie Crust

Makes one 9 inch crust and can easily be doubled

- **1 cup whole sprouted spelt flour**
- **½ cup organic oat bran**
- **¼ teaspoon Nature's Sunshine® sea salt**
- **¼ cup organic butter OR grapeseed oil**
- **4-5 Tablespoons ice cold filtered water**

Directions:

1) In a food processor, combine the flour, oat bran and sea salt by pulsing it 3-4 times.

2) Add in your choice of butter or grapeseed oil and process for 10 seconds or until coarse crumbs form.

3) Remove any ice cubes from your water and measure out the 5 Tablespoons into a cup. Add in the water by tablespoons, while the processor is on, waiting a 3-5 seconds between each addition of water.

4) Process until a soft, moldable dough is formed. It should clean the sides of the food processor bowl.

5) Roll out and use as desired. Remember DO NOT bake it higher than 375 degrees. If your pie requires a hotter temperature, use unrefined grapeseed oil.

For a chilled pudding pie – Place the pie crust in your glass or stoneware pie dish, press to the bottom and to the side walls then finish fluting the edges. Then thoroughly fork the bottom and the sides of the pie crust to poke holes in the crust. Bake in preheated 350 degree oven for 22-25 minutes. Let the pie dish and crust completely cool on a wire rack then fill with pudding pie filling.

For double crust fruit pie – Roll out a thin bottom crust then line your glass or stoneware pie dish. Pour in the thickened fruit. Roll out remaining pastry to fit top of pie. Place over filling. Trim, seal and flute the edges. Make several slits in the top pastry to allow steam to release. Bake in preheated 375 degree oven on bottom rack for 55minutes or until crust is golden brown and filling is bubbly. Cool on a wire rack. (Bake your fruit pie on a piece of parchment paper in case it bubbles over. Once the pie is bubbly, it's done.)

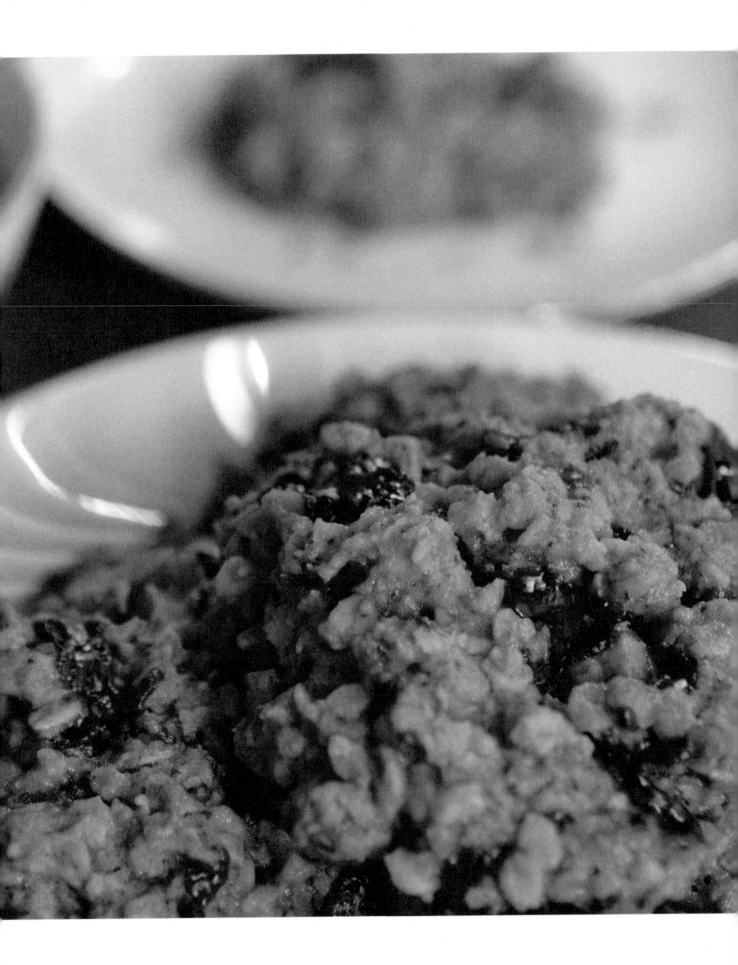

Sea Thief Cookies

·························

The beach is one of my favorite places on Earth. One spring my family and I had ventured to Clear Water, Florida, and despite the cool 60 degree water, my brother and I were determined to swim in the ocean. Mom and Dad strolled across the shore holding our belongings, including a few nut butter chocolate chip cookies we had made. About to take a bite, my mom felt something really hard plunk her on the head. "What was that!?" "My cookie is gone!!" It had vanished from her hand... a feathered sea thief had confiscated her cookie! These cookies serve as great sea gull bait; bake and enjoy them before they're gone!

Nut Butter Choco-Oats Cookies

Gluten Free

·····································

Makes 3 dozen

- 2 organic eggs
- 6 Tablespoons organic butter, no substitutes, softened
- ¾ cup coconut sugar
- ¼ teaspoon stevia
- ¾ cup organic peanut butter OR almond butter, no sugar added and non-hydrogenated

- ½ teaspoon organic pure vanilla extract
- 2 Tablespoons unsweetened applesauce OR canned pumpkin puree
- 2 ½ cups organic gluten free old fashioned rolled oats
- 1 teaspoon baking soda
- 1 cup (5 ounces) 70% or higher dark chocolate, chopped
- ½ cup pecans, chopped
- 1-2 Tablespoons unsweetened almond milk, optional

Directions:

1) In a mixing bowl, beat the eggs on high for 3 to 4 minutes until fluffy. Pour out into a bowl and set aside.
2) In the same mixing bowl, whip the butter, coconut sugar and stevia until creamy.
3) Add the nut butter of your choice and continue to cream.
4) Pour in the eggs, vanilla and your choice applesauce or pumpkin and mix well.

5) Mix in the oats and baking soda until combined.
6) Fold in the chocolate and pecans. Add in the almond milk one Tablespoon at a time and only if needed.
7) Drop batter by spoonfuls onto an unbleached parchment paper lined stainless steel cookie sheet or stoneware baking pan. Bake in preheated 350 degree oven for 10-12 minutes. Remove from cookie sheet to wire racks to cool. Store uncovered slightly.

Did you ever dream that oatmeal cookies could be enjoyed legally? Well, these cookies are not only scrumptious, but guilt free too! My favorite way to savor them is fresh out of the oven with a glass of ice cold almond milk. Happy baking!

Suggestion: Raisins could be substituted for the dark chocolate.

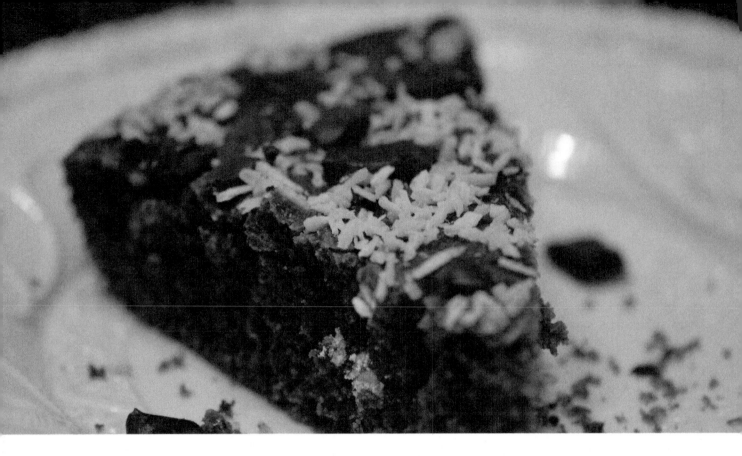

Heirloom Chocolate Cake

Gluten Free
Grain Free

12 servings

- 2 ounces 70% or higher dark chocolate, divided
- 1 Tablespoon extra-virgin coconut oil
- 1 teaspoon organic pure vanilla extract
- ¼ cup prune puree (page 310)
- ¼ cup raw honey OR coconut sugar
- ½-¾ teaspoon stevia
- 1 organic egg, beaten

- ¾ cup unsweetened almond milk
- ¼ cup organic Greek yogurt, plain whole milk
- ¾ cup garbanzo bean flour, sifted
- 2 Tablespoons coconut flour, sifted
- 1 teaspoon baking soda
- 2 Tablespoons unsweetened shredded coconut, optional

Directions:

1) In a 2 quart saucepan, melt 1 ounce of the baking chocolate with the coconut oil.

2) Add to the saucepan, vanilla, prune puree, your choice of honey or coconut sugar and stevia. Stir in the egg, milk, & yogurt and mix well.

3) Sift the garbanzo bean flour, coconut flour and soda into a measuring cup and set aside.

4) Chop the remaining 1 ounce of chocolate into chunks.

5) Add the flour mixture to the saucepan and stir just until combined. Fold in the chocolate.

6) Pour into a 9x9x2 inch glass pan coated with non-stick grapeseed oil spray and sprinkle coconut on top (if desired). Bake in preheated 350 degree oven for 35 minutes.

How to make S'Mores

Meringue makes the marshmallow fluff:
- 3 organic egg whites
- ¼ teaspoon cream of tartar
- 18 drops liquid stevia

- ½ teaspoon pure vanilla extract
- 1- 2 Tablespoons raw coconut nectar OR raw honey, to taste
- ½ teaspoon organic lemon extract
- 2 Tablespoons unsweetened shredded coconut, optional

Directions:

1) In a glass mixing bowl, beat the egg whites and cream of tartar until foamy. Gradually beat in your choice of raw coconut nectar or honey, stevia, vanilla and lemon extract until stiff peaks form.

2) Using a metal spoon immediately spread the meringue onto an unbleached parchment paper lined stainless steel baking sheet. Sprinkle the shredded coconut on the top of the meringue (if desired) and bake in preheated 350 degree oven for 12 minutes or until the meringue is golden brown.

3) While oven is still warm, place a layer of prepared Butter Spritz crispy cookies (page 307) in a single layer in a glass baking dish. Place a 1 inch square of 70% or higher dark chocolate on each cookie. Allow to melt 3-5 minutes with oven on low.

4) Remove from oven. Tear large chunks of the meringue fluff and place on the chocolate, then top with another cookie. Serve immediately. Refrigerate any leftover meringue.

Tips: Use a glass or metal bowl when making meringue. A plastic bowl or plastic utensil may have oil residue on them. Oil, egg yolk and humidity will cause meringue to deflate. Make this meringue and dollop on sliced sweet potatoes for a healthier alternative to candied yams. Tear apart the meringue and use as marshmallows in a fruit salad.

TeTe

My beloved great grandma, TeTe, who lived with us until she was 103 years old, certainly loved cake, and in her honor I named this recipe. We researched her old cookbooks from the 1950's to find "from scratch" recipes. With a few tweaks to the ingredients, we can have our cake, and eat it too!

A truly resilient woman; born 15 years after her only sister, widowed after a year and a half of marriage being left with her 2 month old baby girl (my dad's mother), attended night school 5 years to complete her elementary teaching degree and taught 41 years in the Kansas City school district. After retirement she traveled throughout Europe and Israel. Many of our recipes are pictured on her unique dishes procured from her travels. Later in her life she cared for her older sister until her passing at 101 years and lost her only daughter to brain cancer the following year. When she was 90 years old, she and my PaPa moved in with us and became my best friends and play mates- certainly a gift from the Lord!

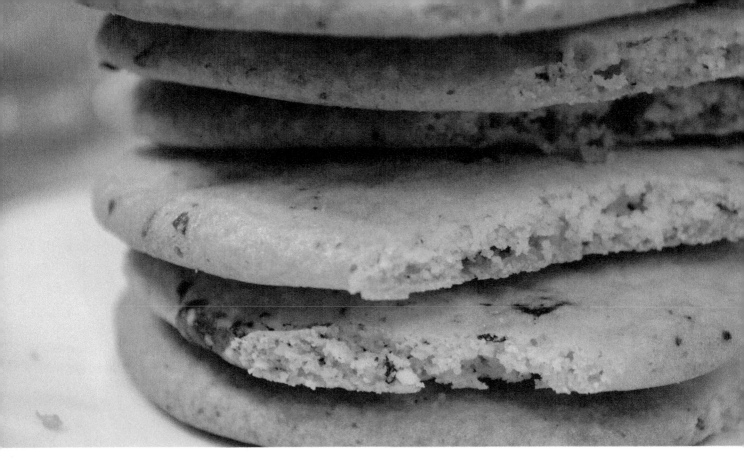

Chocolate Chip Cookies

Gluten Free

Makes 2 dozen

- 1 organic egg
- 6 Tablespoons organic butter, no substitutes, softened
- ½ cup coconut sugar
- ¼ teaspoon stevia
- 1 teaspoon organic pure vanilla extract

- 1 cup almond flour, fluffed not packed
- ½ cup millet flour, sifted
- ¼ teaspoon Nature's Sunshine® sea salt
- ½ teaspoon baking soda
- ½ teaspoon baking powder
- ½ cup pecans, chopped, optional
- ½ cup 70% or higher dark chocolate, chopped

Directions:

1) In a food processor, place the eggs, butter, coconut sugar, stevia, vanilla, flour, sea salt, baking soda and baking powder and process for 1 minute.

2) Pour into a mixing bowl and fold in the pecans (if using) and the chocolate.

3) Drop batter by small spoonfuls onto unbleached parchment paper lined stainless steel cookie sheet or use a stoneware baking pan. Leave plenty of room in between because these cookies spread out and puff up.

4) Bake in preheated 350 degree oven for 14-15 minutes. Remove from cookie sheet to wire racks to cool. Store lightly covered.

Tip: This cookie is great with pecans and wonderful without them! Try it both ways. Cookie Cake: Omit the pecans and spread all the batter onto an unbleached parchment paper lined cookie sheet and bake in preheated 350 degree oven for 23 minutes.

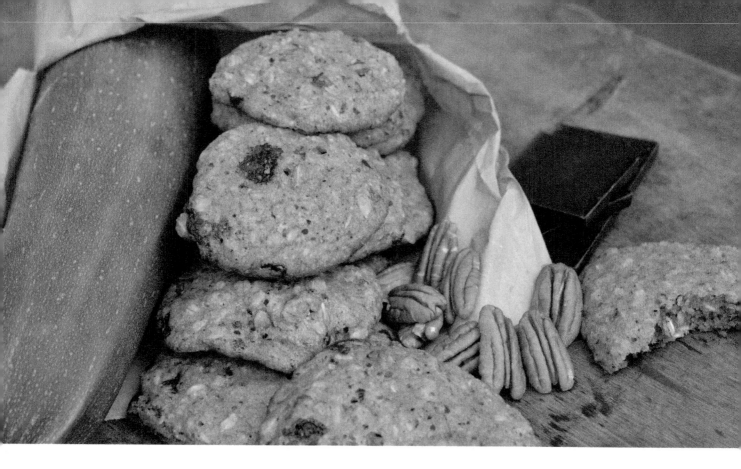

Zucchini Chocolate Chip Cookies

Makes 3 dozen soft cookies

- ½ cup organic butter, no substitutes, softened
- ¾ cup coconut sugar
- ¼ teaspoon stevia
- 2 organic eggs
- 1 teaspoon organic pure vanilla extract
- 1 cup zucchini, shredded and well drained

- ¾ cup millet flour, fluffed
- ½ cup almond flour, fluffed
- 1 teaspoon baking soda
- 1 teaspoon cinnamon
- 1 cup organic gluten free old fashioned rolled oats, dry
- ¾ cup 70% or higher dark chocolate, chopped
- ½-1 cup pecans, chopped

Directions:

1) In a mixing bowl, beat the butter on high until fluffy. Add in the coconut sugar and stevia until creamy. Add in the eggs and beat well.

2) Next, add in the vanilla and the zucchini and mix well.

3) Combine the millet flour, almond flour, baking soda and cinnamon. Slowly add into the batter mixing well. Fold in the oats, chocolate and pecans.

4) Drop batter by spoonfuls onto an unbleached parchment paper lined stainless steel cookie sheet or stoneware baking pan. Bake in preheated 350 degree oven for 10-13 minutes. Remove from cookie sheet to wire racks to cool. Store uncovered slightly

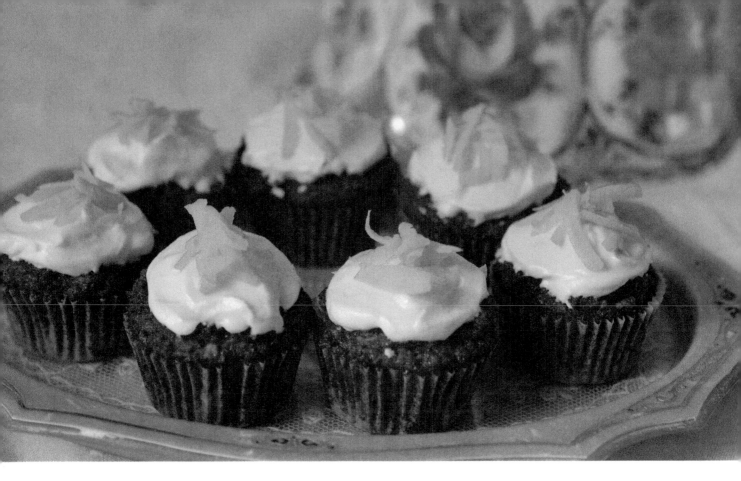

Vanilla Cream Cheese Frosting

Gluten Free
Grain Free

1 cup

- 4 ounces organic cream cheese
- 3 Tablespoons organic butter, no substitutes
- 1 teaspoon unsweetened almond milk
- ¼ teaspoon stevia (21 drops liquid stevia), to taste
- 1 teaspoon organic pure vanilla extract
- 2 Tablespoons raw honey

Directions:

1) Whip cream cheese, butter, almond milk, stevia, vanilla and honey together with a mixer until very smooth and creamy.

2) Frost onto a completely cooled cake and store in the refrigerator.

Lemon Cream Cheese Frosting

Gluten Free
Grain Free

1 ½ cups

- 8 ounces organic cream cheese
- ½ cup organic butter, no substitutes
- 1 teaspoon organic lemon zest
- 2 teaspoons organic lemon juice
- ½ teaspoon stevia
- ½ teaspoon organic pure vanilla extract
- ¼ cup raw honey

Directions:

1) Whip cream cheese, butter, lemon zest, lemon juice, stevia, vanilla and honey together with a mixer until smooth and creamy.

2) Frost onto a completely cooled cake and store in the refrigerator.

Cashew Frosting - Vanilla

1 ½ cups

- 1 cup cashews, soaked
- 3 Tablespoons extra-virgin coconut oil
- ¼ cup unsweetened applesauce
- 3 Tablespoons unsweetened almond milk
- 12-18 drops liquid stevia
- 3 Tablespoons raw honey OR coconut sugar
- 1 ½ Tablespoons arrowroot powder
- ½ Tablespoon organic pure vanilla extract
- ½ teaspoon organic pure almond extract
- ¼ teaspoon guar gum

Directions:

1) Place the cashews in a cup and fill with enough water to cover by one inch. Soak the cashews for 2 hours. Drain and roll up in a towel to soak up any excess liquid.

2) Pour cashews into a high speed blender along with coconut oil, applesauce, almond milk, stevia, your choice honey or coconut sugar, arrowroot powder, extracts and guar gum. Blend on high until smooth and creamy.

3) Frost onto a completely cooled cake and store extra frosting in the refrigerator up to one week.

Frostings (page 315):

- **Blue Frosting** – ½ Tablespoon juice of mashed blueberries per ½ cup frosting.
- **Pink Frosting** – 1/8 teaspoon of beet powder per ½ cup frosting.
- **Purple Frosting** – Combine blue and pink frosting to make purple.
- **Green Frosting** – 5-8 drops Nature's Sunshine® Liquid Chlorophyll ES™ per ½ cup frosting.
- **Yellow Frosting** – Dash of Turmeric spice per ½ cup frosting.

Toppings:

- Green Frosting with Nature's Sunshine® peppermints, crushed.
- Pink Sprinkles – unsweetened shredded coconut, finely minced, mixed with beet powder.
- Yellow Frosting with unsweetened shredded coconut.
- Pink Frosting with cacao nibs.

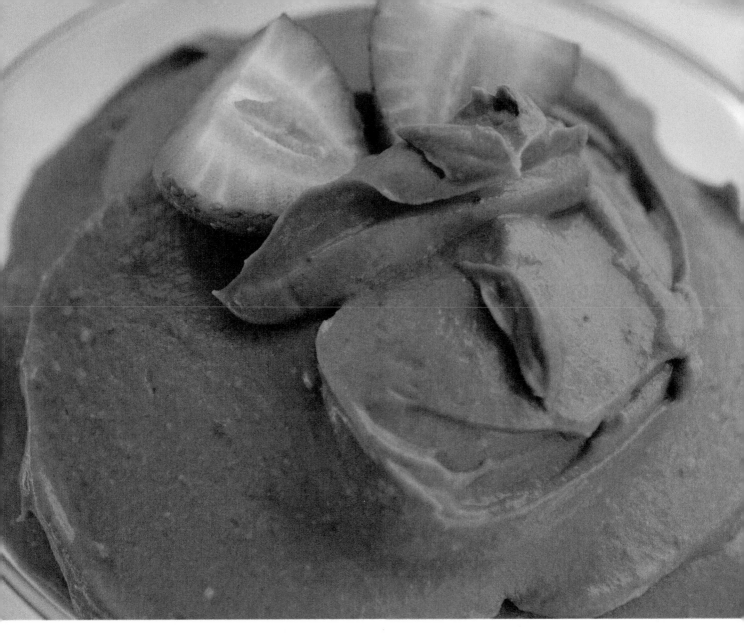

Chocolate Pudding

Gluten Free
Grain Free

2-4 servings

- 1 ½ cups avocado, sliced
- 2 Tablespoons raw honey
- 1 Tablespoon carob powder

- ¼ teaspoon stevia
- 1 ounce 70% or higher dark chocolate, melted
- ½ teaspoon organic pure vanilla extract
- 1 Tablespoon unsweetened almond milk
  OR coconut milk

Directions:

1) In a food processor combine the avocado, raw honey, carob powder, milk, melted chocolate, stevia and vanilla. Process until smooth and creamy.

Scrape down the sides of the bowl if necessary, and process until smooth. Chill in the refrigerator until ready to serve or enjoy immediately.

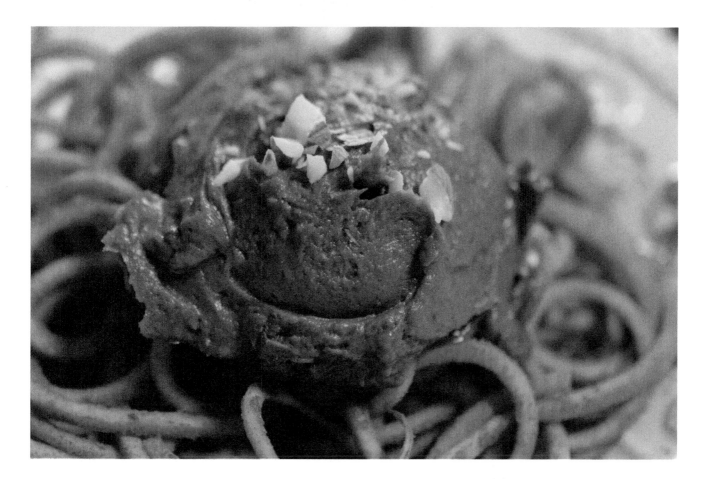

A unique and delicious way to serve this pudding: Spiralize a sweet potato. Dust the snoodles with cinnamon. Plate 1 cup of snoodles for each serving then place ¼-⅓ cup of chocolate pudding in the center. Sprinkle with chopped almonds. Enjoy!

Coconut Pie Crust

Gluten Free
Grain Free

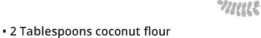

Makes 1 (9 inch) pie

• 1 ¾ cup unsweetened coconut flakes

• 2 Tablespoons coconut flour
• 5 Tablespoons cold organic butter, no substitutes

Directions:

1) In a stainless steel skillet, sauté the coconut flakes, coconut flour and butter for 7 minutes over medium heat, stirring constantly.

2) Remove from skillet and press onto the bottom and up the sides of a 9 inch glass or stoneware pie dish sprayed lightly with non-stick grapeseed oil spray.

3) Bake in preheated 350 degree oven for 7 minutes.

This crust is pictured with the chocolate cream pie filling on page 282-283.

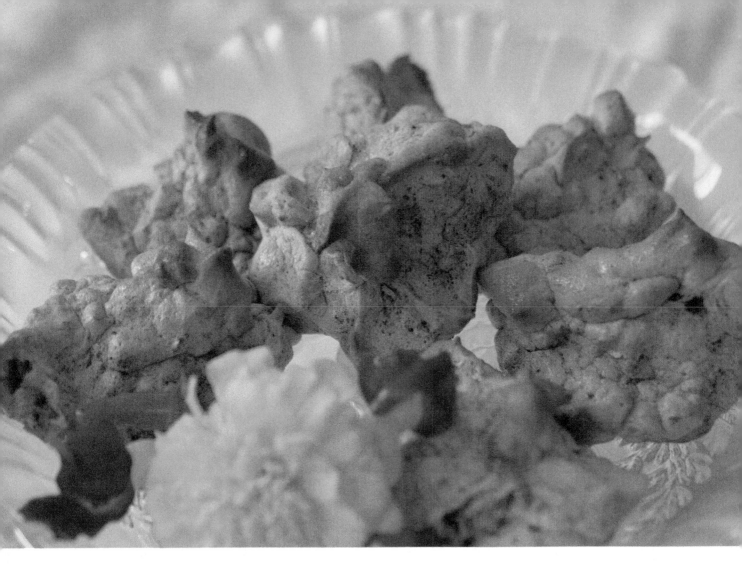

Surprise in the Clouds Cookies

Makes 1 ½ dozen

- ¼ teaspoon cream of tartar
- 3 organic egg whites
- 1-2 Tablespoons raw coconut nectar OR raw honey, to taste
- 18 drops liquid stevia
- 1 teaspoon pure vanilla extract
- 3 teaspoons carob powder
- ½ cup pecans, chopped
- ⅓ cup unsweetened shredded coconut

Directions:

1) In a glass mixing bowl, beat the egg whites and cream of tartar until foamy. Gradually beat in your choice of raw coconut nectar or honey, stevia and vanilla extract until stiff peaks form.

2) Using a metal spoon, fold in the carob powder, pecans and coconut. Then immediately drop the meringue by spoonfuls onto an unbleached parchment paper lined stainless steel baking sheet. Bake in preheated 350 degree oven for 10-12 minutes or until the meringue is golden brown. Cool on a wire rack.

Tips: Use a glass or metal bowl when making these meringue cookies. A plastic bowl or plastic utensil may have oil residue on them which will cause the meringue to deflate.

Key Lime Dream Dessert

2-4 servings

- 1 ½ cups avocado (about 2 medium)
- 6 Tablespoons fresh squeezed organic lime juice
- ½ teaspoon stevia, to taste
- 2-3 Tablespoons raw coconut nectar, to taste
- ¼ cup canned full fat coconut milk
- ½ teaspoon guar gum, sifted
- ¼ teaspoon lemon extract
- 1 Tablespoon Love and Peas® protein powder (Sugar Free)

Directions:

1) In a food processor, process the avocado and lime juice together for 1 minute.

2) Add stevia, coconut nectar, coconut milk, guar gum, lemon extract and Love and Peas. Process until smooth pudding like consistency.

3) For best results, chill 1 hour then serve in fancy cups with your choice of granola sprinkled generously in the bottom or on top. Garnish with unsweetened coconut flakes or a granola topping (page 222, 301).

Tip: The canned full fat coconut milk in this recipe is thick. It is NOT from a carton. One thing we learned while juicing the limes by hand with a citrus juicer, is that if you keep juicing after most of the juice is extracted, you then are grinding too hard on the inside peeling and it will result in the dessert being bitter from the rind.

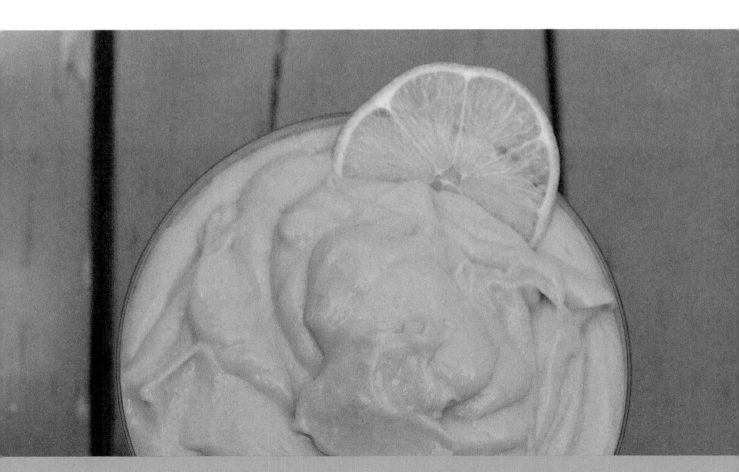

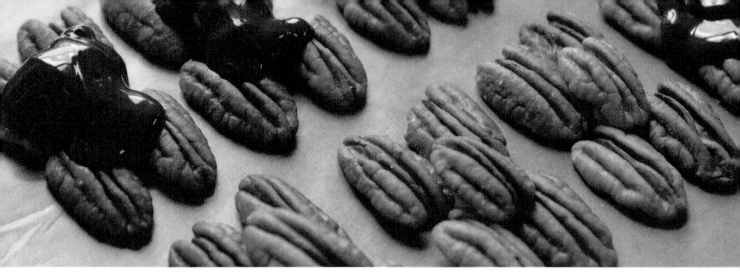

Totally Tasty Turtles

Gluten Free

Grain Free

Makes 2 ½ dozen

- ¾ cup (4.4 ounces) 70%
  or higher dark chocolate, chopped

- 150 pecan halves
- Unsweetened shredded coconut, optional

Directions:

1) Cover a large sturdy cutting board with wax paper.

2) Assemble the pecans on wax paper in clusters of five. Four on bottom and one on top.

3) In a double boiler, melt the chocolate.

4) Drop about one teaspoon full of melted chocolate over each pecan cluster. Make sure you drizzle over each pecan to glue them together as a cluster. Sprinkle with coconut (if desired).

5) Move the board of clusters to a cool place to harden. Once the chocolate cools and hardens, they can be placed on a dish and served. These refrigerate well up to 2 weeks.

Note: Once you are used to dark chocolate, these don't need any sweetener. But, if you do need these sweeter, add 8 drops liquid stevia to the melted chocolate or more to taste.

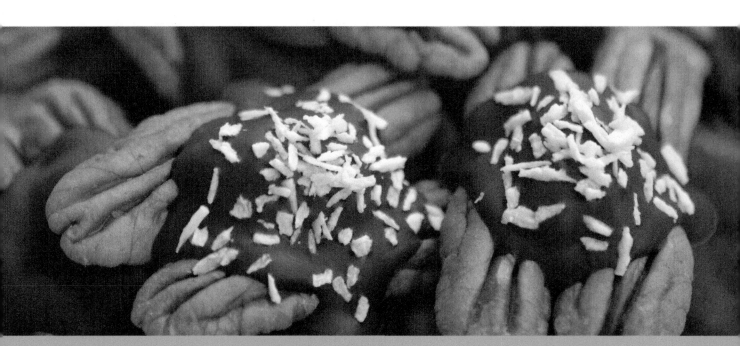

Tasty Granola Topping

6 servings
- ¾ cup organic gluten free old fashioned rolled oats, dry
- ¼ cup organic gluten free oat bran
- 1 Tablespoon coconut flour
- 1 teaspoon cinnamon
- ⅛ teaspoon ground nutmeg
- 3 Tablespoons coconut oil
- 1 Tablespoon unsweetened almond milk
- 1 teaspoon organic pure vanilla extract
- ¼ cup raw honey OR coconut sugar

Directions:

1) Combine all the dry ingredients into a medium sized bowl and stir together until well blended. Pour in the wet ingredients and stir to combine. Spread by spoonfuls on top of your favorite dish and bake.

Cinnamon Apples

6 servings

- 8 organic apples, with peeling
- 1 Tablespoon cinnamon
- 1 ½ Tablespoons raw honey
- ⅓ cup filtered water

Directions:

1) Wash, core and slice the apples into a stainless steel skillet. Add the cinnamon, honey and water. Toss to coat. Cover with lid. Cook over medium heat for 25-30 minutes until apples are tender and bubbly.

> When you're blessed with an abundance of apples, this is a quick way to make a treat.

Vanilla Ice Cream

6 servings

- ¾ cup canned full fat coconut milk
- 1 cup unsweetened almond milk
- ¼ ripe avocado, pit removed and peeled
- ¼ cup raw coconut nectar
- ½ teaspoon stevia
- 1 Tablespoon Love and Peas® protein (Sugar Free)
- 1 Tablespoon organic pure vanilla extract
- 3-4 cups ice

Directions:

1) Collect as much of the thick cream from the coconut milk to make the ¾ cup. Pour into a high speed blender along with the almond milk, avocado, coconut nectar, stevia, protein powder and vanilla. Blend for 15 seconds then add in desired amount of ice.

2) Blend on high until thick and smooth, stopping a few times to stir. Serve immediately in chilled bowls.

> Fudge brownie splurge: Add one 2 ½ x 2 ½ inch square piece of Blissful brownie (page 311) and 1 ½ Tablespoons almond butter. Blend and enjoy immediately.

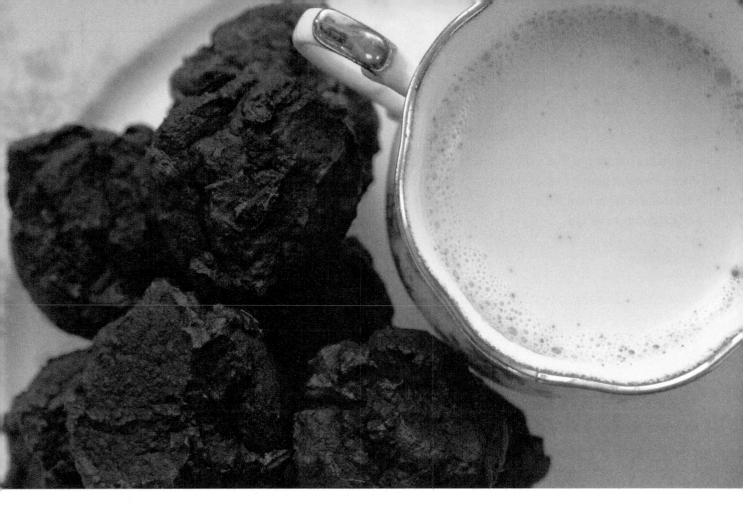

Velvet Deluxe Chocolate Cakes

Gluten Free
Grain Free

2 dozen mini-cakes

- 6 ounces 70% or higher dark chocolate
- 2 Tablespoons extra-virgin coconut oil
- 2 cups canned garbanzo beans
  OR black beans, drained and rinsed
- 4 organic eggs

- ¼ cup prune puree (page 311)
- ½ cup raw honey OR coconut sugar
- ½ teaspoon liquid stevia (chocolate flavor, optional)
- ½ teaspoon baking powder
- ½ cup cocoa powder OR carob powder

Directions:

1) In a double boiler, melt the chocolate and coconut oil over low heat. Remove from burner to cool slightly.

2) In a blender, blend your choice of beans with the eggs on high until smooth and creamy.

3) Add the prune puree, your choice of honey or coconut sugar, stevia, baking powder and your choice of cocoa powder or carob powder to the blender and blend well.

4) Pour in the cooled chocolate and blend well. (Be careful that the melted chocolate is not too hot, it will cook the eggs.)

5) Pour batter into unbleached mini muffin liners in a stainless steel muffin pan or use a stoneware muffin pan only!

6) Bake in preheated 350 degree oven for approximately 12-15 minutes.

Cream Pie Filling

Eat in Moderation

1 (9 inch) pie OR pudding

- **2 cups unsweetened almond milk**
- **¾ cup coconut sugar**
- **⅛ teaspoon Nature's Sunshine® sea salt**
- **5 organic egg yolks, lightly beaten**
- **⅓ cup Love and Peas® protein powder (Sugar Free)**

- **2 Tablespoons organic butter, no substitutes**
- **1 teaspoon organic pure vanilla extract**
- **2 Tablespoons arrowroot powder**
- **½ Tablespoon guar gum**
- **1 pastry shell, baked**

Directions:

1) Pour the almond milk, coconut sugar and sea salt into a 2 quart saucepan and stir to dissolve.

2) Turn the burner on to medium heat and immediately add in the egg yolks and stir constantly for 2 ½ minutes. Turn off burner.

3) Stir in the protein powder, butter and vanilla and continue stirring for 1 minute.

4) Remove from burner and sift the arrowroot and guar gum into the saucepan. Stir to combine. Pour all the filling from saucepan into a high speed blender and blend for 15-20 seconds on high.

5) Pour into prepared pie shell or individual pudding cups and refrigerate at least 2 hours before serving.

This recipe has a thick consistency and tastes really good. However, after the pie has been cut, the filling does tend to flow into the vacant space, so tilt the pie plate in the refrigerator to keep it in place.

- **For a coconut cream pie,** add 1 cup unsweetened shredded coconut in step 7 before pouring into pie shell.
- **For a chocolate cream pie,** add ¼ cup carob powder in step 6.
- **For a banana cream pie,** slice 3 firm bananas into filling in step 7.
- **For a banana coconut cream pie,** slice 3 firm bananas and ¼ cup unsweetened shredded coconut into the filling in step 7.

Cream Pie Filling is pictured on page 282.

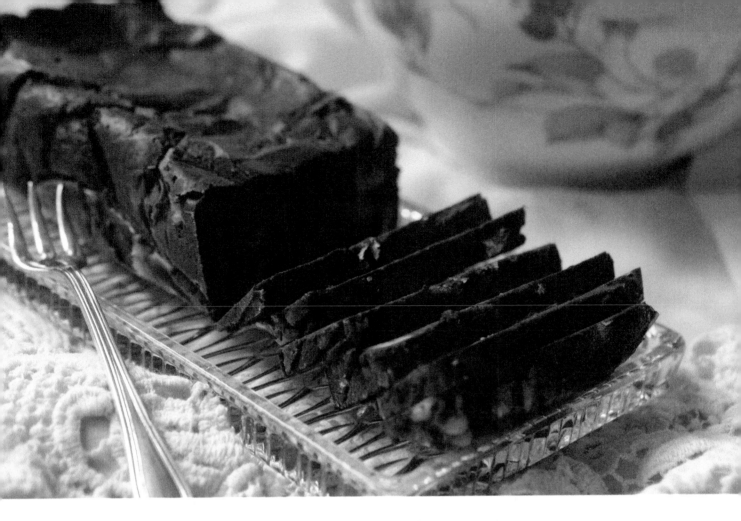

No Pudge Fudge

2 ½ dozen pieces

- ¼ cup extra-virgin coconut oil
- 1 ounce 70% or higher dark chocolate
- ⅓ cup unsweetened canned pumpkin puree
- ¼ cup raw honey OR coconut sugar

- ¼ teaspoon stevia
- ½ teaspoon cinnamon
- ¾ cup unsweetened cocoa OR carob powder
- ½ cup walnuts, chopped

Directions:

1) In a saucepan, melt the coconut oil and dark chocolate on medium-low heat.

2) Add in the pumpkin and stir to combine.

3) Mix in your choice of honey or coconut sugar, stevia, cinnamon and your choice of cocoa or carob powder.

4) Fold in walnuts and sprinkle a few on top. Line a dish with unbleached parchment paper and refrigerate until set. Cover and store in the refrigerator.

ENJOY... in moderation.

Apple Crisp

6 servings

Gluten Free

Grain Free

- 6 cups organic apples, with peeling
- 1 Tablespoon cinnamon, to taste
- 1 Tablespoon coconut flour
- 2 Tablespoons organic butter
- 2 Tablespoons almond milk
- 1 Tablespoon raw honey
- Dash stevia, to taste

Directions:

1) Wash, core and thinly slice the apples into a large bowl. Add the cinnamon to taste, flour, butter, almond milk, honey and stevia. Toss to coat.

2) Pour the apples in a 9x9x2 inch (2 ½ quart) glass baking dish coated with non-stick grapeseed oil spray.

3) Choose a granola topping from page 222, 301 and bake in preheated 350 degree oven for 30-45 minutes until fruit is tender and topping is golden brown.

Peach Crisp

8 servings

Gluten Free

Grain Free

- 8 cups ripe organic peaches, sliced, divided
- 1 Tablespoon guar gum
- 1 Tablespoon organic butter
- ⅓ cup coconut sugar OR raw honey
- ½ teaspoon stevia, to taste
- ⅛ teaspoon almond extract, optional
- ¼ cup fresh squeezed orange juice, optional

Directions:

1) Place 5 cups of fresh or completely thawed peaches in a 2 quart saucepan and sift the guar gum over the peaches. Add the butter, your choice of coconut sugar or honey, stevia, almond extract (if desired) and the orange juice (if needed).

2) Cook for 5-10 minutes, stirring until thickened and bubbly.

3) Pour the thickened sauce over the remaining peaches in a 9x9x2 inch glass baking dish coated with non-stick grapeseed oil spray.

4) Choose a granola topping (page 222, 301) and bake in preheated 350 degree oven for 30-35 minutes until fruit is bubbly and topping is golden brown.

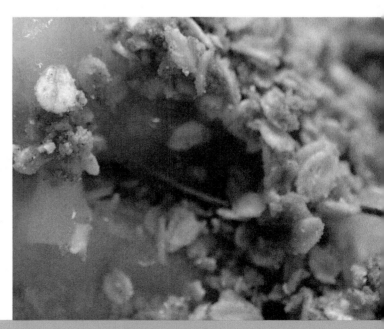

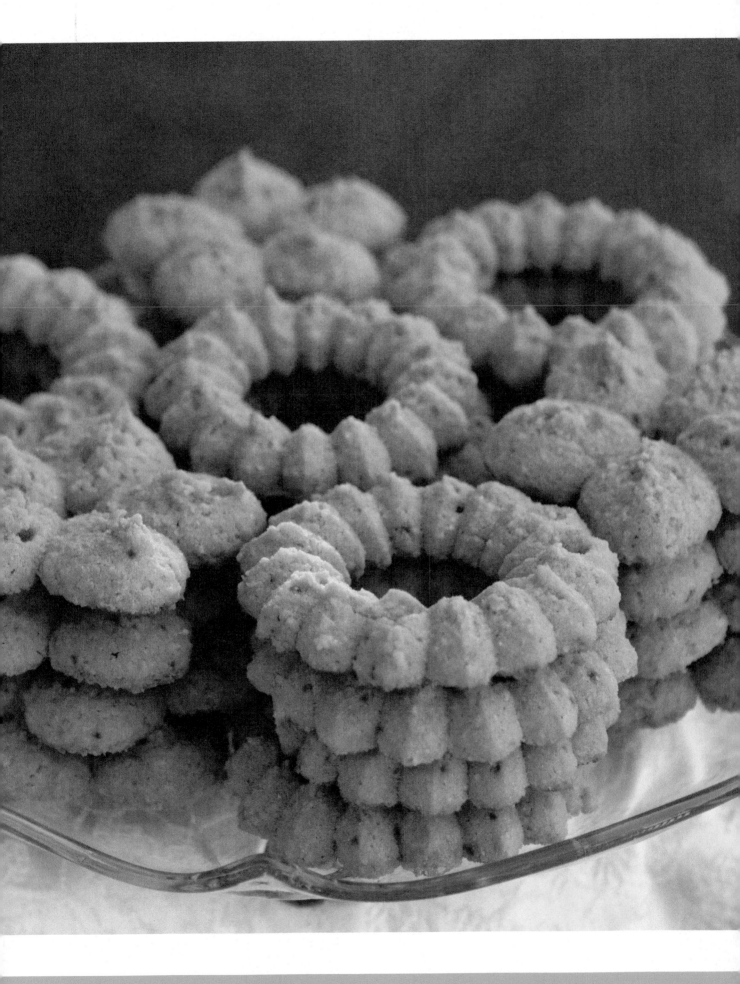

Butter Spritz Cookies

Makes 6 dozen

- 1 cup organic butter, no substitutes, softened
- ½ cup coconut sugar
- ⅛ teaspoon stevia
- 2 small organic eggs
- 1 teaspoon organic pure vanilla extract

- 1 teaspoon unsweetened almond milk
- ⅛ teaspoon Nature's Sunshine® sea salt
- ¾ cup garbanzo bean flour, sifted
- ⅓ cup coconut flour, fluffed, not packed
- ½ cup Love and Peas® protein powder (Sugar Free), fluffed

Directions:

1) In a mixing bowl, cream the butter, coconut sugar and stevia.

2) Add in the eggs, vanilla and almond milk then mix well.

3) Stir together the sea salt, garbanzo bean flour, coconut flour and protein powder. Gradually add to creamed mixture, mixing just until thoroughly combined.

4) Scoop batter into a cookie press and press the cookies out onto an unbleached parchment paper lined cookie sheet, ungreased stainless steel baking sheet or stoneware. No need to leave room because these cookies do not spread out.

5) Bake in preheated 350 degree oven for approximately 12 minutes or until lightly browned around the edges. Remove from cookie sheet to wire racks to cool.

Tip: For crispier cookies – omit one egg.

Flavor options:
- Lemon – replace vanilla extract and the almond milk with 2 teaspoons of organic pure lemon extract and 2 teaspoons organic lemon zest.
- Cinnamon – add 2 teaspoons cinnamon.
- Almond – replace vanilla extract with 2 teaspoons organic pure almond extract.

Use this recipe for a crispy cookie that spreads out-
Follow the exact recipe above except for the flour and protein powder. Use these amounts: 1 cup Garbanzo flour, 1 cup almond flour & ½ cup Love and Peas protein powder. Drop by spoonfuls onto unbleached parchment paper or on ungreased baking sheet. Bake in 350 degree oven for approximately 12-15 minutes.

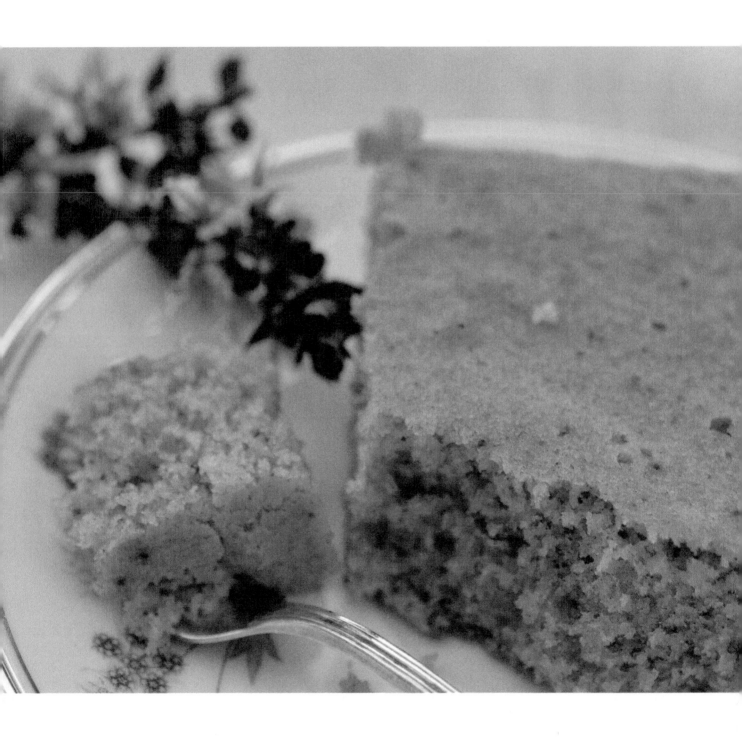

Spice Cake

12 servings

- ½ cup organic butter, no substitutes, softened
- ¾ cup coconut sugar
- ¼ teaspoon stevia
- 3 organic eggs
- ¼ cup organic Greek yogurt, plain whole milk
- ½ cup unsweetened almond milk

- 1 teaspoon organic pure vanilla extract
- 1 cup almond flour, fluffed and measured by spoonfuls
- 1 cup millet flour, sifted twice
- 1 teaspoon baking powder
- ½ teaspoon baking soda
- 1 ½ teaspoons cinnamon
- 1 teaspoon ground nutmeg
- ½ teaspoon ground cloves

Directions:

1) In a mixing bowl, whip the butter for 2 minutes. Add in the coconut sugar and stevia and whip for 1 minute.

2) Add the eggs one at a time, mixing 30 seconds after each addition.

3) Combine the yogurt, almond milk and vanilla. Set aside.

4) Combine the almond flour, millet flour, baking powder, baking soda, cinnamon, nutmeg and cloves. Slowly add in the dry ingredients while alternating with the yogurt mixture until all ingredients are combined. Don't over mix.

5) Pour batter into a 9x13x2 inch glass pan coated with grapeseed oil spray.

6) Bake in preheated 350 degree oven for 25-30 minutes. Test for doneness when a knife inserted comes out clean. Remove from oven to a wire rack to cool completely. Lightly cover to store. Tastes great without frosting.

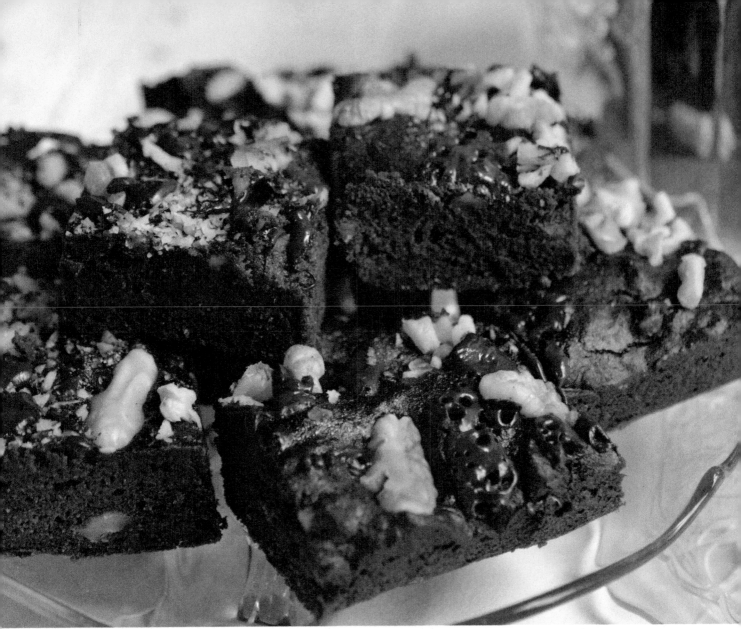

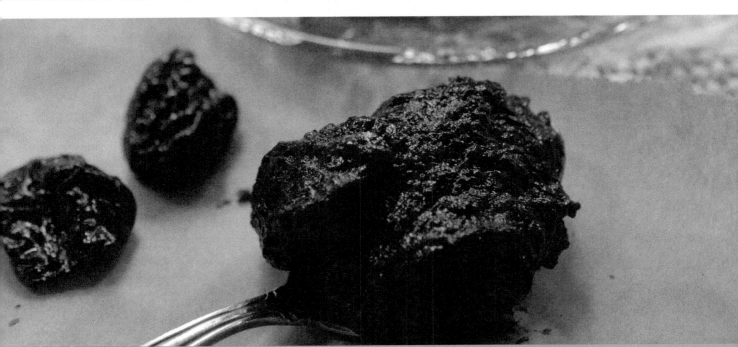

Blissful Brownies

3 ½ dozen (1 inch square servings)

- 3 Tablespoons extra-virgin coconut oil
- 5 Tablespoons organic butter,
  no substitutes, softened
- ¾ cup coconut sugar
- 1 teaspoon stevia (chocolate flavor, optional)
- ½ cup prune puree
- ⅓ cup canned pumpkin puree

- 2 teaspoons organic pure vanilla extract
- 4 organic eggs
- 1 cup garbanzo bean flour, sifted
- 1 teaspoon baking powder
- ½ cup carob powder
- ¾-1 cup walnuts, chopped, divided
- 4 ounces 70% or higher dark chocolate,
  chopped, divided

Directions:

1) In a mixing bowl beat the coconut oil and the butter for 1 minute.

2) Add in the coconut sugar, stevia, prune puree, pumpkin and vanilla. Mix for 1 minute.

3) Add the eggs then mix well. Sift the garbanzo bean flour and baking powder into the mixing bowl, add the carob powder then mix just until blended.

4) Fold in some of the walnuts and chocolate chunks, reserving most of them for sprinkling on top of the batter.

5) Spray a glass pan with grapeseed oil spray. Pour batter into greased pan and sprinkle the remaining walnuts and chocolate on top.

Bake in preheated 325 degree oven for:
Two 8x8x2 inch pans – for approximately 25 minutes for fudgy brownies and 30 minutes for cake-like brownies or until toothpick inserted tests done.
One 9x13x2 inch pan – for 35 minutes.

Remove from oven to a wire rack to cool completely. Lightly cover to store.

How to make Prune Puree

Makes 2 cups

- 2 cups dried organic prunes
- 2 ½ cups warm filtered water
- ¼ - ⅓ cup filtered water

Directions:

1) Soak prunes in warm water for 10 minutes to soften.
2) Drain and rinse the prunes.
3) Place the prunes in a food processor or blender with ¼ cup to ⅓ cup of water and process until it becomes a thick paste. Store in the freezer in a tightly sealed BPA free Ziploc® style freezer bag until ready to use.

Cinnamon Pecan Coffee Cake

12 servings

- 10 Tablespoons organic butter, no substitutes
- 1 cup almond flour, fluffed and measured by spoonfuls
- ¾ cup millet flour, sifted twice
- ¾ cup garbanzo bean flour, sifted twice
- ½ teaspoon stevia (21 drops liquid stevia)
- 1 cup coconut sugar
- ¾ teaspoon baking powder
- 1 teaspoon cinnamon

- ½ cup pecans, chopped
- ⅔ cup organic Greek yogurt, plain whole milk
- ⅓ cup unsweetened almond milk
- 1 teaspoon baking soda
- 1 large organic egg, lightly beaten
- 1 teaspoon organic pure vanilla extract
- ¼ teaspoon Nature's Sunshine® sea salt
- 1 teaspoon cinnamon

Directions:

1) In a food processor, add the butter, almond flour, millet flour, garbanzo bean flour, stevia, coconut sugar and baking powder. Process 20 seconds then pulse 8 times.

2) Remove 1/3 cup of butter batter and place in a small mixing bowl. To this bowl, add 1 teaspoon cinnamon and pecans. Work the butter batter and pecans together by fluffing it with a fork or your fingers, then set aside.

3) In another small mixing bowl, place the yogurt and almond milk then whip in the baking soda. Add to this mixture the beaten egg, sea salt and vanilla extract. Now pour this mixture into the food processor and process 20 seconds.

4) Remove ¾ cup of this mixture from the food processor, place in a small mixing bowl and add 1 teaspoon of cinnamon. Stir to combine and set aside.

5) Spray a 9x13x2 inch glass pan with grapeseed oil spray. Pour in half of the remaining batter from the food processor into glass pan. Then drizzle all of the cinnamon batter over that. Now pour the remaining contents of the food processor over the cinnamon batter.

6) Sprinkle the butter pecan topping all over the top of the cake.

7) Bake in preheated 350 degree oven for 45-50 minutes. Test for doneness when a knife inserted comes out clean. Remove from oven to a wire rack to cool completely. Lightly cover to store.

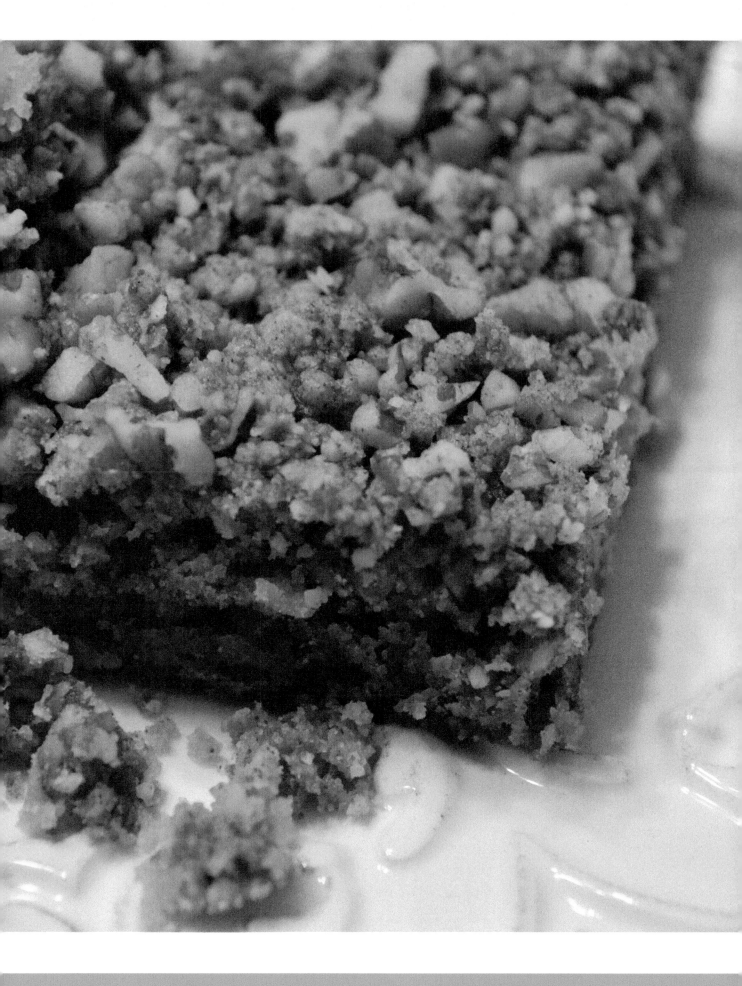

Red Velvet Cupcakes

12 cupcakes

- 1 cup unsweetened almond milk
- 1 Tablespoon fresh squeezed lemon juice
- 1 teaspoon beet powder mixed with 2 teaspoons water
- ½ cup organic butter, no substitutes, softened
- 1 cup coconut sugar
- ½ teaspoon stevia
- 3 organic eggs

- 1 ½ cups almond flour, fluffed
- ⅓ cup coconut flour, fluffed
- 2 ½ Tablespoons carob powder
- 1 ½ teaspoons baking soda
- ½ teaspoon Nature's Sunshine® sea salt
- 1 teaspoon organic pure vanilla extract

Directions:

1) Mix the almond milk and lemon juice together and set aside.

2) Mix the beet powder and water together and set aside.

3) In a large mixing bowl, beat the butter, coconut sugar and stevia together until creamy.

4) Add in the eggs and beat until fluffy.

5) Combine the almond flour, coconut flour, carob powder, baking soda and sea salt. Mix well. Add to the mixing bowl by spoonfuls alternating with the almond milk.

6) Add in the vanilla and beet powder mixture.

7) Pour batter into unbleached muffin liners in a stainless steel muffin pan or use a stoneware muffin pan only!

8) Bake in preheated 350 degree oven for 25 minutes. The cupcakes do not rise very high; they have a sunken in appearance. Allow to cool and frost with cashew vanilla or chocolate frosting. (page 295, 279)

It is a huge concern of the amount of food coloring in red velvet cake. This is my creation using beet powder. The cake is moist and chocolaty; it is delicious right out of the oven without any icing. If you choose to ice it, try the cashew chocolate frosting! Try it with the cashew vanilla frosting, sprinkle on unsweetened shredded coconut and chopped pecans for an almost German chocolate flavor!

Ice Cream Sandwich batter:

Add ¼ teaspoon of guar gum to ½ cup of Red Velvet Cup Cake batter. Mix well and spread onto a stainless steel baking sheet lined with parchment paper in a oval shape measuring 4x2 ½ inches and about ¼ inch thick. Bake in preheated 350 degree oven for about 8-10 minutes. Cool completely. Wafer should be able to peel off the parchment paper and stay together. Slice So Delicious® Dairy Free Coconut Milk non-dairy frozen dessert, No sugar added Vanilla Bean flavored (ice cream) onto one slice of the wafer and top with a second wafer. Wrap in BPA free plastic wrap and place in the freezer. It won't last long!!

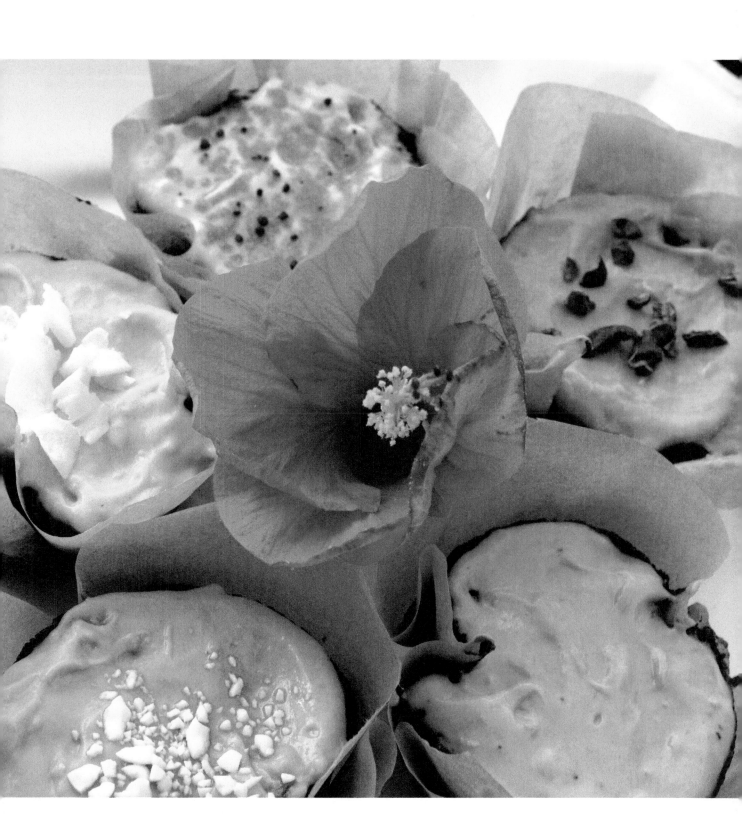

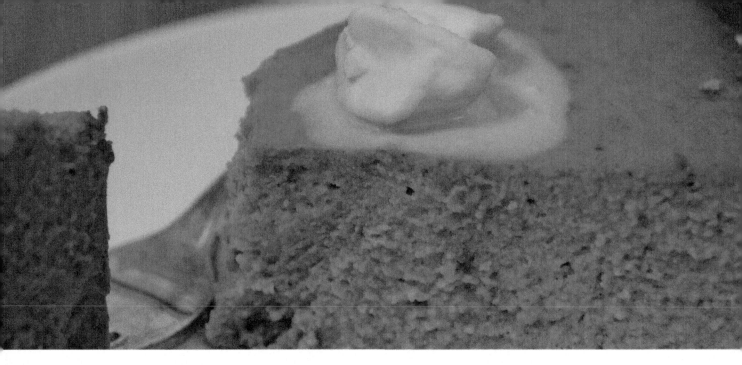

Perfect Pumpkin Pie Filling

1 deep dish or 2 regular 9 inch pies

- 4 organic eggs
- 2 (15 ounce) cans unsweetened pumpkin puree
  OR 4 cups cooked pumpkin•
- 1 teaspoon stevia
- 1 Tablespoon coconut flour, optional
- 1 Tablespoon cinnamon
- ½ teaspoon Nature's Sunshine® sea salt

- 1 teaspoon ground ginger
- ½ teaspoon ground cloves
- ¼ teaspoon ground nutmeg
- ½ cup coconut sugar OR raw honey
- 1 ½ teaspoons organic pure vanilla extract
- 1 (13.5 ounce) canned full fat coconut milk

Directions:

1) In a mixing bowl, beat the eggs until fluffy. Pour in the pumpkin puree and mix well.

2) Combine the stevia, flour, cinnamon, salt, ginger, cloves, nutmeg and coconut sugar (if using) in a small bowl and stir together. Add to the pumpkin and mix well.

3) Add the honey (if using), vanilla and the milk. Mix well.

4) Pour the pumpkin into the glass baking dish coated with non-stick grapeseed oil spray and bake in preheated 400 degree oven for 20 minutes then reduce the heat to 350 degrees for 40-45 minutes or until knife inserted near the center comes out clean.

This recipe is to save time and calories...make the pie and skip the crust!

•Not pie filling! If using fresh cooked pumpkin, increase coconut flour to 2 ½ Tablespoons.
The canned full fat coconut milk in this recipe is thick and NOT in a carton.
Pictured with So Delicious® vanilla bean ice cream (see page 314 box).

Lemon Pie

Eat in Moderation

Makes 1 pie

- ½ cup raw honey
- ½ teaspoon liquid stevia
- 1 Tablespoon guar gum
- 3 Tablespoons arrowroot
- 2 Tablespoons Love and Peas® protein powder
- 1 cup filtered water

- 4 organic egg yolks
- 3 Tablespoons organic butter, no substitutes
- ½ Tablespoon organic lemon zest
- ¾ cup fresh organic squeezed lemon juice
- 1 teaspoon organic pure lemon extract
- 1 pastry shell (9 inches), baked

Directions:

1) In a 2 quart saucepan, pour honey, stevia, guar gum, arrowroot and protein powder. Stir these ingredients with a whisk to thoroughly combine.

2) Turn the burner on to medium-high heat and place the saucepan on the burner. Add the water and eggs and whisk constantly for approximately 2- 2 ½ minutes. The mixture will become thick and frothy.

3) Turn off burner. Stir in the butter until absorbed into the mixture.

4) Pour in the lemon zest, lemon juice, and lemon extract. Stir until all combined.

5) Let the mixture cool for 10 minutes then pour into baked pie shell or pudding cups. Refrigerate for at least 2 hours before serving.

> The Love and Peas® protein powder makes the lemon pudding smooth and creamy. IF you do not have any, coconut flour could be substituted, however it has tiny pieces of coconut in it, so the texture is not smooth; but it tastes really good!

Meringue

Gluten Free
Grain Free
Dairy Free

Makes 1 pie

- 3 organic egg whites
- 1- 2 Tablespoons raw coconut nectar
OR raw honey, to taste

- ¼ teaspoon cream of tartar
- 18 drops liquid stevia
- ½ teaspoon pure vanilla extract
- ½ teaspoon organic lemon extract
- 2 Tablespoons unsweetened shredded coconut, optional

Directions:

1) In a glass mixing bowl, beat the egg whites and cream of tartar until foamy. Gradually beat in your choice of raw coconut nectar or honey, stevia, vanilla and lemon extract until stiff peaks form.

2) Using a metal spoon immediately spread the meringue onto an unbleached parchment paper lined baking sheet. Sprinkle the shredded coconut on the top of the meringue (if desired) and bake in preheated 350 degree oven for 12 minutes or until the meringue is golden brown. Cool on a wire rack.

3) To transfer the cooled meringue to the lemon pie, hold the parchment paper and meringue in one hand while peeling back the paper and rolling it up with the other hand. Lay the meringue on the pie and continue peeling back the paper until all of the meringue is lying on the pie. Serve immediately or refrigerate until ready to serve.

> **Tips:** Use a glass or metal bowl when making meringue. A plastic bowl or plastic utensil may have oil residue on them. Oil, egg yolk and humidity will cause meringue to deflate. If you make this meringue for another flavor of pie, omit the lemon extract and change the pure vanilla extract to 1 teaspoon.

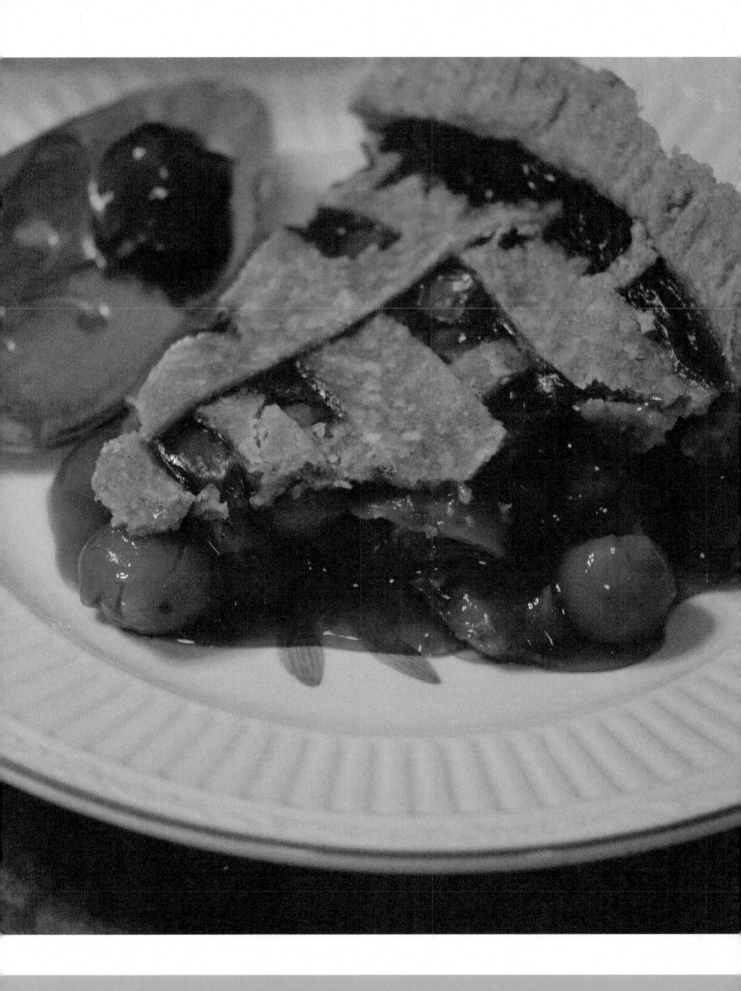

Cherry Pie

1 deep dish pie

Eat in Moderation

- 1 Tablespoon guar gum
- 1 ½ teaspoon stevia
- 1 teaspoon almond extract
- ¼ cup raw honey OR coconut sugar
- 1 cup sweet cherries, frozen
- 3 (14.5 ounce) cans pitted unsweetened tart cherries in water
- Pastry for double-crust pie (9 inches) (page 287)

Directions:

1) Drain the juice from the canned cherries into a 3 quart saucepan, drain well. Sift the guar gum over the juice and stir with a whisk to thoroughly combine.

2) Turn the burner on to medium heat and whisk until thickened and bubbly. Continue whisking as you add the stevia, almond extract and your choice of honey or coconut sugar. Cook for about 2 minutes.

3) Stir in frozen cherries with a spoon. Then gently fold in the canned cherries. Remove from heat and set aside.

4) Line the glass or stoneware deep dish pie plate with bottom crust. Pour in the thickened cherries. Roll out remaining pastry to fit top of pie. Place over filling. Trim, seal and flute the edges. Make several slits in the top pastry to allow steam to release.

5) Bake in preheated 375 degree oven on bottom rack for 55 minutes or until crust is golden brown and filling is bubbly. Cool on a wire rack. (Bake your pie on a piece of parchment paper in case it bubbles over. Once the pie is bubbly, it's done.)

Cherry Crisp: Pour cherries into a glass baking dish coated with non-stick grapeseed oil and sprinkle a granola topping (page 222, 301) on top. Bake in a preheated 350 degree oven for 20-30 minutes until fruit is bubbly and topping is golden.

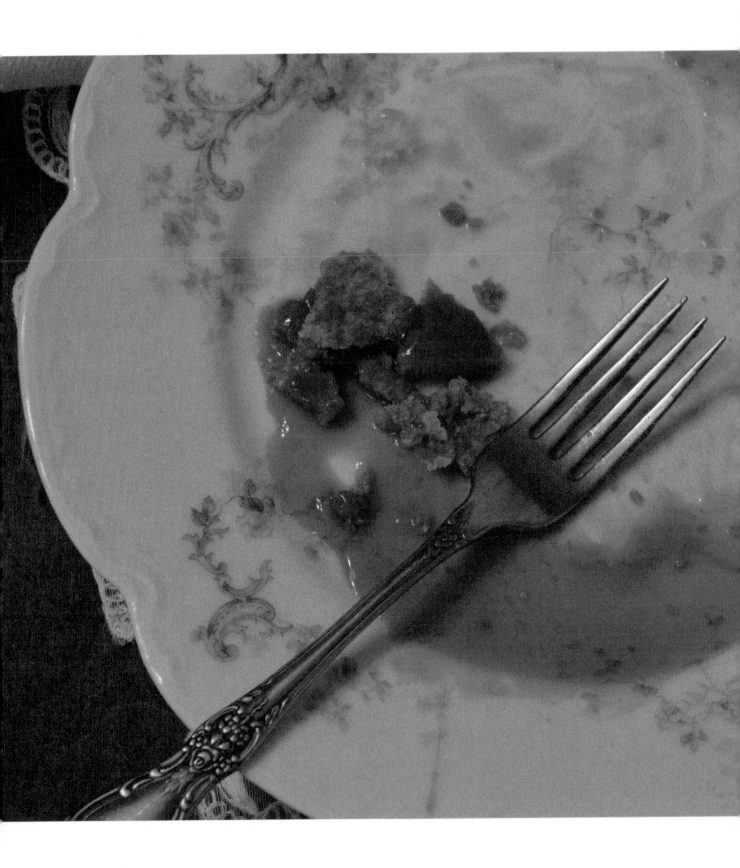

Dad's Cherry Pie

. . . .

Everyone has their favorites, and for my dad, it is this cherry pie. In our less healthier days, my dad and I were "ice cream buddies," but now, we have treats such as this that we can enjoy together. It's just the pits when the pie is gone...

Delicious!

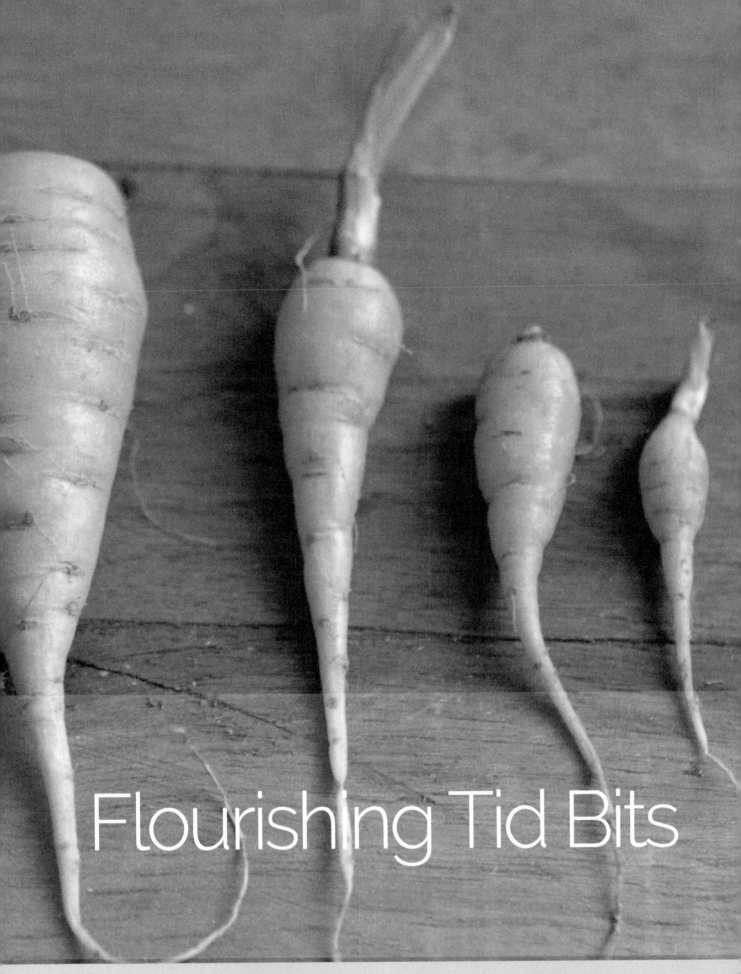

Flourishing Tid Bits

Meals 2 Flourish

Begin 2 Flourish: what to eat when you are new to healthy eating...

	Sample Day 1:	Sample Day 2:
Breakfast:	Blueberry Smoothie	Egg Omelet Muffins
Lunch:	Parade of Flavors salad, cooked chicken breast	Fiesta Quinoa with left over taco meat and beans, carrot sticks
Dinner:	Tacos, Black Beans, Guacamole, sliced Romaine lettuce and shredded carrots	Tender Crockpot Chicken, Garlic Spud Caul-it-Tatoes, Easy Seasoned Broccoli, Orange Courtwarming Salad

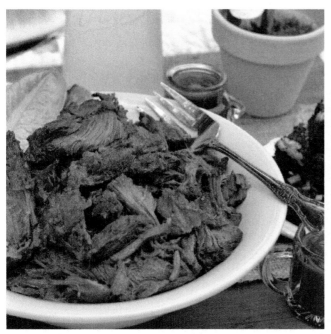
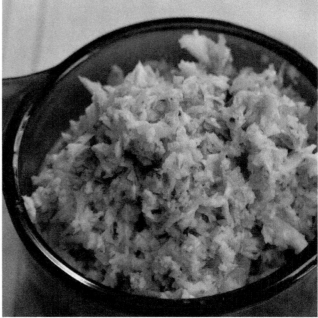

Nourish 2 Flourish:
what to eat for optimized energy, immune strength, and weight management*...

	Sample Day 1:	Sample Day 2:
Breakfast:	Robin's Power Smoothie	Egg Super Food Sauté with sliced avocado and roasted seaweed chips (optional)
Lunch:	Market Me Smile Salad, cooked Spicy Chicken Breast	Favorito Burrito, raw veggies
Dinner:	Perfectly Delicious Salmon, Mild Comforting Spaghetti Squash, Roasted Brussels Sprouts	Baked Chicken, Butternut Curry Soup, Sesame Cashew Crunch Coleslaw

Nourish 2 Flourish - Children:

	Sample Day 1:	Sample Day 2:
Breakfast:	Strawberry Smoothie or Carob Almond Smoothie	Pumpkin Protein Pancakes
Lunch:	Chicken Salad with Whole Grain wrap, veggie sticks with Hunger Hampering Hummus	Marvelous Mexican Dip or Chicken Soup with veggie sticks and Crunchmaster® multi grain crakcers
Dinner:	Italian Chicken Fingers, Sweet Fries, Roasted Green Beans, Strawberry Vinaigrette Salad	Garden Lasagna, Ranch Style Salad Dressing over mixed greens, Kan't Believe It's Not Bread Italian

*Please note that these are suggestions only and are not intended to diagnose, treat, prevent, or cure disease.
Since these statements are not to take the place of a doctor, please consult your doctor prior to altering your diet.

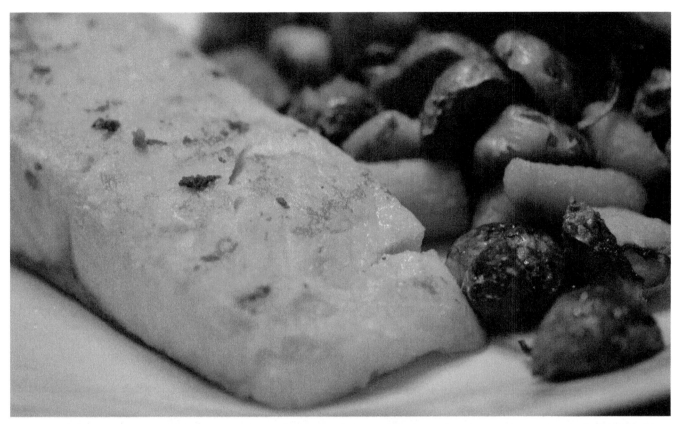

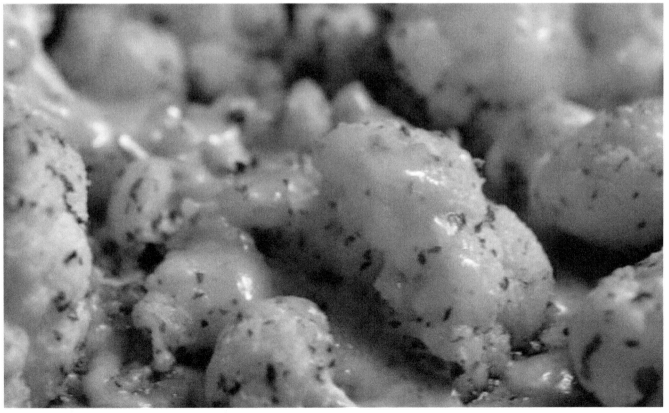

Flourish 4 Meal Formula:

Pick one from each category to comprise your meal. If you do not select a raw vegetable/ salad, a second cooked vegetable can be substituted.

Veggies

1.5 servings = 1.5 cups raw or ¾ cup cooked

- (Steamed/ Roasted/ Stir Fried)
- Green Beans
- Brussels sprouts
- Cauliflower

Healthy Carb

1 serving = ½ cup cooked or 1 slice

- Spaghetti Squash   · Butternut Squash
- Sweet Potato or white (w/ skin)
- Organic Whole Wheat Pasta/ Ezekiel® bread
- Beans

Protein

1 avg. serving = 3-4oz (appx.) or 1 NSP shake

- Wild Salmon (fresh, canned, frozen)
- Wild Cod
- Organic Chicken
- Buffalo/ Grass fed meat
- Hormone Free Turkey
- 1 serving Nature's Sunshine protein shake (Love & Peas) [Sugar Free]

Healthy Fats: avocado, extra virgin olive oil, raw nuts & seeds, organic butter

Raw Salads/Veggies

1 serving = 2 cups greens, 1 cup raw veggies

- Salads: Greek, Sweet Citrus, Italian, Strawberry
- Raw carrot sticks, bell pepper, snap peas, etc. with hummus or guacamole
- Veggie Slaw: shredded carrots, beets, cabbage/ broccoli stems with light dressing
- Broccoli salad made healthy with Vegenaise® or plain Greek Yogurt, honey, sunflower seeds

Other notes: if you want to invest in a juicer, dehydrator, and spiralizer, you will have even more possibilities with the vegetables and fruits! Juicing is a great way to get your veggies in- quickly and in a small volume. Dehydrating foods can turn vegetables into chips! Spiralizing is great for using zucchini to make pasta. Kale can be baked into chips too!

None of these statements have been evaluated by the FDA, nor are they to take the place of a doctor.
The reader assumes full responsibility for his/ her health; this information is not intended to diagnose, treat, prevent or cure disease.

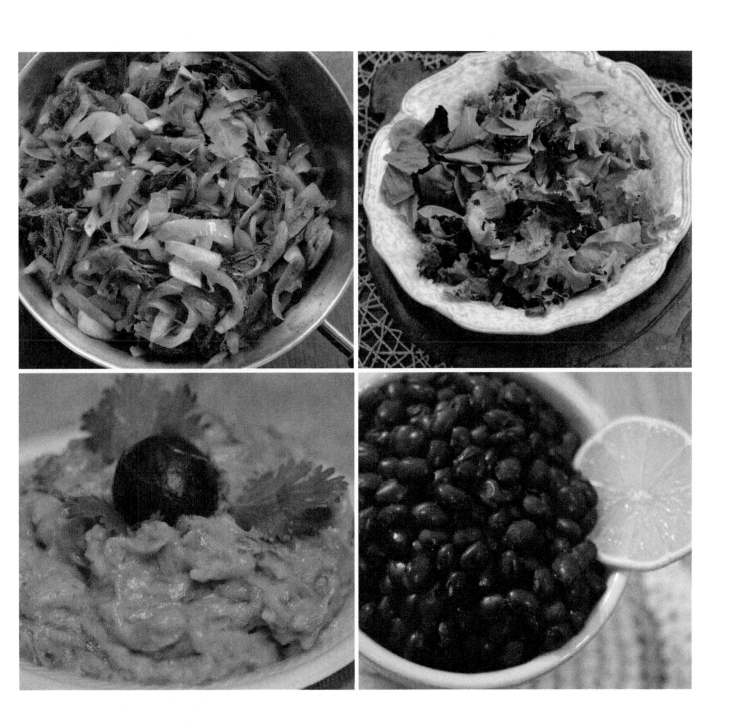

Supplement 2 Flourish

Why Nature's Sunshine®?

With the myriad of supplements on the market and their respective companies, how does one know what ones to choose? My family and I wondered this same thing in 2012. My mom was feeling better after taking some supplements and eating well, but she was not 100%, so she prayed for truth for her health- what was she to do next. Soon after that, I was introduced to Dr. Inge Wetzel, who invested in me and instructed me in Nature's Sunshine and their array of herbs, vitamins, and essential oils. Now, I get to share this health transforming information with you!

What you must have in a supplement company is quality, purity, and efficacy that is not only proclaimed from that company but verified through a third party, such as NSF. Gratefully, Nature's Sunshine embodies each of these. Their manufacturing plant in Utah is open for visits, which is nearly unheard of! Testing for contamination, heavy metals, pesticide residues (and more), Nature's Sunshine only offers the highest quality to their consumers. Your health is worth the best, and Nature's Sunshine makes it affordable. With a $40 purchase through my website www.n2flourish.mynsp.com, you can receive member cost (what I pay), receive a 20% coupon for a future order, and have access to all of the promotions, education, webinars, and even trips if you share Nature's Sunshine with others! You can even participate in their monthly "Sunshine Rewards" auto-ship and receive FREE shipping!

Nature's Sunshine has developed over 500 products over their 43 year legacy so that you have access to nearly any natural health supplement you may need. You will see we mention Nature's Sunshine products throughout this book, and we believe they will be a superb addition to both your kitchen and your health. Some of our favorite products used in this book are:

1. Solstic® Energy
2. Capsicum (shaker bottle)
3. Cordyceps
4. Curcumin BP™
5. Liquid Chloropyll ES™
6. Love & Peas®
7. Maca
8. Mineral Chi Tonic
9. Nature's Harvest
10. Nature's Noni®
11. Nature's Sunshine® flax seed oil with lignans
12. Nature's Sunshine® peppermints
13. Nature's Sunshine® Sea Salt (rich in minerals!)
14. Nutri-Burn®
15. Probiotic 11®
16. Stixated®
17. Thai-Go®

There are so many more that you can use for your personal health goals as well, but these above will get you going on the road to flourishing health with each recipe!

If you are already a member of Nature's Sunshine or have a representative, blessings to you! If you are interested in Nature's Sunshine but you don't have a membership yet, it would be an honor to be your sponsor through www.n2flourish.mynsp.com! Thank you and spread the sunshine! ~Robin Cook

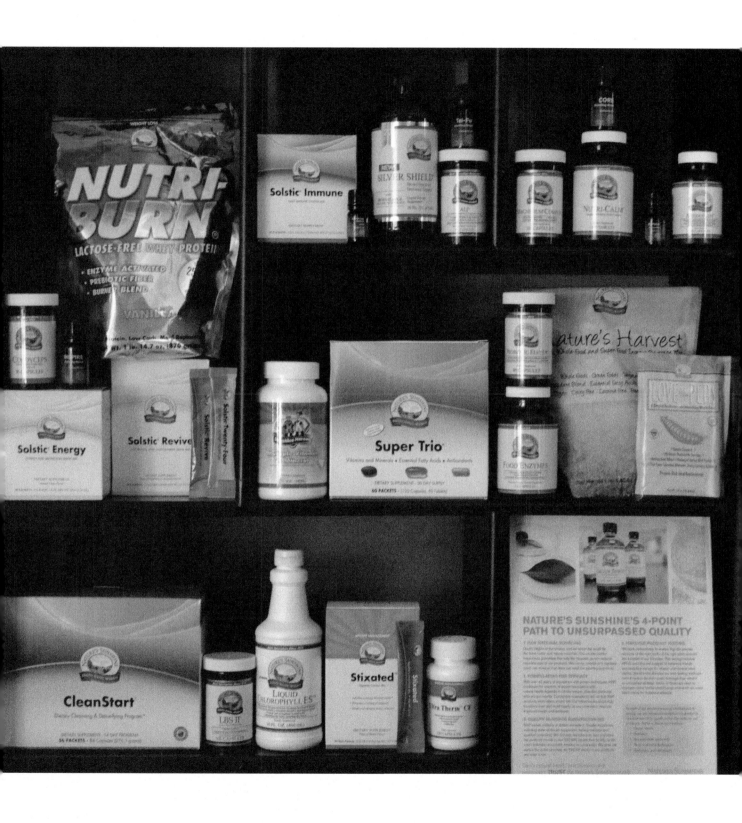

How to make Face Soap

Makes 2 ounces

• 3 drops Nature's Sunshine® Lavender essential oil
• 10 drops Nature's Sunshine® Tea Tree essential oil
• 1 drop Nature's Sunshine® Geranium, Roman Chamomile OR Frankincense essential oil
• ¼ cup (2 ounces) Nature's Sunshine Concentrate®
• 1 teaspoon Nature's Sunshine Silver Shield®
• 1 teaspoon Nature's Sunshine® Nature's Fresh Enzyme Spray

Directions:

1) Place the essential oils in a glass pump bottle OR a BPA free plastic container and shake a second or two to combine the oils. The essential oils have to be added first so that they combine together before any other ingredients are added. Do not mix Nature's Sunshine® essential oils with any other brand of essential oils.

2) Pour in the Nature's Sunshine Concentrate, Silver Shield and the Enzyme Spray. Put the lid on it and shake well.

3) Use about ½ teaspoon to wash face.

* Nature's Sunshine® has glass pump spray bottles available through www.n2flourish.mynsp.com website.

Tip: If you purchase the Nature's Sunshine® Silver Shield 20ppm (4 ounces) glass bottle or the 20ppm (6 ounces) BPA free bottle, you can reuse it for your face soap container.

Eye-makeup Remover

Simply use a tiny bit of extra-virgin coconut oil. Gently rub over eyes and then follow up with face soap above. Rinse with warm water.

How to make Lemongrass Cleaning Solution

Makes 1 cup

- ¼ cup baking soda
- 1 Tablespoon Nature's Sunshine Concentrate®
- 8 drops Nature's Sunshine® Lemongrass essential oil
- 8 drops Nature's Sunshine® Eucalyptus essential oil
- 1 cup filtered water
- 2 Tablespoons 7th Generation® dish soap, optional

Directions:

1) Place the baking soda in a glass jar.

Add in the Nature's Sunshine® concentrate, essential oils, water and if desired, the dish soap.

2) Put the lid on the jar and shake well.

> This solution cleaned 2 shower/tubs, 3 bathroom sinks, kitchen sink, mopped the kitchen floor, mopped the front entry floor and had enough left over to clean 1 toilet! The house smelled so clean!

INDEX

SOURCES

· · · · · · · · · · · · ·

Introduction:
English Standard Version. Bible Gateway. Web. 11 March 2015.
King James Version. Bible Gateway. Web. 11 March 2015.
New Living Version. Bible Gateway. Web. 11 March 2015.
New International Version. Bible Gateway. Web. 11 March 2015.
"Disease Prevention." Harvard School of Public Health: The Nutrition Source. N.p., n.d. Web. 06 Aug. 2015. <http://www.hsph.harvard.edu/nutritionsource/disease-prevention/>.

Anand, Preetha, Ajaikumar B. Kunnumakara, Chitra Sundaram, Kuzhuvelil B. Harikumar, Sheeja T. Tharakan, Oiki S. Lai, Bokyung Sung, and Bharat B. Aggarwal. "Cancer Is a Preventable Disease That Requires Major Lifestyle Changes." The National Center for Biotechnology Information: Pharmaceutical Research. Springer US, 15 July 2008. Web. 06 Aug. 2015. <http://www.ncbi.nlm.nih.gov/pmc/articles/PMC2515569/>.

Hydrogenated oils: "Facts About Hydrogenated Fats and Oils | Ask Dr Sears." Ask Dr Sears The Trusted Resource for Parents. N.p., 09 Aug. 2013. Web. 09 July 2015. <http://www.askdrsears.com/topics/feeding-eating/family-nutrition/facts-about- fats/hydrogenated-fats>.
Hyman, Mark, MD. "Are You Fat Enough? - Dr. Mark Hyman." Dr Mark Hyman. N.p., 05 Jan. 2013. Web. 11 July 2015. <http://drhyman.com/blog/2013/01/05/are-you-fat-enough/>.
"Is Your Salad Dressing Killing Your Weight Loss?." DrAxecom. N.p., 25 Feb. 2013. Web. 11 July 2015. <http://draxe.com/is-your-salad-dressing-killing-your-weight-loss/>.
Additives: "Top 10 Food Additives to Avoid." Food Matters. N.p., 23 Nov. 2010. Web. 09 July 2015. <http://www.foodmatters.tv/articles-1/top-10-food-additives-to-avoid>.
Balch, Phyllis A., CNC. "Threats to Health: When Food, Water, Air, and Earth Get Scary." Prescription for Dietary Wellness. Second ed. New York: Avery, 2003. 195-204. Print.

Wellness Mama, Katie. "How Grains Are Killing You Slowly." Wellness Mama. N.p., 27 June 2015. Web. 8 Aug. 2015. < http://wellnessmama.com/575/how-grains-are-killing-you-slowly/>.
Gluten article: "Is Your Problem Gluten or Faddish Eating?" Fox News. FOX News Network, 01 Aug. 2012. Web. 09 July 2015. <http://www.foxnews.com/health/2012/08/01/is-your-problem-gluten-or-faddish-eating/>.
"What's the Deal with Gluten?" DrAxecom. N.p., 10 Feb. 2010. Web. 09 July 2015. <http://draxe.com/whats-the-deal-with-gluten/>.
Kirkpatrick, Kristin, M.S., R.D., L.D. "10 Things You Don't Know About Sugar (And What You Don't Know Could Hurt You)." The Huffington Post. TheHuffingtonPost.com, 29 Sept. 2013. Web. 11 July 2015. <http://www.huffingtonpost.com/kristin- kirkpatrick-ms-rd-ld/dangers-of-sugar_b_3658061.html>.
Arcidiacono, Biagio, Stefania Iiritano, Aurora Nocera, et al. "Insulin Resistance and Cancer Risk: An Overview of the Pathogenetic Mechanisms." Journal of Diabetes Research 2012 (2012): n. pag. Journal of Diabetes Research. Hindawi Publishing Corporation, 10 Apr. 2012. Web. 11 July 2015. <http://www.hindawi.com/journals/jdr/2012/789174/>.
Pick, Marcelle, OB/GYN NP. "Having a Sweet Tooth Fact or Fiction." Women to Women. N.p., n.d. Web. 08 Aug. 2015. <https://www.womentowomen.com/insulin-resistance/having-a-sweet-tooth-fact-or-fiction/>.
Gill, Colleen, MS, RD, CSO. "Sugar and Cancer." Oncology Nutrition: A Dietetic Practice Group of the Academy of Nutrition and Dietetics. N.p., July 2014. Web. 21 Nov. 2015. <https://www.oncologynutrition.org/erfc/healthy-nutrition-now/sugar-and-cancer/>.
Hardick, B. J., Dr., Kimberly Roberto, and Ben Lerner, Dr. Maximized Living Nutrition Plans. Celebration, FL: Maximized Living, 2010. Print.
Levy, Rob. "Insulin and Colon Cancer Linked." Harvard Gazette. N.p., 7 Nov. 2012. Web. 22 Nov. 2015. <http://news.harvard.edu/gazette/story/2012/11/insulin-and-colon-cancer-linked/>.
Cordain L, Eaton SB, Sebastian A, Mann N, Lindeberg S, Watkins BA, O'Keefe JH, Brand-Miller J. Origins and evolution of the Western diet: health implications for the 21st century. Am J Clin Nutr. 2005 Feb;81(2):341-54.
"Is Sugar Aging Me?" Perricone MD. N.p., n.d. Web. 11 July 2015. <http://www.perriconemd.com/category/is+sugar+aging+me-.do>.
Balch, Phyllis A., CNC. "Sugar By Any Other Name." Prescription for Dietary Wellness. Second ed. New York: Avery, 2003. 205-209. Print.
"Top 10 Natural Sweeteners & Sugar Alternatives - Dr. Axe." DrAxecom. N.p., 26 Apr. 2015. Web. 09 July 2015. <http://draxe.com/natural-sweeteners/>.

New Living Translation. Bible Gateway. Web. 15 March 2015.

Hyman, Mark, MD. "5 Reasons High Fructose Corn Syrup Will Kill You." Dr Mark Hyman. N.p., 13 May 2011. Web. 11 July 2015. <http://drhyman.com/blog/2011/05/13/5-reasons-high-fructose-corn-syrup-will-kill-you/>.

"Tip 6 - Skip the Non-stick to Avoid the Dangers of Teflon." EWG. N.p., n.d. Web. 04 Aug. 2015. <http://www.ewg.org/research/healthy-home-tips/tip-6-skip-non-stick-avoid-dangers-teflon>.

Bauman, Ed, PhD. "Studies Show Microwaves Drastically Reduce Nutrients In Food." Green Med Info. N.p., 22 Aug. 2012. Web. 04 Aug. 2015. <http://www.greenmedinfo.com/blog/studies-show-microwaves-drastically-reduce-nutrients-food>.

Hudson, Kirsten. "What Are Your Dishes Made Of?" Organic Authority. N.p., 12 Feb. 2013. Web. 04 Aug. 2015. <http://www.organicauthority.com/sanctuary/why-avoid-melamine-dishes.html>.

New International Version. Bible Gateway. Web. 23 March 2015.

Chapter 1:

Wetzel, Inge, ND. "Purpose of Protein with Breakfast." HealthStudio.com. N.p., 9 Oct. 2010. Web. 28 Nov. 2015. <http://healthstudio.com/purpsose-of-protein-with-breakfast/>.

Mateljan, George. "Blueberries." The World's Healthiest Foods. N.p., n.d. Web. 03 Feb. 2015. <http://www.worldshealthiestfoods.com/genpage.php?tname=foodspice&dbid=8>.

Herb Allure Inc. Database. HART on CD v 1.93. "Cordyceps" 2001.

Cordyceps Chinese." Nature's Sunshine. N.p., n.d. Web. 27 Nov. 2015. <http://www.naturessunshine.com/us/product/cordyceps-chinese-90-caps/1240/>.

Beaty, Delicia, and Sharon Foutch. "The Benefits of Soaking Nuts and Seeds." Food Matters. N.p., 13 Oct. 2009. Web. 1 Aug. 2015. < http://www.foodmatters.tv/articles-1/the-benefits-of-soaking-nuts-and-seeds>.

"The Chia Cheat Sheet." The Raw Food World News RSS. N.p., 05 Jan. 2015. Web. 02 Aug. 2015. <http://www.news.therawfoodworld.com/chia-cheat-sheet/>.

Harris, Kim. "Soaking Nuts." The Nourishing Gourmet. N.p., 18 July 2008. Web. 02 Aug. 2015. <http://www.thenourishinggourmet.com/2008/07/soaking-nuts.html>.

New Living Translation. Bible Gateway. Web. 12 April 2015. English Standard Version. Bible Gateway. Web. 11 March 2015.

New Living Translation. Bible Gateway. Web. 11 March 2015.

Chapter 2:

Mateljan, George. "Kale." The World's Healthiest Foods. N.p., n.d. Web. 03 Feb. 2015. <http://www.worldshealthiestfoods.com/genpage.php?tname=foodspice&dbid=38>.

Balch, Phyllis A., CNC. "Mom Was Right! Eat Your Vegetables." Prescription for Dietary Wellness. Second ed. New York: Avery, 2003. 80. Print.

Chapter 3:

Herb Allure Inc. Database. HART on CD v 1.93. "Chlorophyll ES" 2014. "Chlorophyll ES, Liquid." Nature's Sunshine. N.p., n.d. Web. 25 Nov. 2015. <http://www.naturessunshine.com/us/product/chlorophyll-es-liquid-16-fl-oz/1483/>. Herb Allure Inc. Database. HART on CD v 1.93. "Solstic Energy" 2011.

"Solstic Energy." Nature's Sunshine. N.p., n.d. Web. 25 Nov. 2015. <http://www.naturessunshine.com/us/product/solstic-energy- 30-packets/6521/>.

Herb Allure Inc. Database. HART on CD v 1.93. "Solstic Revive" 2012.

"Solstic Revive." Nature's Sunshine. N.p., n.d. Web. 25 Nov. 2015. <http://www.naturessunshine.com/us/product/solstic-revive-30-packets/6507/>.

Herb Allure Inc. Database. HART on CD v 1.93. "Stixated" 2014.

"Stixated." Nature's Sunshine. N.p., n.d. Web. 25 Nov. 2015. <http://www.naturessunshine.com/us/product/stixated-30-packets/6540/>.

Herb Allure Inc. Database. HART on CD v 1.93. "Solstic Immune" 2011.

"Solstic Immune." Nature's Sunshine. N.p., n.d. Web. 25 Nov. 2015. <http://www.naturessunshine.com/us/product/solstic-immune-30-packs/6530/>.

"Solstic Twenty-Four." Nature's Sunshine. N.p., n.d. Web. 25 Nov. 2015. <http://www.naturessunshine.com/us/product/solstic-twenty-four-30-packets/6525/>.

Herb Allure Inc. Database. HART on CD v 1.93. "Solstic Cardio" 2011.

"Solstic Cardio." Nature's Sunshine. N.p., n.d. Web. 25 Nov. 2015. <http://www.naturessunshine.com/us/product/solstic-cardio- 30-packets/6520/>.

Webb, Marcus A.,and Richard Craze. The Herb & Spice Companion. New York: Metro, 2004. Print. p.61-62, 85, 101, 105, 110, 156-157

Balch, Phyllis A, CNC.,and Stacey J. Bell. Prescription for Herbal Healing. Second ed. New York, NY: Avery, 2012. Print. Pau d' Arco. p. 111-112

Gunners, Kris, BSc. "10 Proven Benefits of Green Tea." Authority Nutrition. N.p., 02 Sept. 2013. Web. 03 Aug. 2015. <http://authoritynutrition.com/top-10-evidence-based-health-benefits-of-green-tea/>.

Balch, Phyllis A., CNC. "Antioxidants: Powerful Disease Prevention." Prescription for Dietary Wellness. Second ed. New York: Avery, 2003. 46. Print.

Chapter 4:
Mateljan, George. "Sweet Potatoes." The World's Healthiest Foods. N.p., n.d. Web. 03 Feb. 2015. <http://www.worldshealthiestfoods.com/genpage.php?tname=foodspice&dbid=64>.

Balch, Phyllis A., CNC. "Mom Was Right! Eat Your Vegetables." Prescription for Dietary Wellness. Second ed. New York: Avery, 2003. 97. Print.

New International Version. Bible Gateway. Web. 1 Aug. 2015.

Chapter 5:
Kimble- Evans, Amanda. "Heirloom Vegetables: 6 Advantages Compared to Hybrids." Mother Earth News. N.p., 30 June 2009. Web. 04 Aug. 2015. <http://www.motherearthnews.com/organic-gardening/vegetables/heirloom-vegetable-advantages.aspx>.

Chapter 6:
Mateljan, George. "Beets." The World's Healthiest Foods. N.p., n.d. Web. 14 May 2015. <http://whfoods.com/genpage.php?tname=foodspice&dbid=49>.

New International Version. Bible Gateway. Web. 14 Jan. 2015.

Chapter 8:
Mateljan, George. "Brussels Sprouts." The World's Healthiest Foods. N.p., n.d. Web. 03 Feb. 2015. <http://www.worldshealthiestfoods.com/genpage.php?tname=foodspice&dbid=10>.
Balch, Phyllis A., CNC. "Mom Was Right! Eat Your Vegetables." Prescription for Dietary Wellness. Second ed. New York: Avery, 2003. 78. Print.
New American Standard Bible. Bible Gateway. Web. 30 June. 2015.

Chapter 9:
"History of Carrots - A Brief Summary and Timeline." World Carrot Museum, n.d. Web. 01 July 2015. <http://www.carrotmuseum.co.uk/history.html>.
Mateljan, George. "Carrots." The World's Healthiest Foods. N.p., n.d. Web. 03 Feb. 2015. <http://www.worldshealthiestfoods.com/genpage.php?tname=foodspice&dbid=21>.
Balch, Phyllis A., CNC. "Mom Was Right! Eat Your Vegetables." Prescription for Dietary Wellness. Second ed. New York: Avery, 2003. 89. Print.
New King James Version. Bible Gateway. Web. 6 June 2015.
"Nutrition Facts and Analysis for Squash, Winter, Butternut, Cooked, Baked, without Salt." SELF Nutrition Data. N.p., n.d. Web. 25 Nov. 2015. <http://nutritiondata.self.com/facts/vegetables-and-vegetable-products/2648/2>.

Chapter 10:
Balch, Phyllis A, CNC. "Spices and Herbs: Flavor Enhancers That Heal." Prescription for Dietary Wellness. Second ed. New York: Avery, 2003. 146-154. Print.

Shealy, C. Norman., MD, PhD. "Herbalism." Healing Remedies: Over 1000 Natural Remedies for the Prevention, Treatment, and Cure of Common Ailments and Conditions. London: Element, 2002. 118. Print.

"Cinnamon, Ground." The World's Healthiest Foods. N.p., n.d. Web. 02 July 2015. <http://www.worldshealthiestfoods.com/genpage.php?tname=foodspice&dbid=68>.

Balch, Phyllis A, CNC. "Spices and Herbs: Flavor Enhancers That Heal." Prescription for Dietary Wellness. Second ed. New York: Avery, 2003. 163-164 Print.

Shealy, C. Norman., MD, PhD. "Herbalism." Healing Remedies: Over 1000 Natural Remedies for the Prevention, Treatment, and Cure of Common Ailments and Conditions. London: Element, 2002. 139. Print.

Shealy, C. Norman., MD, PhD. "Herbalism." Healing Remedies: Over 1000 Natural Remedies for the Prevention, Treatment, and Cure of Common Ailments and Conditions. London: Element, 2002. 121. Print.

"Parsley." Parsley. N.p., n.d. Web. 02 July 2015. <http://www.whfoods.com/genpage.php?tname=foodspice&dbid=100>. Shealy, C. Norman., MD, PhD. "Herbalism." Healing Remedies: Over 1000 Natural Remedies for the Prevention, Treatment, and Cure of Common Ailments and Conditions. London: Element, 2002. 127. Print.

Shealy, C. Norman., MD, PhD. "Herbalism." Healing Remedies: Over 1000 Natural Remedies for the Prevention, Treatment, and Cure of Common Ailments and Conditions. London: Element, 2002. 135. Print.

Balch, Phyllis A, CNC. "Antioxidants: Powerful Disease Prevention." Prescription for Dietary Wellness. Second ed. New York: Avery, 2003. 46-47. Print.

Mateljan, George. "Avocados." The World's Healthiest Foods. N.p., n.d. Web. 03 Feb. 2015. <http://www.worldshealthiestfoods. com/genpage.php?pfriendly=1&tname=foodspice&dbid=5>.
Balch, Phyllis A, CNC. "Fabulous Fruits and Bodacious Berries." Prescription for Dietary Wellness. Second ed. New York: Avery, 2003. 60. Print.
Chapter 12:
Mateljan, George. "Cauliflower." The World's Healthiest Foods. N.p., n.d. Web. 03 Feb. 2015. <http://www. worldshealthiestfoods.com/genpage.php?tname=foodspice&dbid=13>.
Balch, Phyllis A., CNC. "Mom Was Right! Eat Your Vegetables." Prescription for Dietary Wellness. Second ed. New York: Avery, 2003. 77,79. Print.
New International Version. Bible Gateway. Web. 29 March 2015.
Chapter 14:
"Our Quality." Nature's Sunshine. N.p., n.d. Web. 23 Nov. 2015. http://www.naturessunshine.com/us/company/c1/product-quality/>.

CPSIA information can be obtained
at www.ICGtesting.com
Printed in the USA
LVOW05s1142121215

466410LV00011B/11/P